Introduction to Research
UNDERSTANDING AND APPLYING
MULTIPLE STRATEGIES

Introduction to Research
UNDERSTANDING AND APPLYING MULTIPLE STRATEGIES

Elizabeth DePoy, PhD, MSW, OTR

Professor and Coordinator, Interdisciplinary Disability Studies
Center for Community Inclusion and Disability Studies
Professor, School of Social Work
University of Maine
Orono, Maine

Laura N. Gitlin, PhD

Director, Center for Applied Research on Aging and Health
Professor, Department of Occupational Therapy
Jefferson College of Health Professions
Thomas Jefferson University
Philadelphia, Pennsylvania

THIRD EDITION

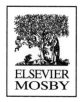

ELSEVIER
MOSBY

ELSEVIER
MOSBY

11830 Westline Industrial Drive
St. Louis, Missouri 63146

W 20.5

INTRODUCTION TO RESEARCH;
UNDERSTANDING AND APPLYING MULTIPLE STRATEGIES
Copyright © 2005, 1998, 1993 by Mosby Inc.

0-323-02853-5

NOTICE

Neither the Publisher nor the Authors assume any responsibility for any loss or injury and/or damage to persons or property arising out of or related to any use of the material contained in this book. It is the responsibility of the treating practitioner, relying on independent expertise and knowledge of the patient, to determine the best treatment and method of application for the patient.

International Standard Book Number 0-323-02853-5

Publishing Director: Linda Duncan
Editor: Kathy Falk
Developmental Editor: Melissa Kuster Deutsch
Publishing Services Manager: Patricia Tannian
Project Manager: Sarah Wunderly
Designer: William Drone

Printed in United States of America

Last digit is the print number: 9 8 7 6 5 4 3 2 1

Photo Credits

To my husband Stephen, who lovingly challenges and thinks with me, and to my family

To my husband Eduardo, my children Keith and Eric, and my mom and dad, all of whom inspire

And to all of our students, from whom we have and continue to learn

Foreword

The third edition of DePoy and Gitlin provides health and human services students and professionals with significantly expanded material for understanding the philosophical foundations of research, the value of systematic inquiry, and the concrete steps for moving through the process of generating and sharing knowledge. What continues to distinguish this text from other research methodological volumes is that readers are exposed to what the authors identify as the 10 essentials of research that involve the fundamental thinking and action processes required for the conduct of either naturalistic or quantitative approaches to research. The authors walk readers through each of the processes involved in framing a research problem, developing a knowledge base, understanding the role of theory, formulating research questions, and sequencing research. Readers will also learn action steps involved in determining the scope or "boundaries" of a study, data collection and measurement, data analysis, and report writing.

Despite its importance to practice, research method courses are often a required upper division or graduate level course that students in the health and human services dread—thinking they will need to memorize facts and figures that have little relevance to their career goals. DePoy and Gitlin offer an antidote to such fears, making research come alive by the generous use of examples throughout the text and a final chapter on "stories from the field." Such examples and stories bring life to the essential thinking and action processes of research, enable practitioners to envision the value of research, and zero in on challenges that they may face in their own research endeavors. Of major significance is that the reader will gain a real appreciation of the research enterprise, be able to read and critique literature, and be guided in the conduct of different research approaches to answer practical and clinically relevant research questions. Of added value, this introductory text provides checklists that will help the researcher get started, as well as a list of references for more in-depth examination. Thus the reader gains greater insight into the role of research in improving practice and an increased appreciation of the science and artistry of research.

Whereas most texts emphasize one research tradition over another, the philosophical underpinnings of experimental and naturalistic inquiry are both presented with the emphasis on the value and importance of each approach. Readers learn about how research questions are framed in each approach and the unique designs and methods appropriate to each research tradition. The take-home message is that both approaches have legitimacy and their own standards of excellence. Rigor is expected whether the approach is experimental or naturalistic, and studies that include both approaches often provide unique insights that go beyond a single approach. This perspective represents an important aspect of this text that contributes as well to the broader debate and discussions as to the role and value of different research traditions and design strategies.

The third edition contains several new sections and chapters that address topics on the cutting edge of the research venture. For example, this edition contains a new chapter on ethics, as well as informed consent documentation. Ethical considerations are paramount these days, and each researcher should be fully aware of requirements for human subject protections and new federal privacy rules that have implications for the type of data that can be collected. This new edition also includes a chapter on seeking financial support for research ideas and practical hints for getting started on writing a research proposal. This is particularly important as health professionals are increasingly expected to seek resources for their programs and related evaluations.

Especially notable in the third edition is the chapter on practice efficacy. The processes of reviewing and rating existing literature and developing consensus around practice guidelines and best practices are delineated. With tight resources for health and human services, there are increasing demands for accountability to demonstrate the worth of different programs and practices. This chapter provides important information for understanding the pros and cons of the evidence-based movement that is gaining popularity among researchers and funding agencies. Although this approach has strong endorsement in the experimental research field, there are cautions in assuming that randomized clinical trials are the gold standard for research. Although such studies are important for maximizing internal validity, they can be criticized for limited generalizability, are difficult to implement in community-based settings, and do not address the full range of questions relevant to clinical practice. Depoy and Gitlin's Evaluation Practice conceptualization makes a substantial contribution to the literature, providing an easy-to-follow model that incorporates both thinking and action processes, including clarification of the problem, reflexive intervention, and outcome assessment. These concepts are critical to understanding the long-term sustainability of a program or

service and offer an innovative approach to integrating research into practice and bridging the research-practice gap.

As in many disciplines, the health and human services field is characterized by a research-to-practice gap. Researchers are generally focused on research theories and designs, data collection, and statistics, which are typically uninformed by practice. On the other hand, practitioners typically rely on clinical practice informed by individual experience independent of a larger theory and research-driven knowledge base. This gap limits the ability of research to translate into meaningful programs and practices that can make a real difference in people's lives.

This book provides a critical bridge between research and practice by having practitioners understand that their clinical intuition can inform research thinking and action processes, and having researchers learn to appreciate the contexts in which systematic thinking and action processes are implemented. It reflects a significant paradigm shift in thinking about and acting on the essential research elements. Its presentation also represents a fundamental shift in the teaching paradigm from a "talking at" approach to engaging text that emphasizes a "listening to" philosophy.

A major joy of this text is the stories woven by two esteemed researchers who draw on a lifetime of practical experiences that have improved the conceptualization, implementation, and evaluation of different research traditions. The passion of DePoy and Gitlin for their research and practice comes through every page of the book and serves to make this book a truly enjoyable reading and learning experience.

Marcia G. Ory, Ph.D., M.P.H.
Professor, Social and Behavioral Health
Director, Active for Life National Program Office
School of Rural Public Health
The Texas A & M University System

Preface

Our main purpose in writing this third edition is to continue our commitment to sharing with the student, health and human professional, and beginning researcher our great enthusiasm and passion for conducting research in health and human services using multiple research strategies. We hope this edition with its conceptual refinements, updated and expanded information, and use of research examples demystifies the research process and provides a foundation from which to critique, understand, and apply multiple research strategies to health and human service concerns. In this third edition, we have further refined and expanded our framework from which to examine and integrate different research traditions in diverse physical, virtual, and conceptual contexts. In so doing, our goal remains to challenge traditional teaching approaches to research processes and to further narrow the gap between quantitative and qualitative paradigms.

Why do health and human service professionals need yet another research text and this third edition? As we stated in the first and second editions of this book, health and human service professions continue to stand at the crossroads of significant megatrends in the delivery and financing of services to clients and families, as well as local, global, and virtual communities. These trends continue at a rapid pace and include the movement from an acute, medical framework to diverse on-site and virtual models of care; a focus on health promotion and disease prevention; the development of new paradigms for

examining the interplay of behavioral, environmental, economic, political, spiritual, and biological interactions; and an increased emphasis on innovative services for underserved and diverse populations.

These new directions in health and human services require innovative approaches to research. The traditional research paradigm taught to students of the social sciences and health professions, referred to as quantitative, empiricist, positivist, or rationalist, represents only one approach to scientific inquiry. Historically, the quantitative or experimental-type approach to research has been upheld as the most scientific, valid, and precise methodology. Unfortunately, this belief still lingers in the health and human service worlds, is well represented in practice models such as evidence-based practice, and has significantly limited the effective use of other research strategies, which, in turn, has restricted knowledge building and use. In light of these limitations and the expanded contexts in which research is being conducted, other research traditions such as discovery-oriented, interpretive, qualitative, naturalistic, participatory, and mixed method, are rapidly gaining importance and recognition as forms of inquiry with their own rules and systematic approaches to understanding human behavior.

The viewpoint we continue to present in this third edition reflects an increasingly accepted school of thought that recognizes and values multiple research strategies. This contemporary perspective proposes that naturalistic and experimental-type research strategies have equal value and contribute in complementary and distinct ways to the science of practice. Knowledge of both of these research traditions presents new opportunities for addressing the complex health and human service research questions that are emerging as a consequence of today's diverse health care environments. Students, professionals, and researchers need a research text that prepares them for using the full range of research traditions to meet the scientific challenges posed by changing service systems. For example, to develop effective health promotion programs for global communities composed of individuals from diverse backgrounds requires understanding specific health beliefs and self-care practices of a range of different groups. Traditional survey techniques have not always been successful in identifying different self-care practices, and existing standardized health belief questionnaires do not necessarily represent the varied values of diverse groups across the globe. Different methodologies and approaches that uncover and accurately represent personal beliefs and practices are required for knowledge building in this area.

Since our second edition was published, many articles and books have discussed and evaluated new methodologies, particularly those from the tradition of naturalistic inquiry and, more recently, mixed methods. However, our approach in this third edition continues to differ significantly from other research texts. Most texts for health and human service professionals still identify quantitative research as the most valid approach to scientific inquiry. Some of these research texts include a discussion of other research traditions but most often in comparison to the gold standard of the experiment. Still other texts explain naturalistic inquiry by using the framework or lens of the experimental researcher. In doing so, the authors assume that naturalistic and experimental approaches differ only with respect to specific procedures. They do not present the essential thinking processes that underlie the activity of qualitative research. Thus the research student cannot come to understand and accurately implement different design strategies from this tradition. There are several new books that focus on mixed methods, which we cite in this third edition. Although these books are greatly welcomed and broaden our under-

standing of the scope of human inquiry, they provide insight into only one type of research approach. The student does not obtain a critical understanding of the truly vast array of research possibilities, nor learn strategies by which to purposively select a particular research approach.

In contrast, this text provides a comprehensive understanding of how researchers think and act across the research traditions and in diverse contexts. It provides a basic introduction to the essential components of a range of approaches. The reader learns how to critically evaluate, respect, and implement each research strategy from its own philosophical perspective, thinking process, language, and specific actions that engage the researcher. In this text we concur with the new wave of qualitative and mixed method books and suggest that it is possible to explain the thought and action processes of these approaches and advance relevant standards by which such research is understood, evaluated, and conducted.

Writing the third edition of *Introduction to Research: Understanding and Applying Multiple Strategies* has given us an important opportunity to reflect on and advance our ongoing conceptualization of the research traditions, their integration, and their use in expanded health and social service contexts. In this third edition we have refined our thinking and present the 10 essential thinking and action processes of research that appeared in the second edition. These highly integrated processes are thought about and solved differently, depending on the particular research tradition being pursued. We have seen from our second edition that a process approach improves our ability to describe and capture the essence of a range of research approaches.

Readers of our second edition will experience the third edition as an improvement. We have updated not only our major discussion of the research traditions and their philosophical foundations but have added new material on clinical, international, and virtual contexts in which research is initiated, conducted, and disseminated. Our underlying assumptions about the purpose and conduct of research and much of the discussion remain intact. We believe all readers will benefit from the clarity that a process approach brings to understanding the fundamentals of conducting research in all research traditions.

The third edition is organized into five major sections. The first four sections move the reader from an understanding of the meaning, elements, and importance of research (Part I) to an examination of the specific thinking processes (Part II), design approaches (Part III), and action processes (Part IV) of distinct research traditions. Each chapter in Parts I to IV focuses on one of the 10 essentials of the research process, all of which are discussed using the language of both experimental-type and naturalistic researchers. We have added a new section (Part V) devoted to using research to improve professional practice and outcome. Throughout the text, many actual and suggested research examples are provided from diverse bodies of literature and our own research experience that are relevant to all service providers. As in the second edition, we end with field stories, real-life snapshots of what it is like to participate in different types of research processes. These brief narrative accounts reveal the hidden side of the research process, how a study unfolds, what it is like to be an investigator, and what really happens after entering the field. Research, after all, is a human endeavor. Too few researchers dare to discuss the personal ups and downs and common blunders that inform knowledge construction.

In this text, we do not intend to solve the controversy over which design approach is best. We urge health and human service professionals to transcend the debate and go beyond attempts of the health care community to polarize research practices. We propose that knowing the strengths and weaknesses of the full range of approaches to thinking and conducting research provides the basis from which to select, combine, and use multiple strategies to answer research questions. Ultimately this text is designed to facilitate the integration of traditions with the belief that integration is the most comprehensive and productive approach to health and human service research. We hope this text advances the movement toward purposive integration that can guide research practices.

Who should use this text? This third edition can be used by undergraduate and advanced students in the health and human service professions. It can also be used by practitioners and beginning researchers who want to broaden their understanding of research traditions to which they have not been previously exposed. Health and human service professionals will continue to experience increasing pressure to initiate research, participate as members of research teams, and use research findings to assess and justify their practice and service programs. This text provides a solid foundation from which to pursue these activities.

Elizabeth DePoy
Laura N. Gitlin

Contents

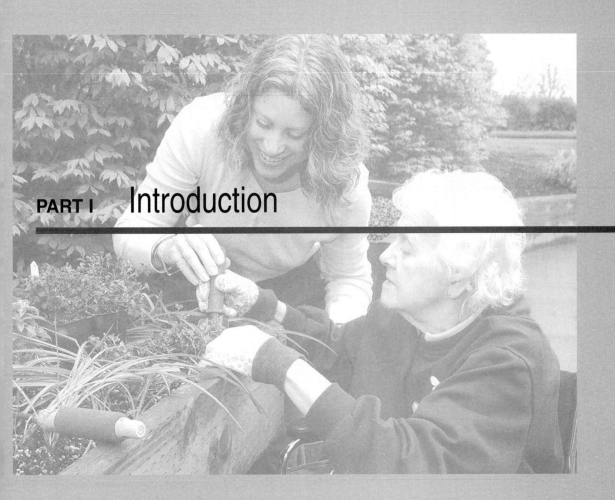

PART I Introduction

Welcome to the world of research!

Conducting research is one of the most challenging, creative, and intellectually satisfying professional activities. Research is an important professional responsibility that develops and advances knowledge from which to base practice. This knowledge is essential if we, as health and human service professionals, are to provide quality services that enhance the lives of our clients, their families, and their communities.

Part I begins with our definition of *research*. We identify and discuss the 10 elements of the *research process* that are essential to the traditions of both experimental-type and naturalistic inquiry.

At this point you may be thinking, "What is research?" "Why is it necessary?" "How does research differ from other ways of learning about things?" "How does one engage in research?" and "What is the process?"

These important questions are examined in the chapters of Part I.

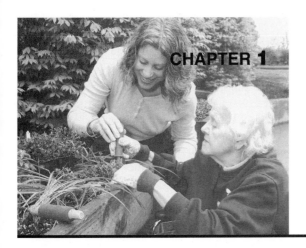

CHAPTER 1

Research as an Important Way of Knowing

KEY TERMS

Abductive reasoning
Action processes
Confirmable
Deductive reasoning
Epistemology
Experimental-type research
Idiographic
Inductive reasoning
Logical
Naturalistic inquiry
Nomothetic
Thinking processes
Understandable
Useful

CHAPTER OUTLINE

A 74-year-old single African American woman with a fractured hip will be discharged shortly from rehabilitation to her home. She appears unwilling to use the self-care techniques you taught her. You wonder if rehabilitation has been effective in meeting its specified goals and what her future capabilities will be once she returns home.

You have learned how to use a new tool to assess the environmental barriers encountered by children with developmental delays. You wonder if this instrument is more accurate and useful than previous ones you have tried.

A research article describes a progressive approach to discharge planning for adults with cognitive impairments. You wonder if you should implement these planning procedures in your own department and if they will be effective in enhancing access to community resources.

You need to initiate a new program to prevent low back injury in migrant farm workers. Existing prevention strategies have not been effective in reducing the incidence of low back injury in this population. You wonder why traditional approaches have failed and how to develop an appropriate knowledge base from which to develop an efficacious program.

You notice in your home care practice that some patients need more visits than others to achieve the same health outcomes. You wonder what factors influence service need. You wonder how to increase health literacy and access to health information for people who cannot see.

WHY IS RESEARCH NECESSARY?

Health and human service professionals routinely have questions about their daily practice. Many of these questions, such as those listed above, are answered best through systematic investigation, or the research process. It is therefore unfortunate that many practitioners do not engage in research. This phenomenon may be caused in part by unfamiliarity with and misconceptions about the research process.

Research is challenging, exhilarating, and very stimulating. As with other professional activities, research can also be time-consuming, tedious, and frustrating. The challenges and frustrations of conducting research occur because it is not a simple activity, particularly health and human service research, in which conducting research in service environments and understanding human behavior are often complex matters. Implementing a research study in the home, community, outpatient clinic, or medical facility can be much more challenging than research conducted in a laboratory or a setting that can be controlled by the investigator. Throughout this book, we discuss the specific dilemmas and design implications posed by research that is implemented in the health and human service practice (particularly in Part V, Improving Your Practice Through Inquiry).

There are many important reasons why you should understand the research process and participate in research activities (Box 1-1).

First, research is a systematic process to obtain scientific knowledge about specific problems encountered in daily practice.[1] Thus it is an important way of finding answers to questions about needed interventions, practice outcomes, and clinical irritations. The fundamental goal of research for health and human services is to develop and advance a body of knowledge to guide professional activity. Research contributes to the development of a scientific body of knowledge in several ways. It generates relevant theory and knowledge about human experience and behavior; it develops and tests theories that form the basis of specific practices and treatment approaches; and it examines, validates, or determines the effectiveness of different practices in attaining their intended and sometimes unintended outcomes.[2]

The second important reason to understand and participate in research is its overall impact on health care policy and service delivery. The knowledge obtained through research is often used directly or indirectly to inform legislators and regulatory bodies about the best health and human service policies and service delivery models. Federal regulatory agencies and other fiscal intermediaries base many of their decisions and practice guidelines on empirical evidence or knowledge generated through the research process. Research models have become increasingly used to identify "best" practices, as described in Chapter 24. Consider managed care; its very foundation uses systematic cost measures and specific outcome measures to yield data that then form the basis for policy, practice decisions, and implementation of treatment guidelines. Additionally, research provides the tools by which to compare practices, health outcomes, and costs across practice settings. Using systematic, standard approaches allows professionals to make comparisons among different patient populations and diverse health and human service contexts, in order to determine their level of efficiency and effectiveness.

BOX 1-1
FIVE REASONS TO LEARN ABOUT THE RESEARCH PROCESS

1. Systematically build knowledge and test treatment efficacy.
2. Impact health policy and service delivery.
3. Participate in research activities.
4. Enhance understanding of daily practice.
5. Become a critical consumer of research literature.

Let us assume that the average length of stay at your facility for stroke patients is 21 days and that within that time, 85% of the patients return home and require minimal assistance to perform activities of daily living. You may consider this an acceptable or even a good outcome. However, comparing your outcomes with other similar institutions, you learn differently. Other institutions that have the same case mix report an average length of stay of only 10 days, with patients achieving the same level of function as your patients. This comparative information enables you to examine the specific clinical practices of your institution critically. By comparing such outcome data as length of stay and functional status, each institution can evaluate and refine its practices to achieve the best or most cost-effective protocols.

The third reason to learn about research is to enable you to participate in research activities in your own practice setting. In many health and human service settings, practitioners establish or maintain a database of clinical information and derive statistical reports on patient outcomes. In some settings, particularly in an academic health science center or teaching hospital, you or other members of your agency will participate in research to advance the research goals of the institution. You may have many diverse roles as a member of a research project. You may initially want to participate in the process as a data collector, chart extractor, interviewer, provider of an experimental intervention, or recruiter of participants into a study. These are all excellent, time-limited roles to learn firsthand—the art and science of the research process. When you feel more comfortable and gain some experience with the process, you may want to serve as a project coordinator and become responsible for the coordination of the detailed tasks and daily activities of a research endeavor; or you may choose the role of the co-investigator and assist in the conceptual development, design, implementation, and analytical components of a study. If you really become hooked on research, you may want to be a principal investigator and assume responsibility for initiating and overseeing the scientific integrity of the entire research effort.

The fourth reason to know about research is that it provides the tools by which you can learn about and be responsive to the experiences and needs of the individuals and groups you help in your professional practice.

The fifth reason to learn about and participate in research is to become a critical consumer of the growing body of research literature that is published in professional journals. Research not only yields a body of knowledge but also provides the evidence and reasoning strategies by which the investigator bases knowledge claims. Thus, research provides the foundation for informed professional decision making and action. By understanding the research enterprise, when you read a research study, you will know not only what an investigator has found, but also how the knowledge was generated and the extent to which it can be applied in practice. Understanding the thinking and action processes of research will provide you with the necessary skills to determine the adequacy of research outcomes and their implications for daily practice.[3] Most important, the knowledge you gain about research findings has the potential to improve your practice and thus improve the quality of life of the people you serve (patients, clients, families) and the health of your community.

As you can see, there are many reasons to learn about the research process. Most important, whether conducting a study or just using systematic techniques in your professional activity, the procedures and methodologies used in research can improve how you think and act in your daily practice. This text offers a range of methodologies and techniques, including case study, analysis of audio or video recordings, single-case design, observation, and in-depth interviewing. As a health care or human service professional, you can use each to gain better insight into a particularly difficult practice situation or, in general, to advance all aspects of your professional practice. For example, if you are experiencing difficulty effectively interacting with and thus treating a child with a developmental disability, borrowing a technique from research (e.g., recording a session and systematically analyzing verbal and nonverbal interactions frame by frame) may provide important insights to better approach this particular individual.

Consider another example:

Let us assume you have been asked to assess the functional ability of a nursing home resident and improve her self-care abilities. You may want to set up a single-subject design to monitor your treatment program and evaluate its effectiveness in producing a desired outcome. The outcome of your intervention will be important to share with staff and administrators. First, take several baseline assessments of the resident's functioning over several days using a standardized functional measure. Second, introduce your strategies to improve self-care. Then, reassess the resident over several days using the same functional assessment. This is a simple and easy approach that allows you to obtain systematic information about your treatment and its outcome.

Consider also the following practice situation:

You work in a hospital setting and participate as a member of a team that is responsible for discharge planning. You and your team need an assessment tool to help identify who is at risk on discharge to home for falling and functional difficulty living alone. The team gives you the responsibility of either identifying an existing tool or creating one. On reviewing the literature for published functional assessments, you find that about 200 tools have already been developed and tested that may be relevant to your purpose.[4] As you can see, knowledge as to how to conduct the literature search systematically and identify appropriate studies, then evaluate the integrity of the research literature and the psychometric properties of existing measures of interest, would be important. If, based on this review, you find that existing measures do not encompass the types of risks of concern to your team, you need to understand how to begin to construct and test an appropriate measure.

Knowing the "essentials" of research is critical. Also, many aspects of the research process can be borrowed and incorporated into your daily practice to improve your knowledge about a clinical question or to systematize your approach in providing health or human services.

One final point should be made regarding the importance of participating in research. As health and human service professionals engage in the research process, they contribute to the development of knowledge and theory and help to validate and improve practice. Through this research activity, health and human service professionals are participating in the advancement and refinement of the research process itself and its application to professional issues and service settings. Health and human service professionals who are involved in research today will make significant contributions to the evolution of research methodologies.[5-7]

WHAT IS RESEARCH?

Research is not "owned" by any one profession or discipline. It is a systematic set of ways of thinking and acting and has distinct vocabularies that can be learned and used by anyone.

Many different definitions of research can be found in texts, ranging from a very broad to a very restrictive understanding of the research endeavor. A very broad definition suggests that research includes any type of investigation that uncovers knowledge. On the other hand, a formal and more restrictive definition of research implies that only one type of strategy, such as a quantitative orientation, is valid. Many researchers use the classic (but we believe restricted) definition offered by Kerlinger, who defines scientific research as "systematic, controlled, empirical, and critical investigation of natural phenomena guided by theory and hypotheses about the presumed relations among such phenomena."[8] Whereas a *broad* definition includes any type of activity as research, a *restrictive* definition, such as Kerlinger's viewpoint, implies that the only legitimate approach to scientific inquiry is hypothesis testing.

In contrast, we define research in such a way as to reflect and allow for a wide range of ways of knowing or systematic approaches to knowledge building. As such, our definition of research is as follows:

Research is multiple, systematic strategies to generate knowledge about human behavior, human experience, and human environments in which the thinking and action processes of the researcher are clearly specified so that they are logical, understandable, confirmable, and useful.

Our definition has three important components (Box 1-2). First, we state that research is more than

---

**BOX 1-2
WHAT IS RESEARCH?**

MULTIPLE SYSTEMATIC STRATEGIES
■ Experimental-type design
■ Naturalistic inquiry

THOUGHT AND ACTION PROCESSES
■ Inductive
■ Abductive
■ Deductive

FOUR CRITERIA
■ Logical
■ Understandable
■ Confirmable
■ Useful

one type of investigative strategy; that is, research is not just hypothesis testing, as suggested by Kerlinger, but rather is represented by a broad range of strategies that are systematically implemented. In contrast to the definition offered by the restrictive view, we recognize the legitimacy and value of many distinct types of investigative strategies. Second, our definition emphasizes that research is composed of *thinking processes* and specific actions *(action processes)* that must be clearly delineated and articulated. We believe that the beauty and efficacy of the research process lie in the explication of how and on what basis a knowledge claim is made. Third, we characterize thinking and action processes as *logical, understandable, confirmable,* and *useful* to meet the criteria of research. That is, in contrast to the broad inclusive definition of research, our approach clearly distinguishes the boundary between research and other forms of knowing (e.g., through trial and error) by establishing these important criteria. Let us examine the three major components of our definition in greater detail.

Research as Multiple Systematic Strategies

The first component of our research definition emphasizes the value of varied systematic strategies to understand the depth and range of research questions asked by health and human service professionals. These multiple research strategies can be categorized as representing either naturalistic inquiry or experimental-type research. These two broad categories of research strategies are based in distinct philosophical traditions, follow different forms of human reasoning, and define and obtain knowledge differently. *Naturalistic inquiry* refers to a wide range of research approaches characterized by a focus on understanding and interpreting human experience within the context in which experience occurs. *Experimental-type research* refers to a range of designs characterized by a focus on prediction and hypothesis testing. Chapter 3 examines the differences between these research traditions, their philosophical roots, and their implications for health and human service research. Naturalistic inquiry tends to be *idiographic;* that is, it focuses on specific phenomena in a context and seeks to highlight the complexity of the phenomenon. Experimental-type approaches examine and characterize what is typical about one or more groups; this is referred to as *nomothetic.*

Our viewpoint, however, reflects a school of thought that has been expressed in numerous professional and academic disciplines. This school of thought proposes that both naturalistic inquiry and experimental-type research strategies have equal importance in establishing a scientific base of health and human service practice and in adequately examining the diversity of human experiences and behaviors. Idiographic and nomothetic understandings each reveal different, valuable, and necessary knowledge.

This viewpoint also firmly asserts that it is not reasonable to critique naturalistic research using experimental language because each approach represents a distinct *epistemology,* or way of knowing and obtaining knowledge.[9,10] As Gareth Morgan, cited by Patton, eloquently claims:

> It is not possible to judge the validity or contribution of different research perspectives in terms of the ground assumptions of any one set of perspectives, since the process is self-justifying. Hence the attempts in much social science debate to judge the utility of different research strategies in terms of universal criteria based on the importance of generalizability, predictability and control, explanation of variance, meaningful understanding, or whatever are inevitably flawed: These criteria inevitably favor research strategies consistent with the assumptions that generate such criteria as meaningful guidelines for the evaluation of research. ...Different research perspectives make different kinds of knowledge claims, and the criteria as to what counts as significant knowledge vary from one to another.[10]

Another implication of our perspective is that combining or mixing methods is an important approach to the study of many of the complex issues of current concern to health and human service professionals. As Bonilla-Silva asserts with regard to the study of contemporary racism, "The research strategy that seems more appropriate for our times is mixed research designs because it allows researchers to cross-examine their results."[11]

Research as Thinking and Action Processes

The second important component of our definition of research refers to thinking and action processes.

Thinking processes and action processes represent the different ways of reasoning and the specific series of actions that distinguish naturalistic and experimental-type investigators in the conduct of their research. Experimental-type research uses primarily a deductive form of human reasoning. Naturalistic inquiry primarily uses inductive and abductive forms of reasoning. Each leads to different types of research action and generates different information or knowledge. Table 1-1 summarizes the major characteristics of these approaches to reasoning.

Deductive Reasoning and Actions

Experimental-type researchers primarily use *deductive reasoning.* This type of reasoning involves moving from a general principle to understanding a specific case. Based on a theory and its propositions, hypotheses are derived and then formally tested. Health and human service professionals use deductive reasoning every day in their practice.[2,12]

TABLE 1-1

Major Characteristics of Inductive/Abductive and Deductive Thinking

Inductive/Abductive	Deductive
No *a priori* acceptance of truth exists	*A priori* acceptance of truth exists
Alternative conclusions can be drawn from data	One set of conclusions is accepted as true
Theory is developed	Theory is tested
Relationships are examined among unrelated pieces of data	Relationships are tested among discrete phenomena
Concepts are developed based on repetition of patterns	Concepts are tested based on application to discrete phenomena
Perspective is holistic	Perspective is atomistic
Multiple realities exist	Single, separate reality exists

Let us assume a physician refers a particular individual to you. You receive the chart, which contains basic information. The individual, who has a diagnosis of possible dementia, is 75 years old and is a widowed woman who lives alone. From this general information and your knowledge about dementia, you begin to conjecture about this individual's future needs and whether she can safely return home alone. You may hypothesize that she will need assistance in performing daily activities of living, and you may hypothesize that she will be unsafe alone at home. When you meet the individual, you apply this general knowledge to understand this specific individual. You begin to test your hypothesis that the person is unable to return home alone. You may use a functional assessment tool to determine the level of personal assistance that is required by the patient. You may evaluate her ability to make judgments as a basis from which to determine home safety risks.

A similar process occurs in research. Using a deductive type of reasoning, the researcher begins with the acceptance of a general principle or belief based on a particular theoretical framework. This principle is then applied or used to explain a specific case or phenomenon. This approach involves "drawing

out" or verifying what is already accepted as true.[13] Consider the following example:

A researcher is interested in testing an intervention to improve the health of caregivers of people with dementia. In this case the researcher may begin from a framework of stress theory that assumes that the characteristics or behaviors of the care recipient are objective stressors that negatively impact the health of caregivers. Accepting this principle as truth, the deductive researcher will be interested in testing the effectiveness of interventions that are designed to reduce objective burden through providing education or teaching behavioral skills management to reduce the impact of the objective stressors.

Inductive Reasoning and Actions

Researchers who work within a naturalistic framework primarily use *inductive reasoning.* This type of reasoning involves moving from a specific case to a broader generalization about the phenomenon under study. In some forms of naturalistic inquiry, inductive reasoning involves fitting data, such as a set of observations or propositions of an existing theory. Health and human service professionals also use this form of reasoning in everyday practice.

> Assume you need to determine the discharge plans for the woman with dementia discussed in the previous example. You have concerns about the ability of the person to live alone, based on your knowledge of dementia as a progressively deteriorating condition. However, you do not know anything about the circumstances of this particular woman, her personal goals or those of her family, or her specific living arrangements. Through observation of the individual in the clinical setting, as well as in-depth interviewing of the client and family members, you discover that an adequate plan for monitoring and caring for the client has been put into place. Thus, you make a discharge decision based on the specifics of this case and the information you uncovered inductively.

A similar reasoning process occurs in research. The researcher searches for general rules or patterns by linking specific observations, which represents an inductive reasoning process. There is no "truth" or general principle that is accepted *a priori* ("from the former") or before the study begins. Consider the example of caregiving previously discussed. To derive an understanding of the nature and scope of stress, one type of inductive research approach could involve examining the daily life experiences of caregivers and their own perceptions of their activities. Using a variety of data collection techniques, such as observation and in-depth interviewing, the researcher might reason inductively by searching for patterns across observations of different caregivers. From this approach the researcher would be able to develop an understanding of the specific situations that cause stress, as well as the types of intervention that would be most useful in promoting caregiver health. The researcher, proceeding inductively, might seek to reveal or uncover a truth based on the perceptions of caregivers. Intervention principles would then be developed based on the researcher's interpretations of the perceptions of caregivers.

Abductive Reasoning and Actions

As we illustrate here, the two research traditions are typically characterized as using deductive and inductive reasoning processes; experimental-type research uses deductive reasoning, and naturalistic inquiry uses inductive reasoning. However, as Agar,

an ethnographer, pointed out in *The Professional Stranger,* this representation is not completely accurate. Some approaches in naturalistic inquiry are best characterized as "abductive."[14] *Abduction* is a term introduced by Charles Peirce[15] and currently used by Agar and other ethnographers to refer to the iterative process of naturalistic inquiry. This process involves the development of new theoretical propositions that account for a set of observations, which cannot be accounted for or explained by a previous proposition or theoretical framework. The new theoretical proposition becomes validated and modified as part of the research process. In this way, ethnography and some other forms of naturalistic inquiry, such as grounded theory,[16] are considered to be "theory generating." In deductive reasoning the data are controlled by the hypotheses. In inductive reasoning an attempt is made to fit the data to a theoretical framework or to a set of identified and well-defined concepts. In *abductive reasoning* the data are analyzed for their own patterns and concepts, which in some cases may relate to available theories and in other cases may not relate.

Differences in Knowledge

Each type of reasoning will result in the generation or production of a different form of knowledge. An inductive or abductive reasoning approach in research is used to "uncover" or "reveal" theory, rules, and processes. A deductive reasoning approach is used to describe, test, or predict the application of theory and rules to a specific phenomenon. Both approaches can be used to describe, explain, and predict phenomena, although only recently has inductive reasoning been valued as contributing to explanation and cause-and-effect relationships.

Let us examine the type of knowledge that is generated by each reasoning approach. The researcher working deductively will assume a truth before engaging in the research process and will apply that truth to the investigation. In the caregiver example, the researcher would assume that all caregivers will experience a form of stress and therefore may benefit from a stress-reduction intervention. The stress-reduction intervention may take the form of group psycho-educational counseling sessions and would be based on existing stress theory. Actual research that has tested this intervention approach has found it to be only mildly effective in reducing caregiver stress and only for some caregiver study participants.[17] Thus the question remains as to why all caregivers do not benefit at the level at which researchers expect.

In a study proceeding inductively or abductively, the researcher might be looking for an intervention approach to emerge from what is learned from those who will receive the intervention. Caregiver research that uses an inductive process may therefore find that caregiver experience cannot be completely understood or explained by stress theory or addressed by stress-oriented interventions alone. New interventions would be suggested by inductively oriented inquiry, such as a broader array of services, based on the specific needs and care issues identified by the study participants.

The deductive approach could show that a stress-reduction intervention benefits some caregivers. The inductive approach could reveal that stress theory is too limited to understand comprehensively the multiple needs of this group and that other theories and types of interventions would be helpful to consider.

As you can see, each type of reasoning and research approach produces important information from which to advance services to caregivers. It is also possible to use both types of reasoning to answer a research problem. For example, you can use an inductive or abductive approach to identify specific areas of caregiver needs and then use a deductive strategy to test systematically the outcome of an intervention that addresses the identified needs. This inductive-abductive-deductive approach is currently being used to develop and test community-based health and human service programs for underserved and culturally diverse populations. First, investigators use inductive strategies to uncover the health and wellness beliefs and needs of the target group. Based on the findings and theoretical frameworks that are refined, intervention strategies are developed, implemented, and systematically evaluated.

The integration of different forms of reasoning makes intuitive sense. In our daily lives we naturally engage in all forms of reasoning. Likewise, health and human service professionals combine knowledge gained from both deductive and inductive reasoning to derive appropriate treatment plans.

Research as Four Basic Characteristics

The third important component of our research definition refers to the criteria we use to characterize the research activity and differentiate it from other ways of knowing about a phenomenon. We have stated that scientific knowledge may be generated by multiple research strategies using inductive or abductive or deductive reasoning. Any research strategy, whether based on inductive or abductive or deductive reasoning, must conform to the four criteria of being logical, understandable, confirmable, and useful.

Logical

In research there is a unique way of thinking and acting that distinguishes it from other ways we use to know, understand, and make sense of our experiences. Charles Peirce,[15] one of the founders of the scientific research process, identified other ways of "knowing" as the following: (1) authority—being told by a respected or trusted source; (2) hearsay—secondhand information that is not verified; (3) trial and error—knowledge gained through incremental doing, evaluating, and modifying actions to achieve a desired outcome; (4) history—knowing indirectly through collective past experiences; (5) belief—knowing without verification; (6) spiritual understanding—knowing through divine belief; and (7) intuition—explanations of human experience based on previous unique and personal organization of one's own experience.

In these other forms, knowledge is gained unsystematically, and it is not necessary to clarify the evidentiary basis or the logical thinking and action processes by which the information is obtained and asserted. Think about how an individual gains knowledge about parenting or providing care to a person who requires assistance. Informal caregivers tend to learn how to provide care through trial and error. Information as to what works and what does not work to achieve a desired goal is gained incrementally, over time, by trying different techniques and informally evaluating their outcome. Many caregivers also use intuition and hearsay or information from other caregivers, family, and friends who may make suggestions based on their own history and experience. Different from this informal set of thinking and action processes, research must be based on systematic thought processes and methodical investigative activities that include documentation, analysis, and drawing conclusions.

By *logical* we mean that the thinking and action processes of a research study are clear, rational, and conform to accepted norms of deductive, inductive, or abductive reasoning. Logic is a science that involves defined ways of thinking and methodically relates ideas to develop an understanding of phenomena and their relationships. The systematic nature of research requires that the investigator proceed logically and articulate each thought and action throughout the research process.

Understandable

It is not sufficient for a researcher to articulate a logical process. This process, the study outcomes, and its conclusions need to be explicit, make sense, be precise, be intelligible, and be credible to the reader or research consumer. If you cannot *understand* the research process, it cannot be used, confirmed, or replicated.

Historically, researchers using naturalistic inquiry did not typically identify the specific steps involved in their investigative process. Currently, however, a significant body of literature describes and makes explicit the thinking and action processes of different forms of naturalistic inquiry.[18,19] Investigators who work out of the naturalistic tradition are advancing the standards of quality by which to judge such research. How are we to distinguish a casual observation of emergency room behavior from a scholarly interpretation of underlying patterns in that setting? Researchers have actively addressed this critical issue.[9,10,19,20]

Confirmable

By *confirmable* we mean that the researcher clearly and logically identifies the strategies used in the study so that others can reasonably follow the path of analysis and arrive at similar outcomes and conclusions. The claims made by the researcher should be supported by the evidence and research strategy and should be accurate and credible within the stated boundaries of the study.

Useful

Research generates, verifies, or tests theory and knowledge for use. In other words, the knowledge derived from a study should inform and potentially improve professional practice and client outcome. Each researcher, consumer, or professional judges the utility of a study based on his or her own needs and purposes. *Usefulness* is a subjective criterion in that it is based on the researcher's judgment about the value of the knowledge produced by a study. However, the value of a study and the usefulness of knowledge become more widely accepted as the new knowledge increasingly stimulates further research and promotes the testing or verification of new or existing theory and practice.

SUMMARY

Our definition of research represents our conceptual framework and guides our subsequent discussions in this book. It is based on a philosophical position that the multiple realities that shape health and human services require an approach to research that is informed by multiple research traditions and design strategies. Our approach to research is practical; that is, the purpose and question of an investigator guide the selection of appropriate methodologies, and in turn the questions asked and the knowledge gained must be useful to the clinical, professional, and consumer communities.

Research is critical to health and human service professionals to advance the knowledge base by which clinical decisions are made. Research informs knowledge development and daily practice, and professionals can participate in this activity in many different ways.

EXERCISES

1. Select a research article in your professional journal. Identify the source from which the investigator obtained the research question. Decide whether the study fits the four characteristics of research as being logical, confirmable, understandable, and useful, and give the reasons for your opinions.
2. Write down three issues that represent a concern to your profession or that have emerged from your daily practice. Determine whether each issue reflects a topic that can and should be researched. How do you currently address these issues?

REFERENCES

1. Yerxa E: Seeing a relevant, ethical and realistic way to knowing for occupational therapy, *Am J Occup Ther* 45: 199-204, 1991.
2. DePoy E, Gilson SF: *Evaluation practice,* Belmont, Calif, 2003, Brooks-Cole.
3. Westerfelt A, Deitz TJ: *Planning and conducting agency-based research,* ed 3, Boston, 2005, Allyn & Bacon.
4. Gitlin LN: *Physical function: a comprehensive guide to its meaning and measurement,* Austin, Tex, 2005, Pro-Ed.
5. Gambrill E: Authority-based profession, *Res Soc Work Pract* 11(2):66-175, 2001.
6. Reason P, Bradbury H: *Handbook of action research,* Thousand Oaks, Calif, 2000, Sage.
7. McTavish DG, Loether HJ: *Social research: an evolving process,* ed 2, Boston, 2002, Allyn & Bacon.
8. Kerlinger FN: *Foundations of behavioral research,* ed 2, New York, 1973, Holt, Rinehart, & Winston.
9. Silverman D: *Doing qualitative research: a practical handbook,* ed 2, Thousand Oaks, Calif, 2004, Sage.
10. Patton M: *Qualitative evaluation and research methods,* ed 2, Newbury Park, Calif, 1990, Sage.
11. Bonilla-Silva E: *Racism without racists: color-blind racism and the persistence of racial inequality in the United States,* New York, 2003, Rowman & Littlefield.
12. Gibbs L: *Evidence-based practice,* Belmont, Calif, 2002, Wadsworth.
13. Hoover KR: *The elements of social scientific thinking,* ed 2, New York, 1980, St Martin's Press.
14. Agar MH: *The professional stranger,* ed 2, San Diego, 1996, Academic Press.
15. Peirce CS: *Essays in the philosophy of science,* Indianapolis, 1957, Bobbs-Merrill.
16. Glaser B, Strauss AL: *The discovery of grounded theory: strategies for qualitative research,* Chicago, 1967, Aldine de Gruyter.
17. Corcoran MA, Gitlin LN: Environmental influences on behavior of the elderly with dementia: principles for home intervention, *Occup Ther Geriatr* 4:5-22, 1991.
18. Berg B: *Qualitative research methods for the social sciences,* ed 5, Long Beach, Calif, 2004, Longman.
19. Denzin N, Lincoln YS: *Handbook of qualitative research,* ed 2, Thousand Oaks, Calif, 2000, Sage.
20. Smith JK: Quantitative vs. qualitative research: an attempt to clarify the issue, *Educ Researcher* 112:6-13, 1983.

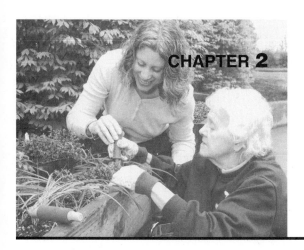

Essentials of Research

Researchers who pursue either naturalistic or experimental-type inquiry confront similar challenges and requirements when conducting research. However, these are interpreted and acted on differently, depending on the type of inquiry pursued. We categorize the challenges and requirements of any type of research endeavor into what we call the *10 essentials* of the research process (Box 2-1).

Each subsequent chapter in this book focuses on one particular research essential and examines its components from the perspectives of both naturalistic inquiry and experimental-type research. Consider this chapter as a brief summary of the entire text. You may want to read this chapter quickly and then refer to it as you make your way through the text as a way of summarizing the meaning of each essential. You can refer to Table 2-1 as a quick guide as well.

TEN ESSENTIALS OF RESEARCH

The 10 research essentials and their order of presentation in this book should not be construed as

---

BOX 2-1
TEN ESSENTIALS OF RESEARCH

1. Identify philosophical foundation
2. Frame a research problem
3. Determine supporting knowledge
4. Identify theory base
5. Develop a specific question or query
6. Select a design strategy
7. Set study boundaries
8. Obtain information
9. Analyze information and draw conclusions
10. Share and use research knowledge

TABLE 2-1

Ten Essentials of Research

Essential	Explanation	Process
Identify a philosophical foundation	Reveal underlying assumptions of ontology and epistemology	Thinking
Frame a research problem	Identify broad topic or problem area	Thinking
Determine supporting knowledge	Review and synthesize existing literature to examine knowledge development in identified problem area	Thinking/Action
Identify a theory base	Use existing theory to frame research problem and interpret result; or construct theory as part of research process	Thinking
Develop a specific question or query	Identify specific focus for research, based on knowledge development, theoretical perspective, and research purpose	Thinking
Select a design strategy	Develop standard procedures or broad strategic approach to answer research question or query	Thinking
Set study boundaries	Establish scope of study and methods for accessing research participants	Action
Obtain information	Determine strategies for collecting information that is numerical, visual, auditory, or narrative	Action
Analyze information and draw conclusions	Employ systematic processes to examine different types of data and derive interpretative scheme	Action
Share and use research knowledge	Write and disseminate research conclusions	Action

representing a step-by-step, procedural, or "recipe"-type approach to the research process. Each essential is highly interrelated and may not necessarily occur in the order in which it is presented in Box 2-1 and in this text. The order depends on the tradition and design that you select.

Experimental-type research is hierarchical in its sequence and approach. It tends to follow the 10 essentials in a precise, ordered, and highly structured manner such that each essential purposely builds on the other in a linear, systematic, and stepwise manner. Figure 2-1 depicts this linear approach, and this graphic is used throughout this book to describe the enactment of the 10 essentials. However, it is important to note that even within experimental-type research, the 10 essentials are not mutually exclusive. As one moves along stepwise, previous steps may be revised as a consequence of new methodological decisions.

Naturalistic inquiry, on the other hand, embodies the 10 essentials using more diverse and complex processes, whereby each essential is related to the other and revisited at different points throughout the

Philosophical Foundation

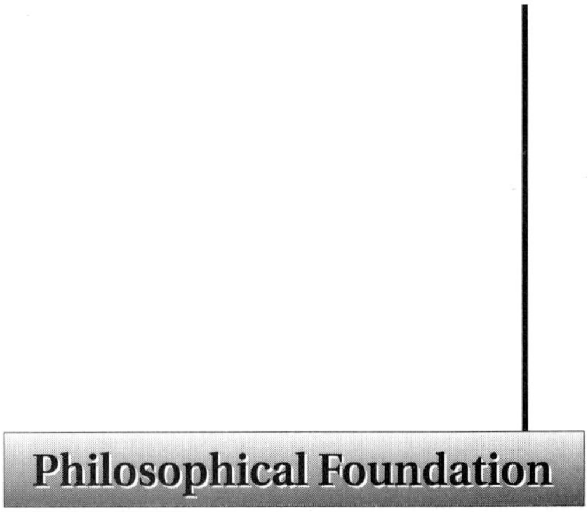

Figure 2-1   Linear approach of experimental-type research.

research process. This spiral image, used throughout this book to depict this type of inquiry (Figure 2-2), links the 10 essentials in different orders, depending on the specific philosophical foundation in which the research is based. The sequences of the 10 essentials within each research tradition in naturalistic inquiry

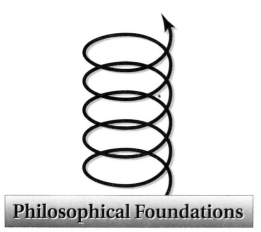

Philosophical Foundations

Figure 2-2   Spiral approach of naturalistic inquiry.

will become clear as you make your way through this book. Let us briefly examine the meaning of each essential.

Identify a Philosophical Foundation

Identifying a philosophical foundation is an important essential that occurs first or in the early stages of the research process. By *philosophical foundation* we mean an individual's particular orientation to how a person learns about human behavior, health, and personal abilities and experiences, or other phenomena of importance in health and human services. In Chapter 3 we classify these orientations into two overarching philosophical categories through which knowledge is viewed and built, each of which gives rise to one of the primary research traditions. Thus the researcher's particular philosophical orientation toward learning about phenomena determines the specific research tradition that is selected: experimentaltype, naturalistic inquiry, or an integration of the two.

In naturalistic inquiry, articulating a philosophical tradition is especially important because of the many distinct philosophical schools of thought that inform this research approach (see Chapter 3).

Researchers who identify their philosophical perspective as symbolic interaction tend to use highly interpretative forms of naturalistic inquiry that focus on the meanings and behaviors of individuals in social interaction. These researchers tend to pursue ethnographical research methodology. On the

other hand, researchers who identify with the philosophical foundation of phenomenology will focus on particular personal experiences of individuals, such as patients living with acquired immunodeficiency syndrome (AIDS), ethnic minorities interacting with health care providers, or how each gender perceives sense of self. Researchers working in a phenomenological tradition tend to pursue methodologies that elicit the telling of a person's personal story or narrative using a variety of sources, including personal interactions, interviews, and diary reviews.

In writing a proposal to conduct a research study or in writing a report of the completed study, the researcher using naturalistic inquiry usually discusses his or her philosophical perspective.

In contrast, experimental-type research is based on one unifying philosophical foundation—logical positivism. Positivism is a broad term that refers to the belief that there is one truth independent of the investigator and that this truth can be discovered by following strict procedures (see Chapter 3). It is not necessary for an experimental-type researcher to identify the philosophical root of his or her research when submitting a research proposal or a published report, because all experimental-type inquiry is based on a single philosophical base. For example, a researcher trained in survey techniques will naturally assume a positivist or empiricist approach to describe a particular phenomenon. Therefore it is not necessary for this researcher to state formally the epistemological assumption embedded in the study.

A philosophical foundation provides the backdrop from which specific methodological decisions in research are made. This does not mean that you first must become a philosopher to participate in research. However, you do need to know that research methodologies reflect different assumptions about human behavior and knowledge and about how we learn about phenomena. By selecting a particular research strategy, you will automatically adopt a particular worldview and philosophical foundation. We believe that, at the very least, you should be aware that you are adopting a specific set of assumptions about human behavior and how people come to understand it. Understanding this philosophical foundation is particularly critical because assumptions about knowledge and their use have major implications for how health and human service professionals understand and respond to the diversity of human characteristics.

Consider the example of a social worker who is hired to design and examine a pregnancy prevention program for Asian American teenagers. From a logical positive tradition, one approach would be to select an existing and validated program, or what is referred to as evidence based practice, and then implement and test it to ascertain its effectiveness in achieving pregnancy prevention for this particular group. In contrast, a naturalistic researcher would begin by discovering the cultural norms and values of Asian American teenagers that are important to informing a prevention program and then, based on this knowledge, construct an intervention tailored to that group. Each research approach has its advantages and limitations.

You probably already have a particular philosophical foundation or preferred way of knowing without fully labeling or recognizing it as such. Sometimes personality, or how one naturally views the world, influences the particular research direction that is adopted. If you prefer to make and follow detailed plans, if you feel uncomfortable with the view that values and biases shape one's worldview, or if you do not like "hanging out" in someone else's world, you may have difficulty with naturalistic inquiry. In contrast, if you are uncomfortable working with and understanding numerical values, you may have difficulty with experimental-type inquiries. Many articles have been written about the personality types of individuals who pursue ethnography versus those who pursue experimental-type research. However, there is nothing definitive about this literature. Certainly, all types of personalities are capable of learning the practices of multiple research paradigms.

Frame a Research Problem

To engage in the research process, the investigator must identify in advance a particular problem area or broad issue that necessitates systematic investigation. Research using any form of inquiry is a focused endeavor that addresses a social issue, theoretically derived prediction, practice question, or personal concern. One of the first thinking processes in which you engage is the identification of the problem area

and the specific purpose for your research. Research topics should come from personal, professional, theoretical, political, and societal concerns. To engage in research, it is important that you identify an area that holds personal interest and meaning to you. The research process is challenging and requires time and commitment. You will quickly lose momentum if you do not pursue a topic of personal intrigue. Some researchers study areas that have been problematic in their own lives. For example, some investigators who pursue disability studies have had a personal encounter with disability, such as growing up with a disabled sibling or parent. Research in an area that has personal significance provides a scholarly forum from which to examine and then personally understand the issues. This is not to say that you have to be an individual with a disability to want to study disability, or that you need to have experienced child abuse to study this phenomenon. However, something about a topic should "grab" you. It has to have personal meaning or some level of importance to your life—intellectually, emotionally, or professionally—for the research endeavor to be personally worthwhile. Since research is a long and engaging process, being passionate about a particular topic area or problem is important.

Once you have identified a topic (e.g., coping strategies of culturally diverse caregivers of dementia patients; impact of maternal alcohol abuse on early childhood development), you can begin to think about your particular purpose in exploring the topic. What do you want to know about the topic? What will be the purpose and use of your particular research? To determine the direction, purpose, and uses of a study, the researcher must read what is already known about the topic.

Determine Supporting Knowledge

Another research essential involves a critical review of existing theory and research that concern your topic or area of inquiry.

> Let us assume, based on your practice with individuals hospitalized with spinal cord injury, that you need to know more about their self-care practices and social supports once they return home. This information will help determine the types of

skills training that would be important to introduce in the hospital and how best to prepare your patients for the challenges they will confront at home. You believe this area of concern is important to investigate. Your first task will be to determine what is known in the published literature. If there is little or no knowledge about the topic, you will need to design a study that describes self-care practices and the role of social networks. If there is some descriptive knowledge of daily practices but little information about whether these practices differ across diverse populations and are associated with availability of social supports, you may want to conduct a study that investigates these aspects of the topic. Suppose there is a body of well-constructed knowledge about gender and ethnic differences in practices of caregivers. This information may lead you to examine the impact of these practices on the general well-being and self-care of individuals who will be discharged to their homes after spinal cord injury. Existing literature should be used to help identify and guide the direction of research that is necessary to build knowledge in your area of interest.

A critical review of the literature initially helps the investigator frame a specific research direction so that the study will systematically contribute to the building of knowledge in the topic or area of concern.

A critical literature review is also used for other purposes throughout the research process. In some forms of naturalistic inquiry, literature review is used as an additional set of data. Literature review may also be used to help the investigator further explore his or her emerging interpretations of observations. In experimental-type research, a critical review using the methodology of meta-analysis is a type of research study in its own right (see Chapter 5). Within any research tradition, the researcher must draw on and place his or her new findings within the context of previous studies when reporting the knowledge developed in a study. The findings of a particular study are always interpreted through or added to other studies to add incrementally to a body of knowledge in the topic area.

Identify a Theory Base

Theory is formally defined as a set of interrelated propositions that provide a framework for understanding or explaining phenomena. (Theory and its relationship with research are described in greater detail in Chapter 6.) The purpose of research is either to construct theory or to test theory. Research that does not contribute to the building of theory or that is not based on theory produces findings that are basically useless. Findings from a study that are not based in or related to a theoretical context cannot be adequately interpreted or understood. Atheoretical collection of data does not contribute to the systematic building of knowledge. Experimental-type researchers tend to test different aspects of a theory; that is, the research begins with a theoretical framework from which specific hypotheses (hunches about what should occur) are generated and tested using different design strategies. Even in a descriptive or correlational study that is not designed to test a specific theory, theory is essential in guiding the research process and interpreting study results.

Naturalistic inquiry generates new theories, expands existing theories, or relates research findings to existing theoretical frameworks. In actual research practice, theory is used by both research traditions for multiple purposes and in many different ways. Thus the use of theory is interjected at different points of the research process, especially in naturalistic inquiry.

Develop a Specific Question or Query

Once a problem area is identified, the researcher must specify a particular research direction. In experimental-type research, this direction takes the form of a highly specified *question* that details the exact factors and the characteristics or phenomena that will be examined.

The experimental-type researcher may pose the question, "What is the relationship between self-care practice and the psychological well-being in individuals with spinal cord injury?" With this question, the researcher identifies two concepts that will be studied: self-care practices and psychological well-being. The researcher will then carefully define these terms and determine how each will be operationalized or measured. A study design is selected that will enable an analysis of the relationship between these two concepts.

In naturalistic inquiry, the research direction is broadly represented and becomes highly specified only through the process of conducting the study itself. In this type of research, the investigator develops a broad working question, or what we call a *query,* that initially identifies the "who, what, and where" of the boundaries of the study, but nothing further.

> The naturalistic-type researcher may pose the question, "What are the experiences of men with spinal cord injury in performing basic self-care activities on their return home?" With this question, the researcher has identified who will be studied (men with spinal cord injuries), where the study will occur (at home), and what the focus of the query will be (how self-care is accomplished). Other concerns may emerge in the course of the study that may lead the researcher to redefine the initial query or consider more specific questions, such as the relationship between specific self-care practices and personal well-being. For example, the researcher may learn in the course of the study that it is important to understand self-care practices by evaluating a broader range of behaviors and underlying values that guide the person's daily routines. The decision to do so is based on initial analyses and formative inter-pretations that occur while the researcher is in the field conducting the study.

Thus, in naturalistic inquiry, the research question is framed broadly and represents a query from which more specific research questions and investigative approaches emerge in the course of learning about a particular phenomenon. The specific questions that arise in the field cannot be anticipated before entering the research setting.

In any type of research approach, however, a broad topic or area of concern must be framed or specified in such a way as to facilitate its exploration.

> Within the broad topic of aging with a physically disabling condition, for example, many subtopics and specific research questions or queries can be formulated.

The level of knowledge development and theoretical understanding of the topic will direct the researcher to the specific research question or query that represents the next logical step to build knowledge in the area.

Select a Design Strategy

Design is perhaps the most fundamental aspect of the research process. Based on one's philosophical posi-

tion, research purpose, theory, and specific research question or query, the researcher will select an action process by which to explore or answer the query. In naturalistic inquiry, research design is fluid and evolves as the investigator gains access to a natural setting and explores the phenomenon of interest. Further, terms that refer to designs can represent both the process and the end product. For example, ethnography is a term that refers to the process of performing fieldwork to understand the cultural patterns of a specified group. Ethnography also refers to the end product: the published report or book about the particular cultural group. Design in naturalistic inquiry means a set of strategies that are employed by the investigator to gain access to a natural setting (e.g., homes of men with spinal cord injury) and to collect and analyze information using a combination of procedures that unfold in the course of conducting the study (e.g., videotape, participant observation, interviewing).

In experimental-type research, design is highly structured with a specified set of procedures that are decided before entering the field and then implemented uniformly and systematically by the investigator. In this tradition a design is similar to a "blueprint" that details each procedure or action process.

> Assume an investigator plans to conduct a survey of high school students to determine their level of knowledge about safe sexual practices. Before conducting the study, the investigator will develop a sampling plan (how subjects will be recruited and selected), will frame a set of questions with a fixed response set, and will identify specific statistical analyses that will be conducted. All these decisions must be decided before beginning the study, then strictly followed.

It is impossible to discuss the vast array of research design strategies in each of the research traditions in one text. We present the most fundamental and useful approaches for health and human service professionals, with a particular emphasis on designs that are amenable to or can be integrated with professional practices.

Set Study Boundaries

Another essential is that a researcher must establish the boundaries or scope of a study. Boundaries are set for a number of reasons, the most important of which is to limit the scope of the study so that it is feasible to conduct or is doable. Ways of setting boundaries include determining the length of study, the participants in the study, the conceptual dimensions that will be examined, and the type and number of questions that will be asked. Setting boundary strategies is different for experimental-type and naturalistic inquiry studies. In experimental-type designs, the boundaries of the study are clearly and precisely defined before entering the field. The researcher establishes a concise plan for identifying and enrolling subjects into the study, determines which questionnaires or data collection strategies to use, and identifies up front the specific conceptual dimensions that are to be included. In naturalistic-type studies, the setting of boundaries is an evolving process that occurs once the investigator enters the research setting. After gaining access to the research setting, the investigator continually makes decisions such as who is interviewed, how and what data are collected, and what conceptual issues are explored.

A major action process in boundary setting is the protection of those boundaries. As discussed in Chapters 11 to 14, protection of human subjects is both an ethical and a legal obligation for all inquiry that directly involves individuals and groups of people.

Obtain Information

A researcher can choose from a wide variety of techniques for obtaining information or data. Later in this text we examine these techniques along a continuum, from unstructured looking and listening techniques to structured, fixed-choice observation and ways of asking questions.

Analyze Information and Draw Conclusions

Analyzing information, the ninth essential of the research process, involves a series of planned activities that differ depending on the specific research tradition in which one works. One of the initial analytical tasks of experimental-type researchers is to reduce numerical data into meaningful and manageable indicators, such as means, mode, and median. Other statistical techniques are then employed depending on the characteristics of the measures, the size of the sample, and the specific research question. The analytical task typically occurs once all the data have been collected and is used to answer the initial research question that was posed.

In naturalistic inquiry, other analytical approaches are used that are appropriate for the analysis of narrative and other nonnumerical types of data. The analytical task has several purposes in naturalistic inquiry. First, it is an ongoing process that occurs throughout the the study and is used to inform field decisions. Second, the analysis systematically applies techniques that can lead to an interpretation of the information that has been obtained.

Share and Use Research Knowledge

Sharing and using research knowledge completes the research process. Reporting conclusions involves preparing a report and disseminating the knowledge gained from the research. Each research tradition approaches this research essential somewhat differently. However, researchers usually describe the purpose of their study; how it contributes to a particular field or topic; the specific procedures that were followed by the researcher, including analytical strategies; and the findings and interpretations of the information obtained. The use of research conclusions may take different forms, including translation of the knowledge gained into specific service programs, as evidence to guide professional practice, or as a step from which other research questions are posed.

ETHICAL CONSIDERATIONS

We have identified 10 essentials or characteristics of any type of research study. Researchers must address each essential at different points in the research process. The application of these essentials in health and human service settings raises special issues and ethical dilemmas. Ethical concerns focus on (1) the rights of human research participants to full knowledge of the purpose of the study and the nature of their involvement, (2) the specific behaviors or conduct of the investigator, and (3) the *ethics* of the question and design procedures. Ethical considerations are explored throughout this book, with specific reference to how they inform each essential.

SUMMARY

All research, regardless of the topic, approach, and use, consists of 10 essentials. In experimental-type research, these essentials are ordered, linear, and performed in a stepwise manner. In naturalistic inquiry, the essentials are carried out in different sequences depending on the particular research tradition and the design used.

Figure 2-3 is used throughout this text to signify the tradition and essential that we are discussing. As you proceed through the world of research with us, you will note that the graphic is also meant to suggest that experimental-type and naturalistic research can be used in tandem or can be integrated. Research integrating experimental-type and naturalistic traditions can occur in any of the thinking processes or action processes that constitute the 10 essentials, as discussed throughout this book.

EXERCISES

1. Select two research articles, and identify the 10 essentials in each.
2. Using both articles, compare and contrast how the essentials are sequenced and described by the investigators.

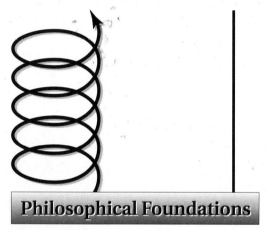

Philosophical Foundations

Figure 2-3   Spiral approach and linear approach to research.

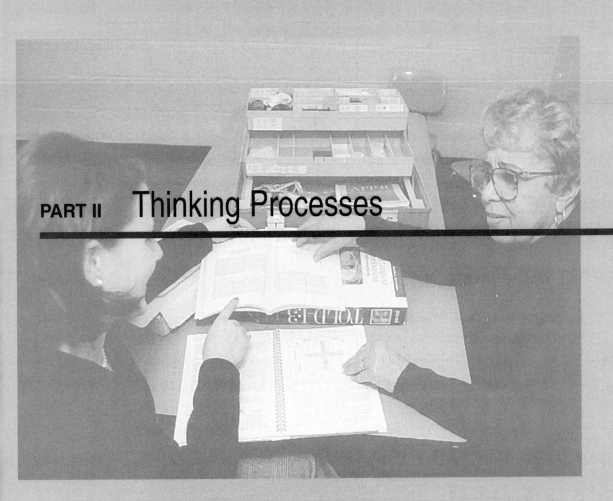

PART II Thinking Processes

In Part I of this text, we introduced the definition, purposes, and essentials of research.

We now delve into Part II, the thinking processes in which all researchers engage to make sound decisions about how to frame, conduct, and use research. These efforts include understanding the philosophical foundations that underpin diverse research traditions, framing the research problem, critically reviewing the literature, linking theory and research, developing a research question or query, and using the appropriate research language to understand and explicate the research process, findings, and interpretations.

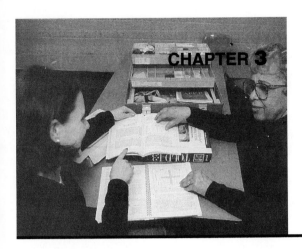

CHAPTER 3

Philosophical Foundations

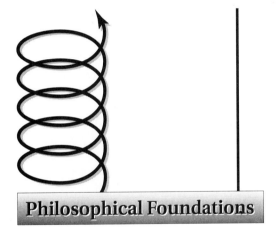

Philosophical Foundations

Although you do not have to be a philosopher to engage in the research process, it is important to understand the philosophical foundations and assumptions about human experience and knowledge on which experimental-type and naturalistic research traditions are based. By being aware of these assumptions, you will be more skillful in directing the research process and in selecting specific methods to use and combine. Also, an understanding of these philosophical foundations will help you recognize that "knowledge" is determined by the way you frame a research problem and the strategies that are used to obtain, analyze, and interpret information.

The questions, "What is reality?" *(ontology)* and "How do we come to know it?" *(epistemology)* have been posed by philosophers and scholars from many academic and professional disciplines throughout

23

history. As we have suggested, in Western cultures there are two primary but often competing views of reality and how to obtain knowledge. These two perspectives reflect the basic differences between naturalistic inquiry and experimental-type research. *Logical positivism* is the foundation for deductive, predictive designs that we refer to as "experimental-type research." On the other hand, a number of holistic and humanistic philosophical perspectives use inductive and abductive reasoning, which form the foundation for the research tradition that we refer to as "naturalistic inquiry."

PHILOSOPHICAL FOUNDATION OF EXPERIMENTAL-TYPE RESEARCH

Experimental-type researchers share a common frame of reference or epistemology that has been called rationalistic, positivist, reductionist, or logical positivism. Although theoretical differences exist between these terms, we use the term "logical positivism" to name the overall perspective on which deductive research design is based.

David Hume, an 18th-century philosopher, was most influential in developing this traditional theory of science.[1] This viewpoint posits that there is a separation between individual thoughts and what is real in the universe outside ourselves. That is, traditional theorists of science define "knowledge" as part of a reality that is separate and independent from individuals and that is verifiable through the scientific method. These theorists believe the world is objectively knowable and can be discovered through observation and measurement that is considered unbiased. This epistemological view is based on the fundamental assumption that it is possible to know and understand phenomena that reside outside ourselves, separate from the realm of our subjective ideas. Only through observation and sense data, defined as information obtained through our senses, can we come to know truth and reality.

Philosophers in subsequent centuries further developed, modified, and clarified Hume's basic notion of empiricism to yield what today is known as logical positivism. Essentially, logical positivists believe that there is a single reality that can be discovered by reducing it into its parts, a concept known

as reductionism. The relationship among these parts and the logical, structural principles that guide them can also be discovered and known through the systematic collection and analysis of sense data, finally leading to the ability to predict phenomena from what is already known. Bertrand Russell, a 20th-century mathematician and philosopher, was instrumental in promoting the synthesis of mathematical logic with sense data.[2] Statisticians, such as Quetelet, Fischer, and Pearson, developed theories to reveal "fact" logically and objectively through mathematical analysis. The logical positive school of thought therefore provided the foundation for what most laypersons have come to know as "experimental research." In this approach, a theory or set of principles is held as true. Specific areas of inquiry are isolated within that theoretical perspective, and clearly defined hypotheses (expected outcomes of an inquiry that investigate only those phenomena) are posed and tested under carefully controlled conditions. Sense data are then collected and mathematically analyzed to support or refute hypotheses. Through incremental deductive reasoning, which involves theory verification and testing, "reality" can become predictable.

Another major tenet of logical positivism is that objective inquiry and analysis are possible; that is, the investigator, through the use of accepted and standard research techniques, can eliminate bias and achieve results through objective, quantitative measurement.[3-6]

PHILOSOPHICAL FOUNDATION OF NATURALISTIC INQUIRY

Another school of theorists has argued an alternative position—individuals create their own subjective realities, and thus the knower and knowledge are interrelated and interdependent.[7-9] In general, these theorists believe that ideas are the lenses through which each individual knows the universe and that we come to understand and define the world through these ideas. Furthermore, within these traditions, there is a range of beliefs about the stability of ideas and the role of language in communicating or even creating ideas and experiences. This epistemological viewpoint is based on the fundamental assumption that it is not possible to separate the outside world from an individual's ideas, language, and perceptions of that world. Knowledge is based on how the individual perceives experiences and how he or she understands his or her world. A number of research strategies share this basic holistic, epistemological view, although each is rooted in a different philosophical tradition.

Although research based on *holistic* perspectives has gained acceptance more recently than logical positivist approaches, the philosophical perspectives are not new. Ancient Greek philosophers struggled with the separation of idea and object, and philosophers throughout history continue this debate.[10] The essential characteristics of what we refer to as "holistic philosophies" are as follows:

1. Human experience is complex and cannot be understood by reductionism, that is, by identifying and examining its parts.
2. Meaning in human experience is derived from an understanding of individuals in their social, economic, political, cultural, linguistic, physical, and virtual environments.
3. Multiple realities exist, and our view of reality is determined by events viewed through individual lenses or biases.
4. Those who have the experiences are the most knowledgeable about them.

In addition to these common characteristics, holistic philosophies encompass a number of principles that guide the selection of particular designs in this category. For example, *phenomenologists* believe that human meaning can be understood only through experience.[8] Thus, a phenomenological understanding is limited to knowing experience without interpreting that experience. On the other hand, interpretive and social "semiotic" *interactionists* assume that human meaning evolves from the context of social interaction.[8,11,12] Human phenomena can therefore be understood through interpreting the meanings in social discourse, exchange, and symbols. Deconstructionists focus on the primacy and fleeting stability of language, and thus research based on that philosophical thought examines how language both forms and undermines what we know.[13] The holistic philosophies therefore suggest a pluralistic view of knowledge; multiple realities can be identified and understood to a greater or lesser extent only within the natural context

in which human experience and behavior occur. To the extent possible, coming to know these realities requires a research design that investigates phenomena in their natural contexts and seeks to discover complexity and meaning. Furthermore, those who "own" or have the experience are considered the "knowers," and they transmit their knowledge through doing and telling.[11]

IMPLICATIONS OF PHILOSOPHICAL DIFFERENCES FOR DESIGN

The previous discussion provides you with the basic elements of different philosophical positions concerning how we think about and develop an understanding or knowledge about human life. Although you do not have to take a position on the ongoing debate between different philosophical positions, it is important that you recognize that by adapting a particular methodology, you are implicitly adhering to a particular way of viewing the world and knowledge development. You may also find yourself gravitating to a particular research approach because you feel more comfortable with it or because it may resonate with how you see the world. How you explicitly or implicitly define and generate knowledge and how you define the relationship between the knower (researcher) and the known (research outcomes or phenomena of the study) will direct your entire research effort, from framing your research question or query to reporting your findings. Let us consider some examples of these important philosophical concepts and their implications for research design.

Suppose that three researchers want to know what happens to participants in group therapy who have joined the group to improve their self-confidence. The researcher who suggests that knowing can be objective may choose a strategy in which he or she defines "self-confidence" as a score on a preexisting, standardized scale and then measures participants' scores at specified intervals to ascertain changes. Changes in the scores suggest what changes the group has experienced.

A second investigator, who believes that the world can be known only subjectively, may choose a research strategy in which the group is observed and the members are interviewed to obtain their perspective on their own progress within the group.

A third investigator, who believes that language shapes individual perception of reality, will focus on analysis of language communication and its multiple uses, contexts, and meanings within the group setting.

A fourth researcher, who believes in the value of many ways of knowing, may integrate the previous three strategies. This researcher tries to understand change from the communication patterns as well as individual perspectives of the participants and from the perspective of existing theory as measured by a standardized self-confidence scale.

RESEARCH TRADITIONS

Thus far we have indicated that there are two primary philosophical traditions that underpin two broad categories of inquiry. We categorize these research approaches as experimental-type and naturalistic inquiry. Within each of these categories are many systematic research strategies. We suggest, however, that research strategies fall within two primary research traditions.

The first tradition shares the philosophical foundation of experimental-type research. In this tradition a prescribed sequence of linear processes (as discussed in detail in subsequent chapters) is designed and implemented.[4,6] Throughout this text we refer to this tradition as "experimental-type research."

On the other hand, strategies that share the principles of a holistic perspective or naturalistic inquiry follow a nonlinear, iterative, and flexible[14] sequence of processes. Throughout this text, we include these strategies in the tradition of "naturalistic inquiry."

Each design tradition has its own language, its own thinking and action processes, and specific design issues and concerns. We use the concept of the two traditions throughout this text as a basis from which to discuss and compare design essentials and research processes within the same philosophical perspective and across philosophical traditions.

Experimental-Type Research

Let us begin with the philosophical foundation of the experimental-type tradition. First, remember that logical positivists believe one can come to know a single reality through a deductive process. This process involves theorizing to explain the part of reality about which the investigator is concerned, reducing theory to observable parts, examining the parts through measurement, and determining the degree to which the analysis verifies or falsifies part or all of the theory. Second, a central principle of logical positivism is that it is possible and desirable to understand the world through systematic objectivity and by eliminating bias in our observations. Given these two critical elements of logical positivism, let us examine how each research essential, as it occurs in a linear sequence, supports the tenets of logical positivist inquiry.

After identifying a philosophical foundation, the researcher begins by articulating a topic of inquiry. We name this step "framing the problem," which identifies and delimits the part of the "real world" that an investigator will examine. Once a research problem is identified, supporting knowledge is obtained by conducting a review of scholarly literature and resources. This research essential discerns how the problem has already been theoretically approached and explained. It examines the extent to which the theory has been objectively and rigorously investigated. The scholarly review of literature and other sources of knowledge therefore provide the researcher with knowledge for developing a theoretical foundation for the inquiry. With this information, the investigator is now ready to propose a specific research question. This question is derived from and builds on previous inquiry, isolates the theoretical material to be scrutinized, and incrementally advances knowledge about the subject under study. The ultimate goal is to predict a part of reality from knowing about other parts. To answer the research question objectively, the investigator selects a research design that answers the research question and controls factors that introduce bias into a study. The design clearly and succinctly specifies all action processes for collecting and analyzing information so that the study may be replicated by other investigators. To ensure that the goals of objectivity and the elimination of bias are met, these actions must be followed exactly as designed. Through data analysis the investigator examines the extent to which the findings have objectively confirmed or raised doubts about the "truth value" of the theoretical tenets and their capacity to explain and ultimately predict the slice of reality under investigation.

Many designs are anchored in the philosophical foundation of logical positivism. Box 3-1 lists the four major categories of design that form the experimental-type tradition, each of which is discussed in detail in Part III of this text.

Naturalistic Inquiry

There is great diversity in the strategies that are categorized as naturalistic inquiry. As indicated in this chapter, designs that fit with this tradition are rooted in different philosophical and theoretical perspectives. The language and thinking processes used by naturalistic researchers vary within the tradition and are significantly different from the language and thinking processes found in the experimental-type tradition. However, all naturalistic approaches have characteristics in common and use qualitative methodologies, although often for different purposes and often to answer distinct types of inquiries.

These designs vary according to (1) the extent to which inquiry involves the personal "essence," language, experiences, and insights of the investigator; (2) the extent to which individual "experience" and meaning versus patterns of human experience is sought; (3) the extent to which the investigator imposes structure in the data collection and analytical processes; and (4) the sequence of the research process.

Neither the point of entry into the spiral of inquiry nor the sequence of the thinking and action processes is prescribed. Thus an investigator may begin with any of the essential thinking and action processes, change the design or specific action strategies in

response to findings throughout the research process, and revisit steps that have already been conducted. Many methodologists use the term iterative to describe the repetitive, flexible, and progressively building process of naturalistic inquiry.[14]

Although there are many design variations, Box 3-2 lists the major categories of design that make up the tradition of naturalistic inquiry, as discussed in detail in Part III.

INTEGRATING TWO RESEARCH TRADITIONS

As briefly discussed, there has been significant and heated debate over which research tradition is most efficacious in advancing our understanding of human experience. Because experimental-type researchers believe that reality can only become known incrementally through implementing objective thinking and action processes, they may not value the naturalistic foundations of *pluralism* and subjectivity. Conversely, many naturalistic researchers question the extent to which human experience can be reduced to a single, observable, and predictive reality. Moreover, because of the philosophical differences between the traditions, many scholars and researchers suggest that the two cannot be integrated because of philosophical incompatibility.

Most recently, however, there is a growing movement in both traditions to recognize the strengths and values of the other. Experimental-type methodologists have begun to recognize that naturalistic inquiry represents a legitimate and logical alternative research strategy to experimental-type inquiry, and naturalistic researchers are giving greater attention to the standardization of analysis and procedures and to the complementary role of experimental-type designs. Consistent with a growing number of methodologists, we believe that the following six points of tension in the health and human service research world have led many investigators to eschew the traditional opposition of qualitative-quantitative research in favor of strategies that overcome or transcend the limitations of each research tradition.

1. The focus on the experimental-type tradition as the only viable research option has been brought into question by findings that repeatedly indicate little or no measurable effects of experimental treatments in health and human service research.

2. There is growing recognition that many of the persistent and unanswered issues that are critical to health and human services cannot be answered by the experimental paradigm alone.

3. There is an increasing realization that quantitative information, in and of itself, does not necessarily provide insight to the various processes that underlie the "hard facts" of a numerical report.

4. There are often great discrepancies in knowledge generated from qualitative and quantitative studies.

5. The increasing emphasis placed on the empirical demonstration of the need for outcomes of health and human services has led naturalistic researchers to consider using replicable strategies.

6. Understanding and eliminating disparities in health and wellness among diverse population groups require the use of multiple discovery and verification strategies.

Both traditions have strengths and limitations; both have value in investigating the depth and breadth of research topics that inform us about human experience; and both can be integrated in a single study or throughout all or some of the parts of a research project involving multiple studies. We suggest that an integrated approach can strengthen health and human service inquiry. An integrated approach involves selecting and combining designs and methods from both traditions so that one complements the other to benefit or contribute to an understanding of the whole.

However, as discussed throughout this text, efficacious integration is contingent on an investigator's firm understanding of the strengths and limitations of the thinking and action processes, the design strategies, and the particular methodological approaches of each tradition. Based on this understanding, the investigator can mix and combine strategies to strengthen the research effort and to strive for comprehensive understanding of the phenomenon under consideration. In their classic work, Brewer and Hunter use the term *multimethod research* and explain the premise of this approach to inquiry in this way:

> Our individual methods may be flawed, but fortunately the flaws in each are not identical. A diversity of imperfection allows us to combine methods not only to gain their individual strengths but also to compensate for their particular faults and limitations. ...Its [multimethod research] fundamental strategy is to attack a research problem with an arsenal of methods that have nonoverlapping weaknesses in addition to their complementary strengths.[15]

The integration of the research traditions as a way to strengthen and advance scientific inquiry has a 35-year history in sociology, anthropology, and education. Only more recently, however, has the integration of the traditions become acceptable and even popular in health and human service research. Many researchers implicitly use one or more forms of integration discussed throughout this text. For example, there is a long history of the use of simple descriptive statistics, such as frequencies and means, in ethnographic research; and quantitative studies frequently use an exploratory, open-ended series of questions before establishing closed-ended and numerically based interview questions.

Several points are important here. First, a multimethod approach enables you to generate more in-depth, nuanced, or complex knowledge about phenomena. Second, although this approach is complex, as in all other forms of inquiry, it requires purposeful and logical development that combines elements of the thinking and action processes from both the naturalistic and the experimental-type traditions for each essential in a research endeavor.

A third important point is that integrated studies transcend the classic philosophical and methodological paradigm debates and enhance scientific inquiry. Integration is based on the philosophical paradigm

TABLE 3-1

Four Distinguishing Characteristics of the Research Traditions

Characteristic	Experimental-Type	Naturalistic	Integrated
Epistemology	Logical positivism	Humanistic or holistic	Multiple
Approach to reasoning	Deductive	Inductive and abductive	All
Theoretical aim	To reduce complexity; test theory	To reveal complexity; develop theory	All
Context	Arranged by researcher	Natural context	Multiple

of pragmatism. As suggested first by Brewer and Hunter[15] and more recently by Tashakkori and Teddlie,[16] contemporary researchers who adopt integrated or mixed methods are not necessarily proceeding from mixed philosophical bases but rather from a single perspective, that of pragmatism. Briefly, *pragmatism* is a school of thought in which concepts such as truth and reality are relative and purposive. Given this philosophical paradigm, the purposive choice of methodology, including mixed methods, is most desirable.

Table 3-1 summarizes the essential characteristics of experimental-type, naturalistic, and integrated inquiries. Examining the differences will help you understand the foundations of each tradition and its integration with the other.

We suggest five distinct ways in which the research traditions can be integrated. Figure 3-1, *A,* shows a study design that initially involves a form of naturalistic inquiry, followed by an experimental-type approach. Usually in this strategy, the purpose of the naturalistic inquiry is to gain an understanding of the boundaries or dimensions of a particular construct or to generate a theory or set of propositions. If the purpose is to define a particular construct or concept, the investigator uses the naturalistic process to inform the development of an instrument or set of measures for use in a quantitative study. If the purpose is to generate or modify a theory using the naturalistic process, this study phase is followed by an experimental-type design, which formally tests an aspect of the theory that has been developed.

Consider the study on women's health by DePoy and Butler.[17] The first phase of the study involved a naturalistic approach in order to derive definitions of health and well-being by rural elder women. The second study phase involved a nonexperimental survey design with a larger cohort of rural elder women to examine the distribution of the constructs that were generated in the first study phase.

Figure 3-1, *B,* presents a strategy for integrating the research traditions that involves the opposite sequence of *A.* In this integration scheme the investigator begins with an experimental-type approach and then introduces naturalistic techniques. Usually in this approach, the quantitative findings suggest the need for more in-depth and complex exploration of a particular phenomenon.

Assume you are conducting an experimental-type study to test the outcome of an acquired immunodeficiency syndrome (AIDS) prevention program for urban teenagers.

Philosophical Foundations

Figure 3-1, A Design strategy that involves naturalistic inquiry followed by an experimental-type approach.

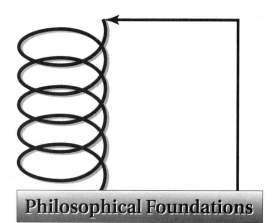

Figure 3-1, B Design strategy that begins with an experimental-type approach and then introduces naturalistic techniques.

Your findings reveal that knowledge about human immunodeficiency virus (HIV) transmission increased. However, actual sexual behaviors did not change. Your initial inquiry is followed with a naturalistic examination of the intervention process to discover why the program did not have an impact on actual behaviors.

In Figure 3-1, *C,* integration occurs at several points throughout the research process. As a naturalistic study unfolds, elements of emerging theory are tested with experimental-type strategies.

In the study conducted by DePoy and Butler, use of health services appeared to be associated with the women's definition of health.[17] To examine this connection systematically, specific experimental-type strategies were introduced.

Similarly, Figure 3-1, *D,* depicts an *integrated design* in which experimental-type inquiry reveals the need to develop insights using naturalistic techniques.

Assume you are testing a preventive AIDS program and you observe that culturally normative values among teenagers appear to influence sexual behaviors. To explore this phenomenon more closely, you may integrate open-ended interviewing techniques or conduct a series of focus groups as one component of your experimental-type testing. This exploration will enable you to gain insights to help you restructure the prevention program to yield a more desirable behavioral change.

In an experimental-type design that examined the frequency of assistive-device use among older adults discharged from rehabilitation, Gitlin et al.[18] found that older adults expressed a range of meanings and personal attributions to devices that were not systematically addressed in the closed-ended questionnaires. They added a naturalistic approach by which the statements of research participants were

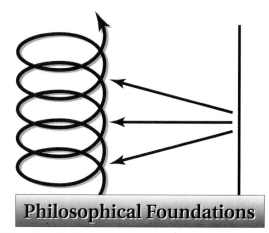

Figure 3-1, C Design strategy in which integration occurs at several points in a naturalistic study.

Figure 3-1, D Design strategy in which integration occurs at several points in an experimental-type study.

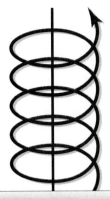

Philosophical Foundations

Figure 3-1, E Design strategy in which integration occurs throughout all thinking and action processes.

recorded, transcribed, and then analyzed using a content and thematic analytical strategy.

Finally, Figure 3-1, *E*, depicts the most fully integrated design. In this scheme the investigator integrates a study from the beginning and throughout all thinking and action processes.

> Consider the study of the service and support needs of adolescents with special health care needs. In this study the investigators integrated participatory action research that used focus group methodology with the administration of a closed-ended, structured survey of service needs. Both approaches were conducted simultaneously and reported as a single study.[19]

SELECTING A RESEARCH TRADITION AND DESIGN STRATEGY

How does one decide which tradition to work from and which particular design strategy to choose? The selection of a design strategy is based on three considerations: (1) what you want to accomplish, or your purpose in conducting the research, (2) the way in which you think or reason about phenomena, and (3) the level of knowledge development in the area to be investigated.

Purpose of Research

Research is a purposeful activity. That is, research is conducted for a specific reason—to answer a specific question or query or to solve a particular controversy or issue. This point is central to the way in which we present the world of research to you throughout this book. The view of research as purposeful is shared by other scientists as well.[16]

Think about what we mean here by "purpose." Purpose drives the decision to engage in research. Assume that you work in a health setting in which you believe the various practices and treatment approaches that you and your colleagues carry out are very important and clinically effective in producing a desired outcome. Your administrator is not convinced, however, and costs associated with your treatment practices are beginning to be questioned. You may need to conduct a research project to validate what you are doing and demonstrate the efficacy of the specific treatment approaches that you use. Alternately, you may need to conduct a research study to help you systematically determine what elements of a new therapeutic approach are most effective in producing the desired outcome, or if the approach is being used with a clinic population for which it was not previously tested. Similarly, assume that you are unsure as to the service needs of a particular clinical group, and you need to obtain a better understanding in order to develop programming for this group.

Consider also the following specific examples of how purpose drives the selection of a design:

> An administrator of a rehabilitation unit in a large teaching and research hospital has just been informed that her social work unit may be closed if she cannot demonstrate the value of the department's programs. The administrator decides that she will implement a research project to demonstrate the value of the service to the patients who are being discharged. She selects three criteria for measurement to define "valuable intervention": (1) patient satisfaction, (2) social work staff time spent with each patient's family in preparation for discharge, and (3) level of daily living skill performance in the occupational therapy clinic before discharge. She selects and measures these three criteria deductively, because she knows that these strengths can be clearly demonstrated by her unit staff. Her purpose in conducting the research

is to improve the chances of survival of her unit. She selects a deductive strategy based on her previous knowledge of the strengths of her programs and the types of positive outcomes she hopes to achieve.

In another hospital, the rehabilitation administrator has been asked to develop new programming for Asian immigrants with AIDS and their families. In the absence of a well-developed body of knowledge in this area, the administrator selects an inductive strategy to find out what type of rehabilitation programming will be most valuable. She conducts in-depth, unstructured interviews with immigrants who have AIDS, their families, and service providers to reveal needs and the culturally relevant methods by which those needs can be addressed within her institution.

As you can see, purpose is a powerful force that drives the selection of a research strategy. In the first example, the administrator selected a strategy that she, as the researcher, could control and one that was based on the *a priori* assumptions she was willing to make. In the second example, the administrator selected a strategy that would uncover information that had not been previously determined. Because patient needs, as perceived by patients and families, were shaping institutional programming, an inductive, naturalistic design strategy was selected.

It is not uncommon to have more than one purpose for your study. Perhaps you already know that your intervention is successful in meeting its aims, but you want to improve a service or obtain an understanding as to why the intervention is effective. This dual purpose may lead to a study that integrates a design from the experimental-type tradition with a design from the naturalistic tradition. The purpose of such an integrated study is to verify what is valuable, as well as to reveal new avenues for programmatic improvement and explanation of effectiveness in achieving desired outcomes.

Preference for Knowing

Your preferred way of knowing is a second important consideration when selecting a particular category of research design. Selecting a design strategy is based in part on your implicit philosophical view, your espousal of the existence and nature of "reality" (ontology), your view of "if we can know" and if so

"how we know what we know" (epistemology), and your comfort level with epistemological assumptions. Typically, we do not consciously reflect on our preferred way of knowing. It is usually demonstrated in which research approach makes the most sense to us and feels the most comfortable. Also, investigator personalities often influence the inclination to participate in one of the two traditions or in integrated inquiry.

Level of Knowledge Development

The third consideration in selecting a research design involves the level of knowledge that has been developed in the particular area of interest. When little or nothing is understood about a phenomenon, a more descriptive and naturalistic approach to inquiry is indicated. When a well-developed body of knowledge has been advanced, predicting designs may be more appropriate and may suit the purposes of the investigator. However, this is not to suggest that naturalistic inquiry is chosen only when little knowledge has been developed. Again, choice is based on a combination of the level of knowledge and the investigator's purpose. We explore the relationship of knowledge to design selection in more detail in subsequent chapters.

Table 3-2 summarizes the criteria for selecting designs across the research traditions.

SUMMARY

We have made the following five major points in this chapter:

1. Experimental-type research is based in a single epistemological framework of logical positivism and involves primarily a deductive process of human reasoning.
2. Naturalistic inquiry is based in multiple philosophical traditions that can be categorized as holistic in their perspectives and involves inductive and abductive processes of human reasoning.
3. Integrated research, which is based on its own philosophical foundation of pragmatism, draws on strategies from both experimental-type and naturalistic inquiry traditions and may involve multiple and varied thinking and action processes.
4. Each tradition has a distinct language and flow of thinking and action procedures.

TABLE 3-2

Criteria for Selecting Designs by Research Tradition

Criterion	Experimental-Type	Naturalistic	Integrated
Practical purpose	Need to control and delimit scope of inquiry	Reveal new understandings	Multiple
Preferred way of knowing	Singular reality, objectively viewed	Multiple, interpreted realities	Multiple
Level of knowledge development	Well-developed theory	Limited knowledge; challenge to current theory	Both

5. The selection of a strategy is based on your preferred way of knowing, your research purpose, and the level of knowledge development in the area of interest.

EXERCISES

1. Select a topic of interest, and determine how you might approach it using experimental-type reasoning and the sequence of the 10 essentials.
2. Using the same topic as above, suggest how you might approach the topic using naturalistic inquiry.
3. Compare and contrast both approaches, and think of how you will approach your topic using integrated strategies.

REFERENCES

1. Hume D: *A treatise on human nature: being an attempt to introduce the experimental method of reasoning into moral,* London, 1974, Longrans, Green, & Co.
2. Russell B: *Introduction to mathematical philosophy,* New York, 1919, Macmillan.
3. Hoover KR: *The elements of social scientific thinking,* ed 2, New York, 1980, St. Martin's Press.
4. Cook TD, Campbell DT: *Quasi-experimentation: design and analysis issues for field settings,* Boston, 1979, Houghton Mifflin.
5. Babbie E: *The practice of social research,* ed 8, Belmont, Calif, 2003, Wadsworth.
6. Campbell DT, Stanley JC: *Experimental and quasi-experimental designs for research,* Boston, 1963, Houghton Mifflin.
7. Denzin N: *Interpretive interactionism,* Newbury Park, Calif, 1988, Sage.
8. Husserl E: *Ideas: general introduction to pure phenomenology,* New York, 1931, Macmillan (translated by WR Boyce).
9. Guba EC: Carrying on the dialogue. In Guba EC, editor: *The paradigm dialogue,* Newbury Park, Calif, 1990, Sage.
10. Randall JH, Buchler J: *Philosophy: an introduction,* New York, 1962, Barnes & Noble.
11. Orcutt BA: *Science and inquiry in social work practice,* New York, 1990, Columbia University Press.
12. Reason P, Rowan J: *Human inquiry,* New York, 1981, John Wiley & Sons.
13. Silverman M: *Facing post-modernity: contemporary French thought on culture and society,* New York, 1999, Routeledge.
14. Anastas JW, McDonald ML: *Research design for social work and the human services,* New York, 1994, Lexington Books.
15. Brewer J, Hunter A: *Multimethod research: a synthesis of styles,* Newbury Park, Calif, 1989, Sage.
16. Tashakkori A, Teddlie C: *Handbook of mixed methods social and behavioral research,* Thousand Oaks, Calif, 2002, Sage.
17. DePoy E, Butler S: Health: elderly rural women's conceptions, *AFFILIA* 11(2):207-220, 1996.
18. Gitlin LN, Luborsky M, Schemm R: Emerging concerns of older stroke patients about assistive device use, *Gerontologist* 38(2)169-180, 1998.
19. DePoy E, Gilmer D: Healthy and ready to work: adolescents with special needs in transition. In Adolescents with disabilities and chronic illness in transition: a community action needs assessment, *Disabil Studies Q,* Spring 2000.

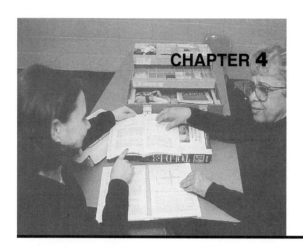

CHAPTER 4

Framing the Problem

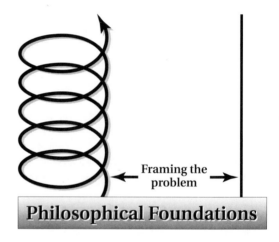

Framing the problem

Philosophical Foundations

Where do you begin now that you are ready to participate in the research process? An important initial challenge in the conduct of research is the selection of a topic and, within that area, a specific problem that is meaningful to study, appropriate for scientific inquiry, and purposeful. By "meaningful" we suggest that the identified research problem should lead to an inquiry that allows the development of new knowledge or verification of existing knowledge that is useful to the individual and/or to

his or her profession or social group. By "appropriate" we mean that the selection of a problem can be submitted to a systematic research process and that the research will yield knowledge to help solve the identified problem. Not all problems relevant to health and human service providers can be addressed through systematic inquiry. By "purposeful" we suggest that health and human service research be designed with purposes that serve investigators, consumers, professionals, funders, policy makers, and others concerned with the delivery of health and human services.

Most beginning researchers are able to identify a topic of interest to them. However, many find that identifying a specific research problem within a topic of interest is a more difficult task. This difficulty is caused in part by the novice investigator's unfamiliarity with problem formulation and its relationship to the research process. It is important to recognize that the way in which a research problem is framed influences and shapes all subsequent thinking and action processes. More specifically, as depicted in Figure 4-1, the way the research problem is framed will lead to the development of a specific research question in the experimental-type tradition of research, or to a line of query in the naturalistic tradition, or to a question and query that integrate both research traditions. Thus, problem identification is not simply a matter of isolating a specific problem statement; one must also have a clear understanding of the relationships among topic, problem formulation, research question/query, and action processes to frame a meaningful, appropriate, and purposeful problem statement.

Problem formulation is also influenced by the personal characteristics of the researcher, including personal interest, perceived need, and preferred epistemology (Box 4-1).

This chapter examines the thinking processes involved in identifying a topic, framing a research problem, and linking design selection to the purpose of the study.

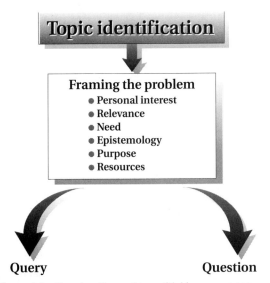

Figure 4-1   Framing the problem: thinking sequence.

BOX 4-1
CONSIDERATIONS IN FRAMING RESEARCH PROBLEMS

■ Personal interest
■ Relevance
■ Need
■ Epistemology
■ Purpose
■ Resources

IDENTIFYING A TOPIC

The first consideration in beginning a research project is to identify a topic from which to pursue a specific investigation. A *research topic* is a broad issue or area that is important to a health and human service professional. One topic may yield many different problems and strategies for investigation.

Examples of topics include posthospital experience, health disparities, health promotion in diverse communities, pain control, community independence, adaptation to disability, drug abuse, hospital management practices, gender differences related to retirement, psychosocial aspects of illness, the disablement process, creativity in aging, and the impact of interventions on specific outcomes.

It is usually easy to identify a topic that is of personal interest or one that is relevant to and important for professional practice.

Where do topics and specific problem areas come from? There are five basic sources helpful to professionals in selecting a topic and researchable problem (Box 4-2).

BOX 4-2
FIVE SOURCES FOR TOPIC IDENTIFICATION

■ Professional experience
■ Societal trends
■ Professional trends
■ Published research
■ Existing theory

Professional Experience

The professional arena is perhaps the most immediate and important source from which research problems evolve. The daily ideas and confusion that emerge from cognitive dissonance, or "professional challenges"[1] (similar to those posed in Chapter 1), often yield significant areas of inquiry. Many of the themes or persistent issues that emerge in case review, supervision, and faculty, student, and staff conferences may provide investigators with researchable topics and ideas. Themes that cut across the diversity of individuals, such as family involvement and consumer perceptions of their experiences in health and human services, provide topics that may ultimately stimulate the framing of specific research problems.

A rehabilitation professional in an inpatient rehabilitation hospital posed to us an observation that she and her staff found intriguing. They observed that many of the adaptive devices for self-care that were routinely issued and used with inpatient training were often left behind by patients in their rooms at discharge. Although she believed patients needed these devices to function independently in their homes, she wondered why patients did not think similarly. When the devices were taken home, she also wondered whether they were used and, if so, whether they enhanced patients' functioning in their environment. Discussions with practitioners in other hospital sites revealed similar observations and concerns. Here then is an identified research problem from which we posed a series of specific researchable questions to examine systematically the issues of device use and abandonment.[2]

Societal Trends

Social concerns and trends reflected in the policies, legislation, and funding priorities of federal, state, and local agencies, foundations, and corporations provide a second and critical area of potential inquiry for health and human service investigation. For example, the report *Healthy People 2010,*[3] a U.S. Public Health Service document, establishes the health-related objectives and priorities for the United States. This document provides a rich foundation for the development of research problems.

Another social arena from which research problems emerge is the set of specific requests for research generated by federal, state, and local governments. Government agencies have numerous established funding streams that provide monetary support to researchers who identify meaningful and appropriate research problems within topic areas relevant to the delivery of health and human services.

In the arena of health promotion and disease prevention, the Centers for Disease Control and Prevention (CDC) issued a call for research that focuses on the identification of risk factors related to secondary disability and the prevention of such. The Department of Health and Human Services (DHHS) has issued requests for research proposals to study the effects of welfare reform on the health of children living in poverty.

To publicize research priorities set by the federal government, the *Federal Register,* a daily publication of the U.S. government (appearing in both hard-copy and on-line formats), lists funding opportunities and policy developments of each branch of the federal government. Most libraries receive the hard-copy publication, and the on-line version can be accessed through the World Wide Web (Internet). The *Federal Register* is an invaluable resource to help identify problem areas and funding sources. Numerous other sources list research grant opportunities, including the *National Institutes of Health (NIH) Guide for Grants and Contracts,* the *Federal Grants and Contracts Weekly,* and the *Chronicle of Higher Education*—just to name a few in the United States. If you are interested in learning about the international and global research issues and questions that are important to grant funders, you can consult the Internet and search your area of interest. Many government sources (e.g., Fullbright Commission) and nongovernmental organizations (NGOs) have specific focal areas and extend recruitment and support efforts to investigators.

Professional Trends

Other resources for identifying important research topics are the on-line or hard-copy newsletters and publications of each health and human service profession. Investigators frequently read these resources to determine the broad topic areas and problems of current interest to a given profession. Also, professional associations establish specific short-term and long-term research goals and priorities for their professions.

> The American Occupational Therapy Foundation identified the need to develop more research in the area of client assessment and intervention outcomes. As a result, the Foundation sponsored funding competitions that supported research addressing these priorities.

More recently, professional associations have been interested in advancing evidence-based practice, so they have sponsored research endeavors to identify the barriers to using this approach and mechanisms for advancing its integration into daily practice. Examining the goals and policy statements of professional associations provides a good source from which to establish a research direction.

Another important resource for identifying problem areas is the reports on health care and practice routinely generated by the Institute of Medicine. For example, their 2001 publication, *Crossing the Quality Chasm: a New Health System for the 21st Century*, outlines the fundamental changes needed in the U.S. health care system. The book provides important data about current health care and raises the many difficult problem areas that must be addressed through research, education, and change in health policy. You may also want to look at the publications of the World Health Organization (WHO) or Rehabilitation International to identify international priorities.

Research Studies

The research world itself also provides a significant avenue from which to identify research topics and problem areas. Health and human service professionals encounter research ideas by interacting with peers, attending professional meetings that report research findings, participating in research projects, and reviewing published research reports. Reading scholarship in print and on-line professional journals provides an overview of the important studies conducted in an area of interest. Most published research studies identify additional research problems and unresolved issues generated by the research findings.

Journals publish current research findings that are useful and relevant to the helping professions; these include the *Journal of Dental Hygiene, Journal of the American Medical Association, Research in Social Work Practice, American Journal of Occupational Therapy, Occupational Therapy Journal of Research, Nursing Research, Medical Care, Physical Therapy, Qualitative Research in Health Care, The Social Service Review, American Journal of Public Health*, and *Social Work Research*.

Routinely reading journals also provides you with an idea of what concerns and issues your professional peers believe are important to investigate, as well as the studies that need to be replicated or repeated to confirm the findings. There are many other journals published by the helping professions and related disciplines that may assist in identifying a topic. Substantive topic journals that cross disciplines, such as *Archives of Physical and Rehabilitation Medicine, Psychiatric Services, Journal of Gerontology, Childhood and Adolescence, Topics in Geriatric Rehabilitation, The Gerontologist*, and *Journal of Rehabilitation*, provide specific ideas for research studies that need to be conducted in topics relevant to health and human service professionals.

Finally, reading articles that provide a comprehensive overview or meta-analysis of a focused body of research is very helpful. Such articles usually summarize the state of knowledge to date and future research needs.

Existing Theory

Theories also provide an important source for generating topics and identifying research problems. As will be discussed in Chapter 6, a theory posits a number of propositions and relationships between and among concepts. To be considered a theory, each specified relationship within the theory must be submitted to systematic investigation for verification or falsification.[4] Inquiry related to theory development is intended to substantiate the theory and advance or modify its development by refuting some or all of its principles.

> Consider the well-known theory of cognitive development put forth by Piaget in the mid-1920s.[5] Piaget developed his theory of the structural development of cognition by

observing his two children. Over 60 years, Piaget, his peers, and other scholars interested in human cognition subjected Piaget's theoretical notions to extensive scientific scrutiny. Hundreds of studies have been conducted to corroborate, modify, or refute Piaget's principles. Further study related to Piaget's theory has been initiated to determine the application of the theory to education and health-related intervention, as well as many other arenas. Another well-known theoretical framework, stress-health process models, has also generated much research to empirically verify the posited linkages between stressors, a person's appraisal of them, and related health consequences.

BOX 4-3
SIX GUIDING QUESTIONS IN FRAMING A PROBLEM

1. What about this topic is of interest to me?
2. What about this topic is relevant to my practice?
3. What about this topic is unresolved in the literature?
4. What is my preferred way of coming to know about phenomena?
5. What societal or professional purpose does knowing about this topic serve?
6. What resources do I have to investigate this topic?

FRAMING A RESEARCH PROBLEM

So now you have some idea as to where and how to identify a topic. Foremost, the topic area must be of keen interest to you because you will be spending a lot of time and energy reading and thinking about this topic. However, you still face the dilemma of identifying a particular problem within a broad topic area. An endless number of problems or specific issues can emerge from any one topic. Thus the challenge to the researcher is to identify just one particular area of concern or specific research problem. A specific research problem provides some boundary to the area to be studied. It identifies the phenomenon to be explored, the reason it needs to be examined, and the reason it is a problem or issue. The way in which you frame and state the problem is critical to the entire research endeavor and influences all subsequent thinking and action processes; that is, the way a problem is framed determines the way it will be answered. Therefore, this first research step should be thought through very carefully.

The questions we pose in Box 4-3 are designed to help guide your thinking as you move from the selection of a broad topic area to the framing of a concrete research problem. By answering these reflective questions, you will begin to narrow your focus and hone in on a researchable problem.

Interest, Relevance, and Need

It is important to be certain that the topic you develop is interesting to you. Research, regardless of the framework and type of methodology used, takes time and can consume your thoughts. Additionally, you should be convinced of the relevance and need for the inquiry. If the problem is not challenging, exciting, relevant, and needed, the process can quickly become tedious and lack meaning to you. Researchers must be passionate about their area of work; otherwise, the effort may seem pointless.

Research Purpose

As discussed in Chapter 3, all research is purposeful. We suggest that there are three levels of purpose that each research project addresses. The first level of purpose is professional. Much of the research in health and human services is initiated to determine empirically the need for an intervention program, to inform professional practice, or to examine the extent to which an intervention is efficacious in achieving its outcome.

The second level of research purpose is personal. Researchers often have personal reasons for conducting research, or they choose topics that resonate personally. Practitioners, administrators, and other health and human service professionals may conduct research for such personal reasons as adding new challenges to their jobs, career advancement, commitment to funding new projects, and a desire for academic collaboration and growth. Furthermore, the topic of interest may reflect a deep personal concern. For example, some researchers who focus on specific diseases choose the disease based on their own family history or encounter with the condition.

The third level of purpose for conducting research is methodological, reflecting issues that emerge from the literature (see Chapter 5). For example, in the experimental-type tradition, the researcher may be interested in describing, explaining, or predicting phenomena, as demonstrated in the following examples of a *purpose statement:*

Descriptive. "Little is known about the nutrition knowledge and beliefs of adults with mental retardation. The present study is a preliminary investigation of nutrition knowledge of persons with mental retardation."[6]

Explanatory. "Although long-term care has been the subject of extensive study, minimal attention has been directed to the role of formal long term care in facilitating employment for women with cognitive disabilities. This study will attempt to fill that gap. Specifically, the study examines the relationship between formal long term care support and nature and degree of employment in women with cognitive disabilities, compared to those who do not receive formal long term care."[7]

Explanatory. "This study, with a relatively large national sample, examines specific coping strategies that caregivers have used to manage their day-to-day responsibilities and how the strategies are related to outcomes of caregiver well-being."[8]

Predictive. "This study was undertaken to examine changes in family functioning from pre-injury to 3 years after pediatric TBI (traumatic brain injury) and to determine those factors that best predict a 3-year family outcome."[9]

In naturalistic designs, the purpose is to understand meanings, experiences, and phenomena as they evolve in the natural setting. The following are examples of purpose statements by investigators using different naturalistic designs:

Ethnography. "The purpose of the study was to 'gain an understanding of the families' demographics, status as immigrants, beliefs about deafness, attitudes toward school and health care professionals, expectations for their children and communication with the deaf child.' "[10]

Ethnography. "The purpose of the study was to gain understanding of the meaning of the family caregiving experience with the hope that greater understanding would assist health professionals in working together with caregivers."[11]

Phenomenology. "The purpose of the study presented here was to evolve a structural definition of health as it is experienced in everyday life."[12]

Grounded theory. "This article discusses the multidimensional relationship that developed between researcher and participants during an exploratory study of enrichment processes in family caregiving to frail elders."[13]

Grounded theory. "The purpose of the present study was to identify processes used by family members to manage the unpredictability elicited by the need for and receipt of a heart transplant."[14]

Heuristic inquiry. The purpose of this study is to examine and understand the meaning of chronic illness in families, from the perspective of all family members.

Participatory action research. The purpose of this inquiry is to assess service needs, as investigated and defined by service recipients themselves.

Meta-analysis. The purpose of this inquiry is to seek universal themes and comparisons in the meaning of culturally competent health care practice in six countries.

Critical theory. This study was conducted to give voice to homeless adolescent women as the basis for understanding need and promoting socially just responses to this set of informants.

Integrated designs can have multiple purposes that reflect both research traditions or only one tradition. Consider the following example in which the purpose combined both traditions:

"The purpose of this integrated study was to reveal the ways in which elder rural women defined health and wellness and then test the accuracy of these definitions in a large cohort of the population."[15]

Epistemology—(Preferred Way of Knowing)

In addition to problem formulation and study purpose, your preferred way of knowing, or epistemology, will also influence either (1) the development of discrete questions that objectify concepts (experimental-type tradition) or a query to explore multiple and interacting factors in the context in which they emerge (naturalistic tradition) or (2) the development of a query that integrates both approaches. The age-old ontological and epistemological dilemmas respectively of "what is knowledge?" and "how do we know?" (discussed in Chapter 3) are active and forceful determinants in how a researcher frames a problem. The researcher's preferred way of knowing is either clearly articulated or implied in each *problem statement.* Reexamine the purpose statements just listed to determine the investigator's preferred way of knowing that is implicitly assumed.

Resources

Resources represent the concrete limitations of the research world. The accessibility of place, group, or individuals and the extent to which time, money, and other resources are necessary and available to the researcher to implement the inquiry are examples of some of the practical constraints of conducting research. These real-life constraints actively shape the development of the research problem an investigator pursues and the scope of the project that can be implemented.

SUMMARY

The many considerations in framing an inquiry include examining the diverse sources and methods through which investigators identify topics for inquiry. Six questions guide the refinement of the topic into a research problem. These questions organize thinking processes along personal, professional, social, ontological, and practical lines. For example, considering your interest in a research topic is a personal thinking process, whereas assessing existing resources available for conducting a project is a practical thinking process. With regard to the purposive aspects of conducting research, investigators organize their research to meet personal, professional, and methodological goals.

Your preferred way of knowing (epistemology) also plays a key role in framing an inquiry. How a researcher frames a problem has significant implications for the selection of design from the experimental-type tradition, the naturalistic tradition, or an integration of the two, as will be seen in subsequent chapters.

Equipped with an understanding of why and how investigators frame research problems, you are ready to begin the thinking process of examining and

critically using literature as a basis for knowledge development.

REFERENCES

1. Schon D: *The reflective practitioner,* New York, 1983, Basic Books.
2. Gitlin LN, Levine R, Geiger C: Adaptive device use in the home by older adults with mixed disabilities. *Arch Phys Med Rehabil* 74:149-152, 1993.
3. U.S. Department of Health and Human Services: *Healthy people 2010.*
4. Wilson J: *Thinking with concepts,* Cambridge, Mass, 1966, Cambridge University Press.
5. Piaget J: *Judgment and reasoning in the child,* New York, 1926, Harcourt Brace (translated by M Warden).
6. Golden E, Hatcher J: Nutrition knowledge and obesity of adults in community residences, *Ment Retard* 35(3):177-184, 1997.
7. Duncan B, Schmidt L: *Linking women with disabilities to employment opportunities and resources,* Oakland, Calif, 2000, World Institute on Disability.
8. Palmore EG: Predictors of outcome in nursing homes, *J Appl Gerontol* 9:1172-1184, 1990.
9. Rivara JB et al: Predictors of family functioning and change 3 years after traumatic brain injury in children, *Arch Phys Med* 77:754-764, 1996.
10. Steinberg AG et al: A little sign and a lot of love: attitudes, perceptions and beliefs of Hispanic families with deaf children, *Qualitative Health Res* 7(2):202-222, 1997.
11. Hasselkus BR: The meaning of activity: day care for persons with Alzheimer disease, *Am J Occup Ther* 46:199-206, 1992.
12. Parse RR, Coyne AB, Smith MJ: Nursing research traditions: qualitative and quantitative approaches. In *Nursing research: qualitative methods,* Bowie, Md, 1985, Brady Communications.
13. Cartwright J, Limandri B: The challenge of multiple roles in the qualitative clinician researcher-participant client relationship, *Qualitative Health Res* 7(2):223-235, 1997.
14. Mishel M, Murdaugh C: Family adjustment to heart transplantation: redesigning the dream, *Nurs Res* 36:332-338, 1987.
15. DePoy E, Butler S: Health: elderly rural women's conceptions, *AFFILIA* 11(2):207-220, 1996.

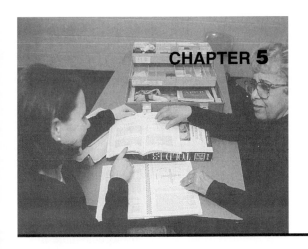

CHAPTER 5

Developing a Knowledge Base Through Review of the Literature

KEY TERMS
Concept/construct matrix
Database
Literature review chart

CHAPTER OUTLINE

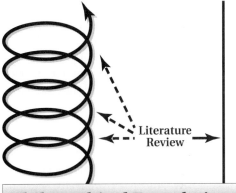

Philosophical Foundations

Most of us have had the experience of spending long hours at the library or on the Internet poring through literature and materials to discover what others have written about a topic of interest. Although you probably have participated in this type of activity for various classroom assignments, reviewing information for research is more systematic and serves more specific purposes.

One important purpose of reviewing the literature for research is to help sharpen the focus of your initial research interest and the specific strategy you plan to use to conduct a study. Discovering what others know and how they come to know it is an important function of the review when conducted at the initial stage of developing a research idea. The review, when conducted at this stage, involves a process by which the researcher critically assesses print material that is directly and indirectly related to both the proposed topic and the potential strategies for conducting the research.

Another purpose of a literature review is to help determine how your research fits within an existing body of knowledge and what your research uniquely contributes to the scientific enterprise. Reviewing the literature for this purpose occurs as you are formulating your research ideas as well as when you are ready to write up your findings.

A literature review also serves as a source of data. For example, in certain forms of qualitative research, literature is brought in at different points of the research process to emphasize, elaborate, or reveal emergent themes. Likewise, a systematic literature review is used in quantitative, or experimental-type, methodologies as data, such as when the review forms the unit of analysis for a meta-analysis or when ranking the level of evidence for a particular issue (see Chapter 9).

Thus, reviewing the literature is a significant thinking and action process in the world of research. However, it is often misunderstood and undervalued.

In this chapter we begin our discussion with a presentation of the different reasons for conducting a literature review. We then detail the specific steps involved in conducting a literature review and share strategies that will help you accomplish this task. Because typically there is so much information directly related to any one topic, as well as literature from related bodies of research that also should be examined, the review process may initially seem overwhelming. However, some "tricks of the trade" can facilitate a systematic and comprehensive review process that is feasible, manageable, and even enjoyable.

WHY REVIEW THE LITERATURE?

There are four major reasons for reviewing literature in research (Box 5-1). Let us examine each reason in depth.

BOX 5-1
REASONS TO REVIEW THE LITERATURE

1. Determine previous research on topic of interest
2. Determine level of theory and knowledge development
3. Determine relevance of current knowledge base to problem area
4. Provide rationale for selection of research strategy

Determine What Research Has Been Conducted on the Topic of Inquiry

Why should you conduct a study if it has already been done and done well or to your satisfaction? Here the key words are "done well" and "to your satisfaction." To determine if the current literature is sufficient to help you solve a professional problem, you must critically evaluate how others have struggled with and resolved the same or a similar question. Most novice researchers think that they are not supposed to be critical of published literature. However, being critical is the very point of conducting the literature review. You are supposed to examine previous studies critically to determine if these efforts were done well and if they answer your question satisfactorily.

An initial review of the literature provides a sense of the previous work done in your area of interest. The review helps identify (1) the current trends and ways of thinking about your topic, (2) the contemporary debates in your field, (3) the gaps in the knowledge base, (4) the ways in which the current knowledge on your topic has been developed, and (5) the conceptual frameworks used to inform and examine your problem.

Sometimes an initial review of the literature will steer you in a different research direction than your original plan.

Suppose you want to examine the extent to which mild aerobic exercise promotes cardiovascular fitness in the elder population. You find several studies that already document a positive outcome, but you question the methodologies used by these studies, including the type of exercise, the research design, and the criteria for inclusion of study participants. Also, you find that many authors suggest further inquiry is necessary to determine the particular exercises that promote cardiovascular fitness, as well as those that maintain joint mobility. Although this area is not what you originally planned, the literature review refines your thinking and directs you to specific problem areas that need greater research attention than the one originally intended. You need to decide if replication of the reported studies is important to verify study findings, whether replication with a different sample (e.g., racially and ethnically diverse elder persons not included in previous studies) would be important, and whether your focus should be modified according to the other recommendations specified in the literature (e.g., need to examine different forms of exercise for a wider range of health outcomes).

Consider another example of how the literature can initially influence the investigator's research direction. Peters[1] was interested in examining the relationship between "victim blaming" and myths about the causes of domestic violence. He performed an extensive literature review to ascertain what studies had been conducted and what instrumentation would be available for his study. Because he was unable to locate instrumentation on myths about domestic violence, he shifted his initial study to developing and validating an instrument to measure the construct of domestic violence myth acceptance. It was necessary for Peters to shift the research focus to instrument construction as a first research step in addressing his initial question.

Determine Level of Theory and Knowledge Development Relevant to Your Project

As you review the literature, not only do you need to describe what exists, but more important, you need to critically analyze the knowledge level, knowledge generation, and study boundaries in each work (Box 5-2).

Level of Knowledge

When you read a study, first evaluate the level of knowledge that emerges from the study. As discussed in Chapter 7, studies produce varying levels of knowledge, from descriptive to theoretical. The level of theory development and knowledge in your topic area will strongly influence the type of research strategy you select. As you read related studies in the literature,

---

BOX 5-2
THREE FACTORS TO REVIEW CRITICALLY

- Level of knowledge
- How knowledge is generated
- Boundaries of a study

---

consider the level of theoretical development. Is the body of knowledge descriptive, explanatory, or at the level of prediction? Typically in general inquiry, and necessarily in experimental-type inquiry, the development of knowledge proceeds incrementally such that the first wave of studies in a particular area will be descriptive and designed to describe the characteristics of the phenomenon. Once the characteristics of a problem are described, researchers search for associations or relationships among factors that may help explain the phenomenon. Based on the findings from explanatory research, attempts may be made to study the phenomenon from a predictive perspective by either testing an intervention or developing causal models to explain the phenomenon further.

Identifying the level of knowledge in the area of interest helps you identify the next research steps.

Over the past 20 years, for example, a rich body of literature on family caregiving has been generated in many disciplines, including family studies, social work, occupational therapy, nursing, and gerontology, at each of the three knowledge levels. Initially, *descriptive* research was necessary to identify the phenomenon of caregiving and describe the physical and psychological concomitants of this activity. *Explanatory* research then showed the role of gender, relationship, culture, and other factors in caregiver appraisals of their experiences. More recently, *predictive* studies have focused on evaluating complex causal models to predict long-term outcomes of caregiving, as well as testing interventions that attempt to reduce the negative consequences of providing extended care.

Even though many studies have been conducted at the descriptive, explanatory, and predictive levels, more research is needed on this topic at each level to fill in important gaps in knowledge. For example, although previous research suggests that caregivers from diverse cultural groups express varying levels of distress and stress from caregiving, we do not know the reasons for this. Also, we do not fully understand the caregiving experience for people from diverse cultural groups or how the experience may differ in urban and rural environments.

How Knowledge Is Generated

Once you have determined the level of knowledge of your particular area of interest, you need to evaluate how that knowledge has been generated. In other words, you need to review the literature carefully to identify the research strategy or design used in each study. Many people tend to read the introduction to a study, then jump to the discussion section or set of conclusions to see what it can tell them. However, it is important to read each aspect of a research report, especially the section on methodology. As you read about the design of a particular study, you must critically examine whether it is appropriate for the level of knowledge that the authors indicate exists in the literature and whether the conclusions of the study are consistent with the design strategy. This is an important critical analysis of the existing literature that you need to feel fully empowered to perform. You may be quite surprised to find that, unfortunately, the literature is full of research that demonstrates an inappropriate match among research question, strategy, and conclusions.

As you read a study, ask yourself the three interrelated questions in Box 5-3. The answers to these questions will help you understand and critically determine the appropriateness of the level of knowledge generated in your topic area. This understanding in turn will help to shape the direction of your research.

Boundaries of a Study

It is also important to determine the boundaries of the studies you are reviewing and their relevance to your study problem. By "boundaries" we mean the "who, what, when, and where" of a study.

If you do not find any literature in your topic area, you may choose to identify an analogous body of literature to provide direction in how develop your strategy.

BOX 5-3
QUESTIONS TO ASK AS YOU READ A STUDY

1. Are the research methods congruent with the level of knowledge reviewed by the investigators in their report?
2. Do the research procedures adequately address the proposed research question?
3. Is there compatibility or fit among literature, procedures, findings, and conclusions?

Suppose you are interested in testing the effectiveness of a hypertension reduction program in a rural setting, and published studies report positive outcomes for a range of interventions. On closer examination, however, you discover that these studies have been conducted in urban areas and include primarily male participants with backgrounds different from the population you plan to include in your study. Therefore, it will be important to examine studies that test health promotion interventions in rural settings and to include participants with characteristics similar to the intended targets of your study. By extending the literature review in this way, you will obtain a better understanding of the issues and design considerations that are important for the specific boundaries of your study. Also, you may discover that the level of theory and knowledge development in hypertensive risk reduction programs is advanced for one particular population (e.g., urban men) but undeveloped in respect to another population (e.g., rural women).

Suppose you are interested in studying communication between mothers of children with disabilities and rehabilitation therapists. Although little information is available on these specific communication patterns, you find numerous studies on patient-physician relationships. It would be important to review this body of research to identify appropriate methodologies and conceptual directions for your study.

Determining the boundaries of the literature helps you to evaluate the level of knowledge that exists for the particular population and setting you are interested in studying.

Determine Relevance of the Current Knowledge Base to Your Problem Area

Once you have evaluated the level of knowledge advanced in the literature, you need to determine its relevance to your idea.

Let us assume you are considering conducting an experimental-type study. In your literature review, you must find research that points to a theoretical framework relevant to your topic and research that identifies specific variables and measures for inclusion in your study. Your literature review must also yield a body of sufficiently developed knowledge so that hypotheses can be derived for your study. In other words, in the experimental-type tradition, the literature provides the rationale and structure for everything that you investigate and for all action processes.

> Suppose you are planning to conduct a study to identify the factors that predict residential placement by family members of older adults with mobility impairment who live in rural communities. You review the literature and find that single predictors, such as the aging member's satisfaction with current living arrangements and the fit between family needs and available community transportation services, are important in determining outcome. This comprehensive review supports the need to conduct a predictive study to examine the interaction of variables.

For each variable you choose to include in your study, even demographics, you must support or justify your inclusion of the variable based in sound literature. Just think of all the extraneous information that could be introduced into a research study. For theoretical, ethical, and methodological soundness, experimental-type approaches require supportive literature for all variables.

> Consider research involving the testing of interventions designed to support family caregivers of persons with dementia. In a study to test an occupational therapy and physical therapy environmental modification, Gitlin et al.[2] first identified research showing that environmental modifications can enhance well-being and safety of persons with dementia, as well as a theoretical framework for this approach. Other research showing that families rearrange their homes as care demands increase also supported the intervention approach. Given the weight of evidence that families experience great distress and express the need to learn new strategies to manage dementia care, particularly as the disease progresses, the intervention approach and use of a randomized trial was well substantiated.

If your literature review reveals a clear gap in existing knowledge or a poor fit between a phenomenon and current theory, you probably should consider a strategy in the naturalistic tradition.

> In their classic work, McCauley et al.[3] pursued their interest in understanding the process by which families choose to institutionalize elder members in nursing homes. In their review of the literature, they presented existing research that laid the foundation for the study. Specifically, they focused on the understanding created by sound inquiry that challenges "the myth that the majority of families abandon or ignore the needs of their older dependent members."[3] However, the authors noted that previous research using survey methodology revealed only a linear process of decision making. They identified a clear gap in the literature that suggested the need for a naturalistic design to fill the conceptual chasm. In other words, their literature review showed that an examination of their topic could not be supported within the experimental-type tradition.

With the addition of foundational work to literature and theory, researchers would have the rationale for selecting more diverse and complex design approaches to subsequent and related studies.

Provide a Rationale for Selection of the Research Strategy

Once you have determined the content and structure of existing theory and knowledge related to your problem area, the next task is to determine a rationale for the selection of your research design. A literature review for a research grant proposal or a research report is written to support directly both your research and your choice of design. You must synthesize your critical review of existing studies in such a way that the reader sees your study as a logical extension of current knowledge in the literature.

We now turn to the mechanics of how to conduct a literature search; then we offer guidelines for developing a written rationale.

HOW TO CONDUCT A LITERATURE SEARCH

Conducting a literature search and writing a literature review are exciting and creative processes. However, there may be so much literature in the area of interest that the review process can initially seem overwhelming. Six steps can guide you in the thinking and action processes of searching the literature, organizing the sources, and taking notes

---

BOX 5-4
SIX STEPS TO CONDUCTING A LITERATURE REVIEW

Step 1: Determine when to conduct a search
Step 2: Delimit what is searched
Step 3: Access databases for periodicals, books, and documents
Step 4: Organize the information
Step 5: Critically evaluate the literature
Step 6: Write the literature review

---

on the references that you plan to use in a written rationale (Box 5-4).

Step 1: Determine When to Conduct a Search

The first step in a literature review is the determination of when a review should be done. In studies in the experimental-type tradition, a literature review always precedes both the final formulation of a research question and the implementation of the study. In the experimental-type tradition, definitions of all variables studied and the level of theoretical complexity underpinning an inquiry must be presented in order for a study to be scientifically sound and rigorous. (We discuss "rigor" in greater detail in subsequent chapters.)

In the tradition of naturalistic inquiry, the literature may be reviewed at different points throughout the project. Although the literature is not critical for defining variables and instrumentation, it serves multiple purposes. For example, the literature may be used as an additional source of data and included as part of the information-gathering process that is subsequently analyzed and interpreted. Another purpose of the literature review in naturalistic inquiry is to inform the direction of data collection once the investigator is in the field. As discoveries occur in data collection, the investigator may turn to the literature for guidance about how to interpret emergent themes and identify other questions that should be asked in the field.

To the extreme are forms of naturalistic research in which no literature is reviewed before or during fieldwork. In a classic study of prison violence using an endogenous research design (discussed in more detail in Chapter 10), the researcher and the research team of prison inmates did not believe that a review

was necessary or relevant to the purpose of their study.[4]

Usually, however, researchers working in the naturalistic-type tradition review the literature before conducting research to confirm the need for a naturalistic approach. For example, in the study by McCauley et al.[3] previously discussed, the literature provided the rationale for their approach.

Although an extensive review of the literature conducted before undertaking any further thinking or action processes refines the research approach and design, investigators are continually updating their literature review throughout their studies.

Step 2: Delimit What Is Searched

Once you have decided when to conduct a literature review, your next step involves setting parameters as to what is relevant to search; after all, it is not feasible or reasonable to review every topic that is "somewhat related" to your problem. Delimiting the search, or setting boundaries to the search, is an important but difficult step. The boundaries you set must ensure a review that is comprehensive but still practical and not overwhelming.

One useful strategy across all traditions is to base a search on the core concepts and constructs contained in the initial inquiry.

For example, suppose you want to determine whether participation in an exercise program for elder nursing home residents improves perceived health status. The concepts and constructs contained in this initial formulation include exercise, nursing home residents, and perceived health status. These terms would be your first keywords, to be used in a computer database or library catalog search. If you are interested in knowing whether a specialized life skills program enhances recovery from brain injury, the concepts include brain injury, life skills, and community reintegration.

Similarly, these lexical concepts (concepts that are expressed as words) would help you begin a search using these variable names as keywords (words or phrases that are used in online searches to identify and categorize work that contains these specific concepts) to seek literature and determine how your topic has already been studied.

Step 3: Access Databases for Periodicals, Books, and Documents

Now that you have determined when the literature search will take place and have established some limits on what will be searched, you are ready to go to the library or search databases of published materials via the Internet. Over the past 15 years, library searches have become technologically sophisticated and are a big advantage over conventional searching mechanisms. However, the most valuable resource for finding references in the library is still the reference librarian. Working with an experienced librarian is the best way to learn how to navigate physical and virtual libraries, find the best search words for your area of interest, and access the numerous databases that open the world of literature to you.

Once in the library, you have choices about how to begin your search. You can access literature through an online *database* or through other indexes and abstracts. Some libraries still have card catalogs, which can be most useful in locating resources offered by the library in which you are searching. However, many libraries have discarded these resources, placing the card catalog on the "endangered species" list or in the antique store. In health and human service research, you will more likely want to search three categories of materials: books, online and paper journal articles, and government documents. You may also find newspapers, news websites, and newsletters useful, especially those from professional associations. In addition, you can construct a literature search based on the references listed in the research studies you obtain. However, do not depend exclusively on what other authors identify as important. References from other articles may not represent the broad range of studies you may need to review or the most current literature. A year or more may pass between submission of a manuscript and its publication; therefore the citations that precede each article may be outdated for your needs.

Searching Periodicals and Journals

Most researchers begin their search by examining online and paper periodicals and journals. To begin your search, it is helpful and time efficient to work with the online databases. Searching databases can

---

> **BOX 5-5**
> **EXPERIENCE OF DISABLED WOMEN WHO EXPERIENCE DOMESTIC VIOLENCE**
>
> *Keywords:*
> disability
> women
> domestic violence

---

be rewarding, but you must know how to use the system. You can search databases by examining subjects, authors, or titles of articles.

Let us first consider a search based on subject. Begin by identifying the major constructs and concepts of your initial inquiry (as discussed earlier). Then, translate these into keywords, which are used to identify works that contain the named concepts. In addition to the title, author, and abstract, most journals require authors to specify and list keywords that reflect the content of their study. Each database groups these studies according to these keywords.

For example, Box 5-5 presents part of a title page of a study on disability and domestic violence. Without these keywords, this study containing disability would not be likely to be identified in a search on domestic violence. This example illustrates how valuable keywords are in adding dimension to a study, ensuring that its future dissemination and use in research can be maximized.

You can obtain help from a reference librarian in formulating keywords, or the computer will help direct you to synonymous terms, if the words you initially select are not used as classifiers. Most online systems are "user friendly" and interactive; that is, the computer provides step-by-step directions on what to do. If you search any of the keywords listed in Box 5-5, you will find significant studies in that topic area. Omit "disability" as a keyword, and see how your search changes.

Let us return to the example of the exercise study to show the importance of keywords. We will begin our search with the keywords "exercise" and "elder." The combination of terms is critical in delimiting and focusing your search. For example, when we searched "Carl's Uncover," a database of journal and newspaper articles available in many university libraries, we first entered the keyword "exercise." The computer indicated 4495 different sources in the past 5 years relevant to the subject of exercise. A review of all these sources obviously would be too cumbersome. We then entered our second keyword, "elder," at a prompt that requested further delimiting. The computer then searched for works containing both topics and indicated a total of 46 articles.

After the computer indicates how many citations are found, the next step is to display the sources. Often you have a choice of examining only the citation or the abstract. If your online system is connected to a printer, you can select a print command and print the citation and abstract. You may also search the system by entering authors' names or words you believe may appear in the titles of sources. This entry expands your search to relevant articles that may not have included the combination of keywords initially used. The computer will search the references and compile a list of sources from which to choose.

In some cases it is more efficient to ask the librarian to conduct a search for you. Large databases, such as the Educational Information Resources Information Center and Medline, although accessible without assistance, can be easily accessed in this manner. If you have to pay for these sources, asking the librarian to conduct an evening search will be less expensive than a daytime search, because the telephone lines that are used to connect the library's computer to the central database charge less in off-peak hours. With the proliferation of free databases, however, such as Medline, Google, and Proquest, you may be able to find even full text citations at no cost.

It is also possible to conduct a more limited search by accessing databases that index or abstract studies in only a specific field or subject. For example, many libraries have a database titled "PsychLIT" that contains sources from psychology and related areas. "Mini-Medline" is another limited database frequently available in universities with health and medical departments. Each database gives user-friendly directions for access and use.

You also may want to do a manual search in the important indexes and abstracts that are not available online, such as some library holdings of *Dissertation Abstracts* and government documents, to ensure that you have fully covered the literature relevant to your

---

BOX 5-6
USEFUL INDEXES AND ABSTRACTS

Social Science Citation Index
General Science Index
Reader's Guide to Periodical Literature
Index to Government Periodicals
New York Times Index
Psychological Abstracts
Medical Psychological Abstracts
Cumulative Index to Nursing and Allied Health
Social Work Abstracts

---

study. In health research, useful indexes and abstracts include those listed in Box 5-6.

You can search these indexes and abstracts by author, subject, or title, just as you have done with the online database. Among the many abstracting and indexing services, *Ulriche's International Periodical Directory* is especially useful because it lists all periodicals and databases in which these periodicals are indexed.

One major directory of abstracts that is not frequently used but is extremely helpful in locating sources is *Dissertation Abstracts International.* We mentioned this source as not always being available online. However, because a literature review in a dissertation is usually exhaustive, obtaining a dissertation in your topic area may provide a comprehensive literature review and bibliography that is immediately available to you. Thus, even if you need to search manually, it is usually worth the extra time and effort.

Searching Books and Other Documents

Most libraries, particularly those in colleges and universities, have computerized listings of their collections of books and documents. As in searching periodicals, online book searching is equally efficient, enjoyable, and rewarding. In these searches, you obtain information about the title, author, and source, as well as the subject, listed by keywords and key concepts. The location of the book and its availability are included in the full citation. If you are unfamiliar with conducting a search, ask the librarian how to use the library system.

Another strategy is to identify whether an article has been published that reviews the literature in your area of interest. A comprehensive literature review or a meta-analysis of studies on a particular area provides an excellent way of beginning your literature search. Also, these reviews usually identify gaps in the literature and make recommendations as to next research steps.

Most beginning investigators are concerned with the number of sources to review. Although there is no magical number, most researchers search the literature for articles written within the previous 5 years. A search is extended beyond 5 years to evaluate the historical development of an issue or to review a breakthrough or classic article. The depth of a review depends on the purpose and scope of your study. Most investigators try to become familiar with the most important authors, studies, and papers in their topic area. You will have a sense that your review is comprehensive when you begin to see citations of authors you have already read, or if you are not finding material that leads to new learning. Also, do not hesitate to contact a researcher who has published in your topic area; ask about the researcher's recent work (which may not be published yet) and recommendations on specific current articles for you to review.

Step 4: Organize Information

With your list of sources identified by your searches, you are ready to retrieve and organize them. We usually begin by reading abstracts of journal articles to determine their value to the study. Based on the abstract, we determine if the study fits one of four categories, as suggested by Findley.[5] If a study is highly relevant, it goes into what Findley calls the "A" pile—those studies that absolutely must be read. If the study appears somewhat relevant, it is placed in the "B" pile—those studies that probably will be read, depending on the direction taken. If the study might be relevant, it goes into a "C" pile—those studies that may be read, depending on the direction taken. Finally, if a study is not relevant at all, it is put into an "X" pile—those studies that will not be read but will be kept, just in case. With books, do the same type of categorizing based on the table of contents and the preface.

Next, begin with the "A" pile, and classify the articles according to the major subjects or concepts.

It is helpful to pick a reading order to outline a preliminary conceptual framework for your literature review.

Because it is not possible to remember all the important information presented in reading, note taking is critical. There are many different schemes for note taking. Some find that taking notes on index cards is effective because index cards can be shuffled and reordered to fit into an outline. Others take notes on a database or word-processing system. In general, your notes should include a synopsis of the content, the conceptual framework for the work, the method, and a brief review of the findings. Whatever method you use, always be sure to cite the full reference. All researchers have had the miserable experience of losing the volume or page number of a critical source and then spending hours to find it later.

Although investigators organize and write notations in their own way, we offer two strategies—using a chart and using a concept/construct matrix—to help you organize your reading. These two organizational aids will also assist in the writing stage of your review.

Charting the Literature

For a *literature review chart,* you select pertinent information from each article you review and record it using a chart format. To use a chart approach, you need to determine the categories of information you will extract from each article to record or place on the chart. The categories you choose should reflect the nature of your research project and how you plan to develop a rationale for your study. For example, if you are planning an experimental exercise study for elder patients with diabetes, your review may need to highlight the limited number of adequately designed exercise studies with this particular population. Therefore the categories of your chart might include the designs of previous studies and the health status of the samples. Table 5-1 shows an excerpt from such a chart. This chart would be used to structure a review of literature on exercise intervention studies for healthy older adults and to evaluate research designs and specific outcomes of previous studies.

Charting research articles in this way allows you to reflect systematically on the literature as a whole and critically evaluate and identify research gaps.

TABLE 5-1				
Excerpt from Literature Review Chart				
Author (Date)	**Sample Boundaries**	**Design**	**Dependent Constructs**	**Claims**
Blumenthal et al[6] (1982)	24 elder adults from retirement homes (mean age 69 years)	No control group	Mood (profile of mood)	No change
			Temperament (Thurstone scale)	No change
			Self-report of Improvement	40% Improved
			Personality type	No change

TABLE 5-2					
Excerpt from Butler's Concept/Construct Matrix					
	Concept 1	**Concept 2**	**Concept 3**	**Concept 4**	**Concept 5**
Concept	Homelessness	Gender	Middle age	Pathology	Poverty
Source	Hosp and Com 1100-1100	Miller	Hunter and Sundrel	DSM-IV	Axinn and Levin

From Butler SS: *Middle-aged, female and homeless: the stories of a forgotten group,* New York, 1994, Garland.

Concept/Construct Matrix

The *concept/construct matrix* organizes information that you have reviewed and evaluated by key concept/construct (the x axis) and source (the y axis). Table 5-2 shows an excerpt from a concept matrix.

In this naturalistic study of homeless, middle-aged women, Butler[4] began her literature review by searching three major constructs: homelessness, gender, and middle age. Two other constructs, pathology and poverty, were also identified in the literature on homeless persons. Butler integrated these constructs into her theoretical discussion of existing knowledge, and they were added to the concept matrix.

As you begin to write the literature review, the concept/construct matrix facilitates quick identification of the articles that address the specific concepts/constructs you need to discuss. This approach also provides a mechanism to ensure that you review each core construct of your area of inquiry in the literature and systematically link to the others.

Step 5: Critically Evaluate the Literature

Several guiding questions can help you critically evaluate the literature you read. Use the questions in Table 5-3 to guide your reading of the research literature and the questions in Box 5-7 to assist your evaluation of nonresearch literature. Your responses to these evaluative questions will inform your research direction.

An evaluation of nonresearch sources involves examining the level of and support for the knowledge presented. Nonresearch sources include position papers, theoretical works, editorials, and debates. As mentioned earlier, another important resource is work that presents a critical review of research in a particular area. These published literature reviews provide syntheses of research as ways of summarizing the state of knowledge in particular fields and identifying new directions for research.

Step 6: Write the Literature Review

Now that you have searched, obtained, read, and organized your literature, it is time to write the actual review. You need to summarize your review for a proposal to seek approval from your institution's office for protection of human subjects, for a proposal to seek funding to support your research, or to justify the conduct of your study for a manuscript that describes the completed research project. A good literature review presents an overview of the

---

TABLE 5-3

Evaluating Research Articles

Experimental Type	Naturalistic Inquiry
_____ Was the study clear, unambiguous, and internally consistent? _____ What is (are) the research question(s)? Are they clearly and adequately stated? _____ What is the purpose of the study? _____ How does the purpose influence the design and the conclusions? _____ Describe the theory that guides the study and the conceptual framework for the project. Are they clearly presented and relevant to the study? _____ What are the key constructs identified in the literature review? _____ What level of theory is suggested in the literature review? Is it consistent with the selected research strategy? _____ What is the rationale for the design found in the literature review? Is it sound? _____ Does the design of the project fit the level of theory? Is relevant knowledge presented in the literature review? _____ Diagram the design. _____ Does the design answer the research question(s)? Why or why not? _____ What are the boundaries of the study? How are the boundaries selected? _____ What efforts did the investigator make to ensure validity and reliability? _____ What data collection techniques were used? Is the rationale for these techniques specified in the literature review and/or in the methods section? _____ How does data collection fit with the study purpose and study question? _____ How are the data analyzed? Does the analysis plan make sense for the study? How does the analysis plan fit with the study purpose and study question? _____ Are the conclusions supported by the study? _____ What are the strengths of the study? _____ What level of knowledge is generated? _____ What use does this knowledge have for health and human service practice? _____ Are there ethical dilemmas presented in this article? What are they? Did the author(s) resolve the dilemmas in a reasonable and ethical manner?	_____ Was the study clear, unambiguous, and credible? _____ What is (are) the research query(ies)? Are they clearly and adequately stated? _____ What is the purpose of the study? _____ How does the purpose influence the design and the conclusions? _____ Describe the theory that guides or emerges from the study. _____ What are the key constructs identified in the literature review or emerging from the study? _____ What level of theory is suggested in the literature review? Is it consistent with the selected research strategy? _____ What is the rationale for the design found in the literature review? Is it sound? _____ Does the design of the project fit the level or acceptability of theory? Is relevant knowledge presented in the literature review? _____ Does the design answer the research query(ies)? Why or why not? _____ What are the boundaries of the study? How are the boundaries selected? _____ What efforts did the investigator make to ensure trustworthiness? _____ What information collection techniques were used? Where is the rationale for these techniques specified and is it sound? _____ How does information collection fit with the study purpose and study query? _____ How are the data analyzed? Does the analysis plan make sense for the study? How does the analysis plan fit with the study purpose and study query? _____ Are the conclusions supported by the study? _____ What are the strengths of the study? _____ What level of knowledge is generated? _____ What use does this knowledge have for health and human service practice? _____ Are there ethical dilemmas presented in this article? What are they? Did the author(s) resolve the dilemmas in a reasonable and ethical manner?

relevant work on your topic and a critical evaluation of the works. There is no recipe for writing a narrative literature review. Most investigators, whether working in an experimental-type or naturalistic tradition, include in their narratives the categories of information shown in Box 5-8. One suggested outline for writing the narrative of a literature review is presented in Box 5-9.

SUMMARY

The literature review is a critical evaluation of existing literature that is relevant to your study. Because it is a critical evaluation, reviewing the literature is a thinking process that involves piecing together and integrating diverse bodies of literature. The review provides an understanding of the level of

---

BOX 5-7
GUIDING QUESTIONS FOR EVALUATING NONRESEARCH SOURCES

1. What way of knowing and level of knowledge are presented?
2. Was the work presented clearly, unambiguously, and consistently?
3. What is the purpose of the work? Is the purpose implicit? It is stated? How does the purpose influence the knowledge discussed in the work?
4. What is the scope and application of the paper?
5. What support exists for the claims being made in the source?
6. What debates, new ideas, and trends are presented in the work?
7. What are the strengths and weaknesses of the work?
8. What research queries, or questions, emerge from the work?

BOX 5-9
SUGGESTED OUTLINE FOR WRITING NARRATIVE

I. Introduction (overview of what the review covers)
II. Review of specific concepts
III. Description of how each concept has been studied
IV. Overview of studies
V. Design
VI. Results
VII. Critical evaluation
VIII. Critical summary of current knowledge and gaps in literature
IX. Integration of concepts; relationships proposed in studies
X. Identification of research needs
XI. Rationale for study and design
XII. Overview and niche for proposed study

BOX 5-8
ELEMENTS OF WRITING A LITERATURE REVIEW

■ Introduction
■ Discussion of each related concept, construct, principle, theory, and model in current literature
■ Brief review of related study designs and their results
■ Critical appraisal of current related research and knowledge
■ Integration of various works reviewed
■ Fit of investigator's study with the collective knowledge related to topic under investigation
■ Overview and justification for study and design

---

theory and knowledge development that exists about your topic. This understanding is essential so that you can determine how your study fits into the construction of knowledge in the topic area.

The literature review is also an action process whereby concepts are organized and sources are logically presented in a written review. The literature review chart and concept/construct matrix are two organizational tools that will help you conceptualize the literature and write an effective review. An effective written review convinces the reader that your study is necessary, and it represents the next step in knowledge building. Remember, the primary

purposes of writing a literature review and including it in the written report of your research are to establish the conceptual foundation for your research, establish the specific content of your study, and, most important, provide a rationale for your research design.

Also, keep in mind that a systematic review of the literature can also function as a research methodology. Chapter 10 describes two methodologies that use published literature as the unit of analysis.[7]

EXERCISES

1. You are interested in studying the effectiveness of a joint mobilization program to increase the range of motion of the lower extremities of children with spinal cord injuries. Identify the keywords you will use to conduct a search for relevant literature.
2. Select a research article and develop a concept/construct matrix from the literature presented. What level of knowledge and theory development is presented for each concept/construct? For each study, was the selected design appropriate for the level of knowledge in the literature?
3. Identify a specific area of research that interests you and the specific related constructs. Conduct a keyword search for each construct using a relevant database. How many articles do you identify for each construct searched? How would you refine your keyword search?

REFERENCES

1. Peters J: The domestic violence myth acceptance scale: development and psychometric testing of a new instrument. Dissertation, 2003, University of Maine.
2. Gitlin LN: Conducting research on home environments: lessons learned and new directions, *The Gerontologist* 43(5):628-637, 2003.
3. McCauley W, Travis SS, Safewright MP: Personal accounts of the nursing home search and selection process, *Qualitative Health Res* 7(2):236-254, 1997.
4. Butler SS:.*Middle-aged, female and homeless: the stories of a forgotten group,* New York, 1994, Garland.
5. Findley TM: The conceptual review of the literature or how to read more articles than you ever wanted to see in your entire LIFE, *Am J Phys Med Rehabil* 68:97-102, 1989.
6. Blumenthal JA et al: Psychological and physiological effects of physical conditioning on the elderly, *J Psychosom Res* 26:505-510, 1982.
7. Denzin N, Lincoln Y: *Handbook of qualitative research,* Thousand Oaks, Calif, 2000, Sage.

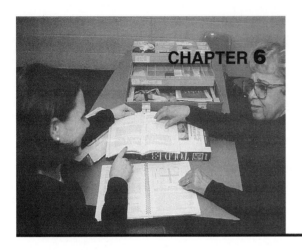

CHAPTER 6

Theory in Research

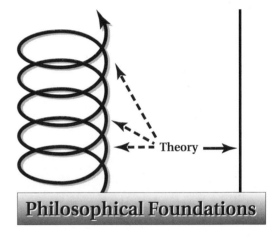

Theory

Philosophical Foundations

Think of a particular field of inquiry or a particular research question or query of interest to you, and ask yourself the following two questions:

- What do we know about this phenomenon?
- What theories have been developed to explain the phenomenon?

You will want to keep asking these basic questions as you engage in the research process and explore different problems of interest. For each research question or query that you pose, the way in which you answer these basic questions will largely determine the type of research actions (e.g., design strategy, analysis, and reporting) that you will implement. As discussed in previous chapters, the level of knowledge and theory development in a particular field shapes how a research question or query is framed and a design strategy is implemented. The role of theory in experimental-type and naturalistic research is critical.

WHY IS THEORY IMPORTANT?

When people hear the word *theory*, they often feel overwhelmed and assume that the term is not relevant to their daily lives or is too abstract and complicated to understand. However, think about how difficult life would be without theory. Theory informs us each day in many aspects of our lives, from knowing how to prepare for the weather to guiding our professional practice. For example, predicting the weather is based on existing theory. The meteorologist looks at present weather conditions and past weather patterns and makes a prediction in the form of a forecast.

In health and human service delivery, you make a decision about which intervention to use based on theory. You use a theory to guide your decisions, even though you may not be fully cognizant that you are actually doing so.

Assume you are a health or human service professional in a psychiatric hospital. A new member comes to your group therapy session with a diagnosis of a major depressive disorder. Theoretically, you know that this diagnosis is associated with a set of symptoms and behaviors, particularly self-degradation, faulty thinking, and melancholia. Based on this cognitive-behavioral theoretical understanding of the symptoms,[1] as well as the prediction of the individual's behavioral outcomes, you approach this client with support and engage him or her in a cognitive-behavioral program in which self-degrading ideation is incrementally decreased. Without the theory, you would not know how to work skillfully with this client.

As discussed in Chapter 1, a primary purpose of research is directly linked to theory. In experimental-type designs a primary purpose of research is to test theory using deduction, whereas in naturalistic inquiry the purpose is to generate theory using induction or abduction. This chapter introduces another important aspect in the relationship between research and theory: you must have a theoretical framework to conduct adequate research.

As discussed throughout this text, thinking and action processes are equally important parts of research. Critical to the thinking processes are the set of human ideas that can be organized to understand human experience and phenomena. As described later in this chapter, these ideas are theories or parts of theories. Even though we may not realize it, theory frames how we ask, look at, and answer questions. Theory provides conceptual clarity and the capacity

to connect the new knowledge obtained through data collection action processes to the vast body of knowledge to which it is relevant. Without theory, we cannot have conceptual direction. Data that are derived without being conceptually embedded in theoretical contexts do not advance our understanding of human experience and ultimately are not useful. As Neuman states, "[T]heory helps a researcher see the forest instead of just a single tree."[2]

Let us examine more closely why theory must inform or shape research actions by considering the meaning and use of common terms such as "race" and "ethnicity."

Every 10 years the United States government conducts a national census in which characteristics of individuals, families, and neighborhoods are ascertained by collecting information. Over the last 3 decades, there has been a significant debate about the need and rationale for recording race and ethnicity.[3] However, there is no consensus about a clear, theoretically based definition and thus a measure of race and ethnicity in the census. That is, no one really knows what the terms race and ethnicity mean; there is great conceptual confusion. As Ahmad and Sheldon state, "[T]he 'ethnic' question in the census is both rigid and externally imposed. It uses a culturalist, geographic, and 'nationalist' notion of race dressed up as ethnicity."[3] As such, some have argued that the gathering of race and ethnicity data is *atheoretical* and thus can be dangerous; it may lead to inaccurate analysis and development of policies or social actions that are consequently inappropriate.[4]

Nevertheless, given our present social structure and how health and social policy is formulated, knowledge about racial and ethnic categories can be important for program planning. Thus, collecting information about race and ethnic categories must be based first on a careful consideration of the definition and use of these terms as theoretical constructs, then on appropriate ways to *operationalize* or measure the theoretically based definition. Only a theoretically based approach can avoid the potential harm to significant numbers of people by ungrounded and vague usage of these important terms.

WHAT IS THEORY?

By now you might be asking, "So what is theory?" Definitions range from traditional views of theory as systems to organize, describe, and predict a single reality; to abstract systems of language symbols that provide multiple interpretations and ideas of phenomena; to ideological foundations for social action.[5]

We draw on Kerlinger's classic definition of theory because we believe it is the most comprehensive and useful for investigators and students of research. Kerlinger defines theory as "a set of interrelated constructs, definitions, and propositions that present a systematic view of phenomena by specifying relations among variables, with the purpose of explaining or predicting phenomena."[6] In this definition, theory is a set of related ideas that has the potential to explain or predict human experience in an orderly fashion, and it is based on data. The theorist develops a structural map of what is observed and experienced in an effort to promote understanding and facilitate the ability to predict outcomes under specific conditions. Through deductive research approaches or empirical investigations, theories are either supported and verified or refuted and falsified. Through inductive approaches, theories are incrementally developed to explain and give order to observations of human experience.

As implied in Kerlinger's definition, four interrelated structural components are subsumed under theory and range in degree, or level, of abstraction. Although numerous taxonomies for the parts of a theory have been proposed,[7] we suggest that the four basic structures of theory are concepts, constructs, relationships, and propositions or principles. Let us first examine the meaning of abstraction and then discuss each level.

Levels of Abstraction

Abstraction often conjures up a vision of the ethereal, the "not real." In this book, however, we use the term abstraction as it relates to theory development, to depict a symbolic representation of shared experience. For example, if we all see a form that has fur, a tail, four legs, and barks, we name that observation a "dog." We have shared in the visual experience and have created a symbol (the word dog) to name our sensory experience.

All words are merely symbols to describe and communicate experience. Words are only one form

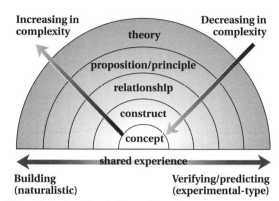

Figure 6-1 Levels of abstraction.

of abstraction; different words represent different levels of abstraction; and a single word can represent multiple levels of abstraction.

Figure 6-1 displays the four *levels of abstraction* within theory and their interrelationships. Shared experience is the foundation on which abstraction is built. It is important to recognize that we do not use the term reality as the foundation. "Reality" implies that there is only one viewpoint from which to build the basic elements of a theory. In contrast, this text is based on the premise that humans experience multiple realities and multiple perspectives about the nature of reality. As such, levels of abstraction must be built on shared experience, defined as the consensus of what we obtain through our senses. For experimental-type researchers who work deductively, shared experience is usually thought of as sense data, or that which can be reduced to observation and measurement. For researchers working inductively and abductively in the naturalistic tradition, shared experience may include meanings and interpretations of human experience.

Let us use the example of the "furry being with four legs and a tail that barks" to illustrate the multiple meanings that can be attributed to shared experience. Shared experience tells each of us that this is a dog, but the word "dog" may also carry with it diverse meanings, such as fear and happiness.

Each type of experience is equally important to acknowledge, as are the different meanings attributed to a single word.

Concepts

As depicted in Figure 6-1, a *concept* is the first level of abstraction and is defined as a symbolic representation of an observable or experienced referent.[8] Concepts are the basic building blocks of communication because they provide us with the means to tell our experiences and ideas to one another. Without concepts, we would not have language.[8] In the case of the "furry being," the word "dog" can function as a concept. At this basic level of abstraction, the term dog describes an observation shared by many. The words "furry," "tail," "four legs," and "bark" are also concepts because they are directly sensed.

In experimental-type research, concepts are selected before a study is started and are defined so as to permit direct measurement or observation. In naturalistic research, concepts are derived primarily through direct observations and continual engagement with the phenomenon of interest in the context in which it occurs.

Constructs

A *construct,* the next level of abstraction, does not have an observable or a directly experienced referent in shared experience. Meanings become important to consider at this level of abstraction, because two individuals who articulate the same construct may attribute disparate meanings to it. If we look again at the term *dog* as a construct rather than a concept, the word "dog" may mean "fear" to some and "happiness" to others. Although we stated above that dog is a concept, in this case "dog" functions as a construct because what is observable is not the communicated meaning. Rather, the meaning of the term dog takes on the feelings evoked by "dog," such as fear and happiness.

Fear and happiness are also examples of constructs. What may be observed are the behaviors associated with fear or happiness, that is, someone who sweats, shakes, and turns pale at the site of a dog or someone who smiles, approaches, and pets the dog, respectively. These observations of both feelings are synthesized into the constructs of fear and happiness. Thus, fear and happiness are not directly "observed" but are surmised by observations of human behavior and are based on a constellation of behavioral concepts.

Categories provide additional examples of constructs. The category of "mammal" or "canine" is an example of a construct. Although each category or construct is not directly observable, it is composed of a set of concepts that can be observed.

Other examples of constructs relevant to health and human service inquiry include quality of life, health, wellness, life roles, rehabilitation, poverty, illness, disability, functional status, and psychological well-being. Although not directly observable, each is made up of parts or components that can be observed or submitted to measurement. Think about the construct of "quality of life"; what concepts is this construct composed of? If you consider that even this relatively low level of abstraction can be complex, you begin to understand why health and human service research is so complex.

Relationships

So far, we have been discussing single-word symbols or units of abstraction. At the next level of abstraction, single units are connected and form a relationship. A *relationship* is defined as an association of two or more constructs or concepts. For example, we may suggest that the size of a dog is related to the level of fear that a person experiences. This relationship has two constructs, "size" and "fear," and one concept, "dog."

Propositions (Principles)

A *proposition* is the next level of abstraction. A proposition, or principle, is a statement that governs a set of relationships and gives them a structure. For example, a proposition suggests that fear of large dogs is caused by negative childhood experiences with large dogs. This proposition describes the structure of two sets of relationships: (1) the relationship between the size of a dog and fear and (2) the relationship between childhood experiences and the size of dogs. It also suggests the direction of the relationship and the influence of each construct on the other.

A theory related to the "furry being" may be that "fear of large dogs derives from childhood experiences." Therefore the fear can be cured by psychoanalysis that aims to reverse the negative effects of childhood experiences.

This theory explains the phenomenon "fear of dogs"; it is verifiable and can lead to prediction. If, through research, we can support a positive relationship between childhood experiences and fear of dogs and the effectiveness of psychoanalysis in reducing that fear, we can predict this relationship in the future and control its outcome.

Design Selection and the Four Levels

We conclude our discussion of levels of abstraction with principles that relate these levels to the selection of a particular research design or approach to studying a phenomenon of interest. We view abstraction as the symbolic naming, representation, and frequent communication of shared experience. The further a symbol is removed from shared experience, the higher the level of abstraction. Each level of abstraction moves farther away from shared experience (see Figure 6-1). The higher level of abstraction, the more complex your design becomes. This principle is based on common sense. If the scope of your study is to examine a construct, a complex investigation may not be necessary, such as that required for the development or testing of a full-fledged theory.

Suppose you are interested in determining the level of cognitive recovery in a group of persons with head injuries. This type of investigation is an inquiry into the construct of "cognitive recovery" and requires that one construct be defined and measured in your population. Complexity is encountered in the research process with the lexical definition of the construct, which describes its meaning in words. Once you select a definition, the rest of the research process is relatively straightforward.

However, suppose you want to move into the realm of propositions and determine the extent that the person's age at the time of injury affects recovery rate. In this type of investigation, you need to define the construct lexically (in words), define "recovery," and state the nature of the relationship between recovery and the concept of "age." As you add more constructs, such as "level of severity of injury" and "status before injury," your design increases in complexity.

Let us consider another example that requires a different type of inquiry.

Assume you are interested in understanding the behaviors that place rural teenagers at risk for contracting human immunodeficiency virus (HIV). Because most knowledge on HIV risk in the adolescent population focuses on urban teenagers, you have limited theory, or sets of constructs, to investigate. Consequently, you simply collect data through asking questions and observing behaviors of the referent group. As your observations proceed, however, you find many factors emerging that impact rural teenage behavior and risk. The complexity of your research approach increases as you focus on discovering and interpreting the meaning of specific patterns or relationships among constructs that you observe.

Although concepts, constructs, relationships, and propositions or principles provide the basic language and building blocks of any research project, each research tradition handles the levels of abstraction differently.

ROLE OF THEORY IN DESIGN SELECTION

How does theory shape the selection of research design strategies? When theory is well developed and conceptually fits the phenomenon under investigation, deductive studies will likely be implemented, as in the tradition of experimental-type research. When theory is poorly developed or does not fit the phenomenon under study, inductive and abductive studies that generate theory may be more appropriate, as in the tradition of naturalistic inquiry. The degree of knowledge development and relevance of a theory for the particular phenomenon under investigation determines in part the nature and type of research that needs to be conducted.

The relationship of theory and design can be illustrated by considering the classic theory of moral development advanced by Lawrence Kohlberg, a well-known scholar. He suggested three basic levels of moral reasoning that develop and unfold throughout the life span: preconventional, conventional, and postconventional.[9] Briefly, in the preconventional reasoning stage, individuals develop notions of right and wrong, based on reward or punishment; in conventional reasoning, individuals use accepted norms of right and wrong to guide their moral decisions; and in postconventional reasoning, humans use their own intrinsic notions of morality to formulate decisions and actions. Many investigators have accepted this theory as truth and have attempted to characterize and predict the moral reasoning of different populations. Scales to measure moral reasoning have been developed based on Kohlberg's theory and have been used with different groups of people representing diverse socioeconomic, age, and gender groups. Based on these studies, populations and individuals have been categorized according to the level of moral reasoning they exhibit. This information has been extremely valuable in promoting our understanding of morality in humans. The characterization of moral reasoning based on Kohlberg's theory is an example of a deductive relationship between theory and research; that is, the theory has been accepted as true, and subsequent studies intend to verify and advance the application of the theory in varied populations.

In most studies of moral reasoning in adults based on Kohlberg's theoretical framework, however, women had been reported to reason at a lower level than men. Researchers therefore concluded that women were not as morally advanced as men. Although this conclusion makes no sense, this type of deductive illogic is common practice, particularly when a theory is developed for one group and automatically applied to another without consideration of its "fit."

Recognizing this illogic with regard to women, researchers using different theoretical frameworks began to tackle the issue. Carol Gilligan used a feminist framework and did not accept Kohlberg's theory as true for women because it was intuitively contrary to what she experienced and believed. She argued that although knowledge had been well developed in this area, the theory did not seem to fit or to be relevant to the experiences of women. She therefore chose to approach the investigation of moral reasoning in women by applying inductive research strategies. Through extensive interviews, Gilligan found that women were not less moral than men but rather based their moral decision making on criteria that were substantially different from those identified by Kohlberg's theory and those operationalized in the scales developed to reflect his theory.

This example shows extensive theory development. However, Gilligan's research suggested that Kohlberg's notions did not explain moral reasoning for a particular group—women. By using inductive strategies, Gilligan was able to identify and show the processes by which women reason and function, and thus develop theory that reflected their thought processes. Not surprisingly, Kohlberg had developed his theory of moral reasoning by studying men. Therefore the deductive strategy was most valuable in expanding knowledge of the moral reasoning in men, but not necessarily in women. Gilligan's research strategy illustrates the relationship between theory and naturalistic inquiry; in other words, naturalistic inquiry is extremely valuable as a *theory-generating* tool, but it also can be used to verify or refute a theory.

Another example more relevant to health and human service practice involves the newly revised *International Classification of Functioning, Disability, and Health* (ICF).[10] In response to the difficulties encountered by experimental-type researchers in creating and identifying how best to use previous editions of the ICF in diverse populations, the World Health Organization and National Institutes of Health jointly implemented Cultural Applicability Research (CAR). This is an innovative mixed-method approach to developing instrumentation across global cultures and groups. CAR identifies the contextual, multilevel consequences of diagnostic conditions and provides empirical knowledge to inform the tenth ICF revision of this important taxonomy.[11]

This example shows how the limitations of applying theory and knowledge developed on one group to other diverse groups are met with inductive and deductive systematic inquiry in current health and human service research.

Now that you have a good sense of the meaning of theory and how theory relates to research knowledge development and design strategy selection, let us consider the role and relationship of theory and research in each of the research traditions.

THEORY IN EXPERIMENTAL-TYPE RESEARCH

Experimental-type researchers begin with a theory and seek to simplify and reduce abstraction by making the abstract observable, measurable, and predictable (see Figure 6-1). This process of *theory testing* typically involves specifying a theory, then developing

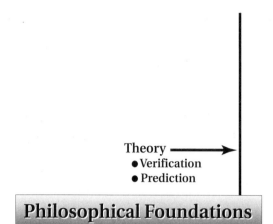

Theory ⟶
● Verification
● Prediction

Philosophical Foundations

hypotheses. A *hypothesis* is linked to a theory and is a statement about the expected relationships between two or more concepts that can be tested. A hypothesis indicates what is expected to be observed and represents the researcher's "best hunch" as to what may exist or may be found, based on the principles of the theory.

As an example, defensive attribution theory, building on general attribution theory, has been used as an important theoretical foundation in investigating individual and community responses to victims of sexual assault. Defensive attributions are unconscious, self-protective mechanisms[12-15]; when invoked, they function subconsciously to reduce the observer's fear and threat by attributing character and behavioral blame to the victim. Based on this theory, a major hypothesis suggests a positive association between similarity with the victim and victim blaming.[16] That is, the more an individual feels at risk, the more likely she is to accept explanations that attribute blame to the victim on the basis of some fault of her own. The hypothesis is based on the theoretical tenet that victim blame identifies the circumstance, which can be avoided and thus can diminish the perceived threat of assault.

Hypotheses can be written in two forms, nondirectional or directional (see Chapter 7). The following nondirectional hypothesis is derived from defensive attribution theory:

• There is a relationship between perceived similarity with the victim and victim blaming.

A hypothesis can also indicate the direction or nature of a relationship between two concepts or constructs, as in the following example of a directional hypothesis:

• As the perceived similarity among respondent and victim increases, victim blaming will increase.

Now consider another example. Personal control theory is based on the premise that control over one's immediate life space or personal environment is an important human invariant that transcends cultural groups.[17] This theory suggests that humans, by their nature, must achieve some level of control in everyday life. Applied to the field of rehabilitation, the theory suggests that persons with physical difficulties resulting in limitations in performing daily activities may be threatened by or experience loss of control. This threat of or actual loss of control may in turn result in feelings of anxiety, which may lead to depression unless strategies, either cognitive or behavioral actions, are implemented to help the person achieve a sense of efficacy and control. By enhancing control, persons experience a sense of enhanced self-efficacy and personal mastery.

Based on this theory, what do you think are some of the hypotheses that may be generated and tested? One directional hypothesis might be that use of adaptive technology enhances self-efficacy in people who have activity limitations resulting from physical impairments. This hypothesis has been tested by various researchers. Now, can you think of other meaningful hypotheses based on this theory?

Consider the hypotheses you thought of and those we suggested. What can you conclude about a hypothesis? As shown in Figure 6-2, a hypothesis is the initial reduction of theory to a more concrete and observable form. Based on the hypothesis, the researcher develops an operational definition of a concept so that it can be measured by a scale or other instrumentation. The operational definition of the concept further reduces the abstract to a concrete, observable form. An operational definition of a concept specifies the exact procedures for measuring or observing the phenomenon. In the example of attribution theory, the investigator needs to operationalize identification with the victim and victim blaming. The process of operationalizing a concept is not easy or straightforward. Likewise, in the example of personal control theory, the investigator needs to operationalize self-efficacy. Each researcher may

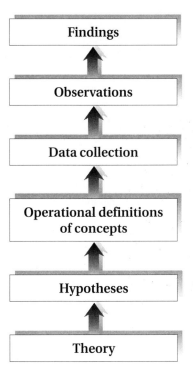

Figure 6-2 Using theory in experimental-type research.

develop his or her own way of operationalizing key concepts. This process is discussed in greater detail in Chapter 16, where we examine issues related to measurement and instrument construction.

Using an operational definition, the researcher makes observations that result in data points, which are then analyzed. Analysis determines if the findings verify, refute, or modify the theory. This is the fundamental premise of the scientific process. Reducing abstraction to measurable components is used primarily to test relationships among concepts of a theory, and it is used ultimately to determine the adequacy of a theory in order to make predictions and thus control the phenomenon under study.

Box 6-1 lists the basic characteristics of the use of theory by experimental-type researchers. The process, referred to as logical deduction, begins with an abstraction and then focuses on discrete parts of phenomena or observations. Constructs are defined and simplified, then operationalized into concepts that can be observed to allow measurement.

BOX 6-1
SIX CHARACTERISTICS OF USE OF THEORY IN EXPERIMENTAL-TYPE RESEARCH

1. Logical deductive process.
2. Primarily uses theory testing.
3. Movement from theory to lesser levels of abstraction.
4. Assumes unitary reality that can be measured.
5. Assumes knowledge through existing conceptions.
6. Focus on measurable parts of phenomena.

This process moves from a more abstract to a less abstract level, or to a more concrete and observable level.

THEORY IN NATURALISTIC INQUIRY

Whereas theory testing is the primary goal of researchers in the experimental-type tradition, researchers working in the naturalistic tradition usually are developing theory from observations. Thus, in naturalistic inquiry, the researcher begins with shared experience and then represents that experience at increasing levels of abstraction. In this approach, definitions of concepts and constructs are not necessarily set before a study is begun; rather, definitions emerge from the data collection and analytical processes. In many of the orientations of naturalistic research, the aim is to "ground" or link concepts and constructs to each observation or datum. This theory-method link,[18] or grounded-theory approach, is described in a classic work by Glaser and Strauss in this way:

> Generating a theory from data means that most hypotheses and concepts not only come from the data, but are systematically worked out in relation to the data during the course of the research. Generating a theory involves a process of research.[19]

As discussed later in this text, each strategy classified as naturalistic inquiry is based on a different set of assumptions about how we come to know human experience. However, all researchers in the naturalistic tradition tend to use qualitative

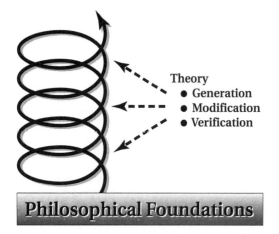

Theory
- Generation
- Modification
- Verification

Philosophical Foundations

methodologies to ground theory in observations. That is, definitions of concepts and then constructs emerge from the investigative process and analysis of the documentation (the data) of shared experience.[18] Based on emergent concepts and their relationships, the investigator develops theory to understand, explain, and give meaning to social and behavioral patterns.

Although each design structure describes this process somewhat differently, Figure 6-1 illustrates the basic idea of the inductive process.

In some naturalistic inquiries, theory is used in a similar manner to experimental-type research. Once immersed in observations, the investigator frequently draws on well-established theories to explain these observations and make sense of what is being observed. Consider how the previous discussion of victim blaming might provide the ethnographer with an understanding of cultural views of sexual assault victims. In the process of observing how groups perceive, describe, and respond to sexual assault victims, the ethnographer may be reminded of a defensive attribution theory that seems to fit with the data set. Thus the theory is applied to the data set as an explanatory mechanism. However, the use of theory in this example occurs after the data have been collected and analyzed. When an investigator is proceeding inductively, theory does not guide data collection and is not imposed on the data; rather, the data may suggest which theory, if any, might be relevant.

This is not to say that naturalistic inquiry is atheoretical. Theory use, however, has a different function than in experimental-type research. All research begins from a particular theoretical framework based on assumptions of human experience and reality and how we can come to know them. This theoretical framework is not substantive or content specific, but it is structural and process oriented and frames the research approach assumed by the investigator.

Theory can be used in naturalistic inquiry in many ways. For example, the researcher may also begin within a substantive theoretical framework to explore its particular meaning for a specific group of people or in specified situations. An investigator might examine how a group of feminist scholars responds to defensive attribution theory as a force that shapes social services for sexual assault victims. In this case, as in most naturalistic traditions, the function of the substantive theory is to place boundaries on the inquiry rather than fit the data into the theoretical framework by reducing concepts to predefined measures.

Box 6-2 summarizes the basic characteristics of the use of theory in naturalistic inquiry. As we illustrate, the treatment of theory occurs primarily within inductive and abductive processes that move from shared experience to higher levels of abstraction. Theory generation in the naturalistic tradition serves primarily to reveal the multiple meanings and subjective understandings of the phenomena under study. In this process, knowledge emerges from informants or study participants.

Table 6-1 presents an overview of the use of theory in both experimental-type and naturalistic research traditions, as well as how theory can be used in an integrated research design.

BOX 6-2

FIVE CHARACTERISTICS OF THEORY IN NATURALISTIC INQUIRY

1. Inductive and abductive processes.
2. Primarily generates theory.
3. Movement from shared experience to higher levels of abstraction.
4. Assumes discovery of meaning through multiple subjective understandings.
5. Focus on depicting complexity.

TABLE 6-1

Use of Theory Among Research Traditions

Experimental-Type	Naturalistic	Integrated
Deductive	Inductive and abductive	All
Theory testing	Theory generating Theory validating	Both
Decrease level of abstraction	Increase level of abstraction	Both

SUMMARY

In this chapter we have discussed the following five major points:

1. Theory is fundamental to the research process.
2. Theory consists of four basic components that reflect different levels of abstraction. These levels are concepts, constructs, relationships, and propositions (principles).
3. The level at which a theory is developed and its appropriateness to your phenomenon under study determine in part the nature and structure of research design.
4. Experimental-type research moves from greater levels of abstraction to lesser levels of abstraction by reducing theory to specific hypotheses and operationalizing concepts to observe and measure as a way of testing the theory.
5. Naturalistic inquiry moves from less abstraction to more abstraction by grounding or linking theory to each datum that is observed or recorded in the process of conducting research.

EXERCISES

1. Select an experimental-type article, and determine the level of abstraction presented in the literature review. Identify all parts of the theory that are presented in the article.
2. In the same article, search for the important constructs (those that have been subjected to measurement), find their lexical definitions, and determine how the authors have operationalized them.
3. Select a naturalistic article, and examine the use of theory in the study. What level of abstraction is developed in the article?

REFERENCES

1. Beck A: Cognitive therapy: past, present & future, *J Consult Clin Psychol* 61(2):194-198, 1993.
2. Neuman WL: *Social research methods: qualitative and quantitative approaches,* ed 3, Boston, 1997, Allyn Bacon.
3. Ahmad W, Sheldon T: Race and statistics. In Hammersley M, editor: *Social research: philosophy, politics and practice,* Newbury Park, Calif, 1992, Sage.
4. Rodriguez R: *Brown: the last discovery of America,* New York, 2003, Penguin.
5. Seidman S: *Contested knowledge: social theory in the postmodern era,* ed 2, Malden, Mass, 1998, Blackwell.
6. Kerlinger FN: *Foundations of behavioral research,* ed 2, New York, 1973, Holt, Rinehart & Winston.
7. Mosey AC: *Applied scientific inquiry in the health professions: an epistemological orientation,* Rockville, Md, 1992, AOTA.
8. Wilson J: *Thinking with concepts,* Cambridge, Mass, 1966, Cambridge University Press.
9. Kohlberg L: *The psychology of moral development,* New York, 1984, Harper & Row.
10. *International classification of functioning, disability, and health,* ed 10, Geneva, 2004, World Health Organization.
11. Ustun TB, Catterji S, Rehm J, et al: *Disability and culture: universalism and diversity,* Seattle, 2002, Hogrefe & Huber.
12. Heider F: *The psychology of interpersonal relations,* New York, 1958, Wiley.
13. Fiske ST, Taylor SE: *Social cognition,* ed 2, New York, 1991, McGraw-Hill.
14. Shaver KG: Defensive attribution: effects of severity and relevance on the responsibility assigned for an accident, *Journal of Personality and Social Psychology* 14:101-113, 1970
15. Thorton B, Ryckman R, Robbins M: The relationship of observer characteristics to beliefs in the causal responsibility of victims of sexual assault, *Human Relations* 35:321-330, 1982.
16. Peters J: *Validation of the domestic violence myth acceptance scale,* 2002, University of Maine (unpublished dissertation).
17. Schulz R, Heckhausen J, O'Brien AT: Control and the disablement process in the elderly, *Soc Behav Personality* 9(5):139-152, 1994.
18. Patton MQ: *Qualitative evaluation and research methods,* ed 2, Newbury Park, Calif, 1990, Sage.
19. Glaser B, Strauss A: *The discovery of grounded theory: strategies for qualitative research,* New York, 1967, Aldine.

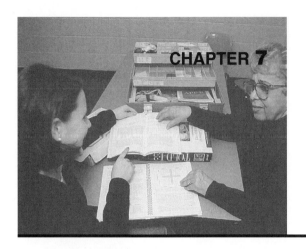

CHAPTER 7

Formulating Research Questions and Queries

KEY TERMS

Breakdowns
Descriptive questions
Directional hypothesis
Hypotheses
Integrated designs
Nondirectional hypothesis
Predictive hypotheses
Predictive questions
Query
Question
Relational questions

CHAPTER OUTLINE

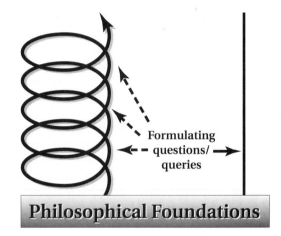

Formulating
questions/
queries

Philosophical Foundations

Up to now you have learned about specific thinking and some action processes, such as the role of theory in research (Chapter 6), ways to identify and frame research problems (Chapter 4), and the purpose of and methods for conducting the literature review (Chapter 5). All these processes are part of the important work of refining the structure and content of any type of inquiry. Now you are ready to move beyond these initial starting blocks as we examine how to develop specific questions within the experimental-type tradition and queries within the naturalistic tradition. Developing a question or query represents the first formal point of entry into a study.

We have just used two distinct terms, *question* and *query,* to describe the initial formal points of entry into a study. These terms reflect the different approaches to research used in each tradition. Your research question or query will guide all other subsequent steps and decisions, such as how you collect information and what other types of procedures you will follow.

RESEARCH QUESTIONS IN EXPERIMENTAL-TYPE DESIGN

In experimental-type research, entry into an investigation requires the formulation of a very specific question with a prescribed structure. That is, from a broad topic of interest to you, you must articulate a specific question that will guide the conduct of the investigation. This question must be concise and narrow and must establish the boundaries or limits as to what concepts, individuals, or phenomena will be examined in the study. The question also must be posed *a priori,* or before engaging in the research process. The question becomes the foundation or basis from which all subsequent research action processes are developed and implemented.

The purpose of the research question in the experimental-type tradition is to articulate not only the concepts, but also the structure and scope of the concepts that will be studied. The research question leads the investigator to highly specified design and data collection action processes that involve a form of observation or measurement to answer the ques-

tion. Research questions are developed deductively from the theoretical principles that exist and are presented in the literature.

Each type of question reflects a different level of knowledge and theory development concerning the topic of interest. Questions that seek to describe a phenomenon, referred to as Level 1 questions, are asked when little to nothing is empirically known about the topic. Level 2 questions explore relationships among phenomena and are asked when descriptive knowledge is known but relationships are not yet understood. Level 3 questions test existing theory or models and are asked when a substantial body of knowledge is known and well-defined theory is developed.

Level 1: Questions That Seek to Describe Phenomena

Level 1 questions are *descriptive questions* designed to elicit descriptions of a single topic or a single population about which there is theoretical or conceptual material in the literature but little or no empirical knowledge. Level 1 questions lead to exploratory action processes with the intent to describe an identified phenomenon. Consider the following examples of studies based on Level 1 questions.

Let us assume that a body of knowledge exists regarding the attitudes of kindergarten to grade 12 teachers toward the inclusion of children with disabilities in regular education classrooms. However, little is known about the attitudes of occupational therapy educators toward including students with disabilities in professional occupational therapy education. A research study based on a Level 1 question would be meaningful and appropriate to describe the attitudes of a specific professional group (i.e., occupational therapy faculty) toward accepting and teaching students with diverse disabilities in occupational therapy classes.

Much research has been conducted on falls in the elder population, with extensive knowledge about the risk factors associated with falling and interventions that may be helpful. However, many clinicians note that older people, whether fallers or nonfallers, may also experience "near-falls," or a stumble, trip, or imbalance, without falling to the ground. Because near-falls are frequently reported by older people but

Research question ⟶

Philosophical Foundations

no research has been conducted on this phenomenon, it would be important to start a program of inquiry with a Level 1 question to describe this potentially important phenomenon and whether it represents a preclinical sign of frailty.

You are a therapist working in a rehabilitation center. One of your responsibilities is to introduce patients to a range of adaptive equipment that they may need or may find useful in the hospital and on their return home. You notice, however, that some of your older patients appear hesitant to use this equipment, and you are not convinced that they continue to use the issued assistive devices once they are home. Since this has important practice, policy, and cost implications, you and your department consider this concern important enough to investigate.

Your first step is to conduct a comprehensive literature review. You might start with a keyword search, such as "adaptive equipment," "assistive devices," and "rehabilitation." The literature review shows only a limited body of knowledge regarding adaptive equipment use and little theoretical development to explain patterns of use, particularly among elders discharged from rehabilitation. Thus, based on this review, you realize that the first step is to design a Level 1 study to describe patterns of equipment use in the home after rehabilitation and identify reasons for use and nonuse among clinical populations, such as older people with recent strokes or hip fractures, who would benefit from the use of equipment over time.[2] Your initial Level 1 research questions may be as follows:

What is the frequency of use of adaptive devices by older individuals who have been diagnosed with strokes and discharged to their home after rehabilitation?

What are the reasons for use and nonuse of assistive devices by this clinical population at 3, 6, and 9 months after discharge?

Think about the basic, descriptive research question in the previous example. What is the main concept or variable that will need to be measured? It is the use of adaptive equipment. What is the primary population that will need to be recruited? It is older adults with a stroke who will be discharged to their home with one or more assistive devices. As you can see, the focus of a Level 1 question is on "the what" (Box 7-1).

> **BOX 7-1**
> **LEVEL 1: DESCRIPTIVE RESEARCH QUESTIONS**
>
> ■ What are the attitudes of occupational therapy faculty toward including students with disabilities in professional occupational therapy education?[3]
> ■ What are student enrollments, numbers and types of faculty, and student-faculty ratios in accredited Master's of Social Work (MSW) programs of the past 18 years?[4]
> ■ What is the prevalence of fear of falling among community-dwelling older persons with impaired mobility?[5]

Level 1 questions focus on the description of one concept or variable in a population. A variable can be defined as a characteristic or phenomenon that has more than one value. To describe a variable, you must first derive a lexical definition of the concept (description of the term in words) from the literature and then operationalize it (define a concept by how it will be measured).

Level 1 questions focus on measuring the nature of a particular phenomenon in the population of interest. These types of questions use the stem of "what are" or "what is" and refer to one population. As shown in the examples, only one population is identified, such as occupational therapy faculty, near-fallers, and individuals discharged to home following rehabilitation. Also, single concepts are examined in each study: attitudes toward inclusion, fear of falling, and reasons for use and nonuse of equipment. Each of these concepts can be defined in such a way to permit their measurement; that is, they can be examined empirically.

Level 1 questions describe the parts of the whole. Remember, the underlying thinking process for experimental-type research is to learn about a topic by examining its parts and their relationships. Level 1 questioning is the foundation for clarifying the parts and their specific nature. In the scheme of levels of abstraction, Level 1 questions target the lowest levels of abstraction: concepts and constructs (see Chapter 6).

As discussed in later chapters, Level 1 questions lead to the development of descriptive designs, such as surveys, exploratory or descriptive studies, trend designs, feasibility studies, need assessments, and case studies.

Level 2: Questions That Explore Relationships Among Phenomena

Once a "part" of a phenomenon is described and there is existing knowledge about it in the context of a particular population, the experimental-type researcher may pose questions that are relational. Level 2 reflects *relational questions* and builds on and refines the results of Level 1 studies. The key purpose of Level 2 type of questioning is to explore relationships among phenomena that have already been identified and described. Here the stem question asks, "What is the relationship?" or a variation of this (e.g., "association"), and the topic contains two or more concepts or variables.

> You are involved in establishing exercise programs for adults as part of their cardiac care. Although you know there is much evidence to support the cardiovascular benefits of aerobic exercise in general, you do not know much about the exercise capacity of middle-aged men, and this group has become your primary clinical population. Thus, you may be interested in asking a Level 2 question such as, "What is the relationship between exercise capacity and cardiovascular health in middle-aged men?" In this case the two identified variables that are measured are exercise capacity and cardiovascular health. The specific population is middle-aged men. As you can surmise, Level 1 research must have been accomplished for the two variables to be identified, defined, and operationalized.

Let us revisit the Level 1 examples and see how they can be modified to become Level 2 questions. Suppose we have conducted studies to address the Level 1 questions in Box 7-1. If we continue our research agenda in each of these areas of inquiry, we would be ready for the relational questions in Box 7-2.

Level 2 questions address relationships between variables. Studies with this level of questioning represent the next level of complexity above Level 1 questions. These questions continue to build on knowledge in the experimental-type framework by examining their parts, their relationships, and the nature and direction of these relationships. Level 2 questions primarily lead to research that uses passive observation design, as discussed later in the text. Refer to the

---

BOX 7-2
LEVEL 2: RELATIONAL-TYPE QUESTIONS

- What is the relationship between the attitudes of occupational therapy faculty and the number of students with disabilities admitted into occupational therapy education programs?
- What is the relationship between student learning and student-faculty ratio in MSW programs?
- What is the relationship between fear of falling and incidence of falls in African American elders who live alone in community-based settings?

---

levels of abstraction in Chapter 6 and see where Level 2 questions fit in the schema of building knowledge in the experimental tradition.

Level 3: Questions That Test Knowledge

Level 3 questioning builds on the knowledge generated from research conducted in Level 1 and Level 2 investigations. A Level 3 question asks about a cause-and-effect relationship among two or more variables, with the specific purpose of testing knowledge or the theory behind the knowledge.

> At Level 2 we asked the question, "What is the relationship among the attitudes of occupational therapy faculty and the number of students with disabilities admitted into occupational therapy education programs?" Assume that in conducting this relational-type study, we find an association between faculty attitudes and number of students with disabilities. That is, our study shows that programs that have occupational therapy educators with positive attitudes have a higher enrollment of students with disabilities than programs with faculty having negative attitudes. Building on this knowledge, you can now ask a Level 3 question such as the following: "To what extent do faculty attitudes influence the number of students with disabilities who are accepted into occupational therapy programs?" Such a study would test the theory behind the reasons that positive attitudes promote opportunity for students with disabilities. Also, the study would be able to predict the opportunity for disabled students to be accepted into occupational therapy programs on the basis of faculty attitudes.

At this level of questioning, the purpose is to predict what will happen and provide a theory to explain the reason(s). Based on a Level 3 question, specific *predictive hypotheses* are formulated; that is, statements are generated that predict the outcome of one variable on the basis of knowing another variable. In the example, knowledge generated from this type of Level 3 study would provide guidance to identify specific strategies for promoting educational opportunities. In other words, it would provide knowledge regarding where, why, and how to intervene.

Now consider another type of Level 3 question.

> For the past 15 years of research on family caregiving, many Level 1 studies have described the experience of caregiving by families of children and older adults with a wide range of physical and cognitive impairments. Also, based on Level 1 findings, there is a rich body of knowledge at Level 2. For example, numerous studies show that women and spouses tend to show more distress and burden with caregiving than other family members. Given the knowledge of stress associated with caregiving and different relational patterns that have emerged, more recent research has tested Level 3 type of questions. These studies, using basic stress theories, have sought to predict caregiving outcomes over time and to test specific theory-based interventions to alleviate the burden associated with the role of caregiver. Such Level 3 questions include the following:
>
> To what extent does a home-based skills-training intervention improve communication patterns between children with physical impairments and their mothers?
>
> To what extent does participation in a telephone support group reduce emotional burdens among women caring for family members with dementia?

Level 3 questions assume that two concepts are related, based on findings from previous Level 2 research studies. The main purpose of Level 3 studies is to test these concepts in action by manipulating one to affect the other. Level 3 is the most complex of experimental-type questioning. Once the foundational questions formulated at Levels 1 and 2 are answered, Level 3 questions can be posed and answered to develop knowledge of not only the parts and their relationships, but also how these parts interact and why they interact to cause a particular outcome. Level 3 questions examine higher levels of abstraction, including principles, theories, and models (see Chapter 6).

To answer a Level 3 question, research action processes capable of revealing causal relationships among variables must be implemented. A true experimental design or a variation would need to be conducted.

Developing Experimental-Type Research Questions

As you see, question formulation for experimental-type research is relatively straightforward. You can refer to Table 7-1 as a basic guide in helping you develop research questions at the three levels. Also, Box 7-3 provides helpful rules for developing questions at the appropriate level.

Keep in mind that one challenge in developing an experimental-type research question, particularly for new researchers, is proposing a question that is (1) very specific, (2) not too broad, and (3) feasible to study. One tendency is to develop a question that is too "big." If your question can be broken down into subquestions, you know you have not yet developed an appropriate research question.

Hypotheses

As discussed in previous chapters, experimental-type researchers frequently engage in studies that involve *hypotheses*. A classic definition of hypothesis is "a proposition to be tested or a tentative statement of a relationship between two variables."[6]

TABLE 7-1

Questions at Three Levels in Experimental-Type Research

Level	Stem	Level of Abstraction	Design Possibilities
1	What is...? What are...?	Concepts and constructs	Survey Exploratory Descriptive Case study Needs assessment
2	What is the relationship...?	Relationships	Survey Correlational, passive Observation Ex post facto
3	Why...?	Principles Theories Models	Experimental designs Quasi-experimental designs

BOX 7-3
HELPFUL RULES IN DEVELOPING A RESEARCH QUESTION

1. At Level 1, examine a variable in one population.
2. At Level 2, examine the relationship between a minimum of two variables.
3. If there is a cause or effect to be investigated, pose the question at Level 3.
4. If the words "cause," "effect," or any of their synonyms appear in the question, eliminate these words, or specify what they are and how they vary.
5. All variables must be written so that they vary.
6. At Level 3, there must be two variables that specify a cause and effect.
7. If a Level 3 question is written, make sure it is both ethical and possible to manipulate the causal variable. If not, rewrite the question at Level 2.

From Brink PJ, Wood MJ: *Basic steps in planning nursing research: from question to proposal,* ed 3, Boston, 1998, Jones & Bartlett.

As the definition implies, hypotheses are primarily necessary and developed for Level 2 and Level 3 questions. For a Level 1 question, the experimental-type researcher usually has a "hunch" about the expected distribution of a single variable; however, a statement about a single variable is not a hypothesis. By definition, a Level 1 question does not have the essential elements of at least two variables and a statement of expected relationship.

Although a hypothesis is a researcher's best hunch about a phenomenon, this "guess" does not emerge from thin air. Rather, it must be based on existing literature and theory and must stem from the research question guiding the study.

Hypotheses serve important purposes in experimental-type research. First, they form an important link between the research question and the design of the study. In essence, hypotheses rephrase the research question and turn it into a testable or measurable statement. Second, hypotheses may identify the anticipated direction of the proposed relationship between stated variables. Information regarding directionality of a relationship between variables is usually not contained in the actual research question.

The two types of hypothesis are *directional hypothesis* and *nondirectional hypothesis.*

Consider this research question, "What is the relationship between the attitudes of occupational therapy faculty and the number of students with disabilities admitted into occupational therapy education programs?" In this study the investigator may hypothesize that there will be an association between faculty attitudes toward inclusion and the number of students with disabilities admitted into programs. However, the direction of this expectation is not stated. If the investigator formulates a directional hypothesis, it may appear as follows: "It is hypothesized that positive faculty attitudes will be associated with a greater number of admissions of students with disabilities."

Notice that this statement does not suggest or state an expected cause but rather states a positive direction in a proposed relationship.

Now consider the hypothesis for the following Level 3 question: "To what extent do faculty attitudes influence the number of students with disabilities who are accepted into occupational therapy programs?" The researcher is interested in predicting admission rates as a result of faculty attitudes. The researcher may structure a project in which programs and faculty with positive attitudes are compared with programs and faculty with unfavorable attitudes. If other variables are controlled and a design is developed in which causal relationships are ascertained, the following hypothesis may be stated:

There will be a significant difference in admission rates between programs with and programs without positive faculty attitudes toward inclusion of students with disabilities.

Based on a literature review and prior empirical findings, the researcher may choose to state the directional hypothesis as follows:

There will be significantly fewer students admitted to programs with unfavorable faculty attitudes than to programs with favorable faculty attitudes toward inclusion.

As discussed later in this text, a third and critical purpose of hypotheses is that these purposefully constructed statements "set the stage" for the type of statistical analyses that will be used.

Table 7-2 provides examples of hypotheses for each type of experimental-type research question.

TABLE 7-2

Examples of Hypotheses by Level of Question

Level	Question	Nondirectional Hypothesis	Directional Hypothesis
1	What is the pattern of use and reasons for nonuse of mobility aids among elders with ambulation difficulties?	No hypothesis is possible.	*Expected distribution:* Older adults with ambulation difficulties will use mobility aids with high frequency.
2	What is the relationship between the attitudes of faculty toward disability and the actual number of admissions of students with disabilities?	There will be an association between attitudes and the number of student admissions.	Positive faculty attitude will be associated with a greater number of admissions of students with disabilities.
2	What is the relationship between gender and depression in spousal caregivers of elders with physical disabilities?	The level of depression in female spouses will be different from the level of depression in male spouses.	Female spouse caregivers will be more depressed than male spouse caregivers.
3	To what extent do faculty attitudes influence the number of students with disabilities who are accepted in occupational therapy programs?	There will be a significant difference in admission rates between programs with and programs without positive faculty attitudes toward inclusion.	Significantly fewer students are admitted to programs with faculty who have unfavorable attitudes than to programs with faculty who have favorable attitudes toward inclusion.
3	What is the effect of psycho-educational counseling for family caregivers with depression?	The level of depression in family caregivers who attend psycho-educational sessions will differ from those who do not attend sessions.	Depression will be lower among caregivers who attend psycho-educational sessions than among those who do not attend.

RESEARCH QUERIES IN NATURALISTIC INQUIRY

Now we turn to a completely different approach to formulating research. In naturalistic inquiry, formal entry into a study requires the initial development of a broad query. Although various philosophical perspectives inform inquiry within naturalistic research, as previously discussed, and although the task of framing the problem and query are somewhat different among varied approaches, there is some underlying similarity to problem development.

Researchers in the naturalistic tradition generally begin by identifying a topic and a broad problem area or specifying a particular phenomenon from which a query is pursued. We thus use "query" to refer to a broad statement that identifies the phenomenon or natural field of interest.

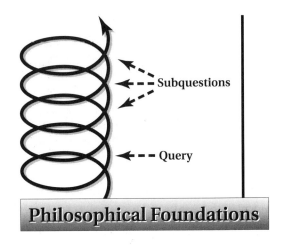

Philosophical Foundations

The natural field where the phenomenon occurs forms the basis for discovery from which more specific and limited questions evolve in the course of conducting the research. Thus the initial entry into the field is based on a query statement that identifies the phenomenon of interest and the location and popula-

The phenomenon of interest may refer to symbolic patterns of interaction in a cultural group, the experience of disability, or the meaning of pain.

tion or community that will be the focus. Then, once in the field and as new insights and meanings are obtained, the initial problem statement and query are reformulated. Based on new insights and issues that emerge in the field, the investigator formulates smaller, concise subquestions that are subsequently pursued in the field. These smaller questions are contextual; that is, they are derived inductively from the context itself and are rooted in the investigator's ongoing efforts to understand the broad problem area. In turn, each smaller question that is posed may lead the investigator to use a different methodological approach. This interactive questioning–data gathering–analyzing–reformulating of the questions and initial query represents a critical and core action process of naturalistic inquiry.

Let us examine the process by which a research query is developed and then reformulated in three different qualitative methodological approaches within the naturalistic tradition. As you read on, think about what is similar and what is different about the formulation and reformulation of queries.

Classic Ethnography

As the primary research approach in anthropology, ethnography is concerned with describing and interpreting cultural patterns of groups and understanding the cultural meanings people use to organize and interpret their experiences.[7] In this approach the researcher assumes a "learning role" to interpret and experience different cultural settings. The information gathered bridges the world and culture of the researcher to that of the researched.[8] Once the ethnographer has identified a phenomenon and cultural setting, a query is pursued. Agar explained the process in this way:

When you stand on the edge of a village and watch the noise and motion, you wonder, "Why are these people [here] and what are they doing?" When you read a news story about the discontent of young lawyers with their profession, you wonder, "What is going on here?"[7]

As you can see, experimental-type questions and hypotheses stand in stark contrast to the interpretative-opened query posed initially by the ethnographer.

As the processes of data gathering and analysis proceed in tandem, specific questions emerge and are pursued. These questions emerge in the field as a consequence of what Agar labels as *breakdowns,* or disjunctions. "A breakdown is a lack of fit between one's encounter with a tradition and the schema-guided expectation by which one organizes experience."[7] A breakdown represents the difference between what the investigator observes and expects to observe. These differences stimulate a series of questioning and further investigation. Each subquestion is related to the broader line of query and is investigated to resolve the breakdown and develop a more comprehensive understanding of the phenomenon in its entirety. An ethnographic query therefore establishes the phenomenon, the setting of interest, or both. The query also sets up the thinking and action processes necessary to understand the boundaries.

To summarize, once a query has been posed, questioning occurs simultaneously with collecting information and making sense of it. One process drives the other. The interactive questioning, data gathering, and analytical processes result in the reformulation and refinement of the problem and the structuring of small subquestions. These subquestions are then pursued in the field to uncover underlying meanings and cultural patterns.

Health and human service professionals have used ethnographic methods, such as interviewing and participant observation (discussed more fully in subsequent chapters), to examine cultural variations in response to disability, adaptation, health services utilization, health care practices, and other related areas.

> The health or human service professional conducting an ethnography may start with a general query such as, "How is pain expressed differently by men and women?" or "How are individuals with severe disabilities able to live independently, and what are their patterns of adaptation to community inclusion?"

Phenomenology

The purpose of the phenomenological line of inquiry is to uncover the meaning of human experience through the description of those experiences as they are lived by individuals.[8] The first research step from this perspective is to identify the phenomenon of investigation.

For example, pain, resilience, wellness, homelessness, and sadness may be phenomena that are relevant to the helping professions. From the articulation of the phenomenon, a research query is generated, such as the following:

What is the meaning of being homeless for middle-aged women?

What is the meaning of fear for persons with traumatic injury?

What are the common elements in experiencing a feeling of well-being among poor, rural, elder persons?

BOX 7-4
EXAMPLES OF GROUNDED-THEORY QUERIES THAT GENERATE THEORY

■ What theoretical principles characterize the experience of women who become homeless?
■ What similarities and differences can be revealed among ways in which traumatically injured individuals experience their acute care hospitalization?
■ How do Native Americans residing in a rural New England community define and maintain their health?

BOX 7-5
EXAMPLES OF GROUNDED-THEORY QUERIES THAT MODIFY THEORY

■ How can the current theory of moral development be expanded or modified to explain the moral development of Native American children and adolescents?
■ What is the relevance of current theory on career development in white middle-class male children and black middle-class female children?

This approach is different from ethnography in that phenomenological queries focus on experience from the perspective of the individual and do not seek to understand group or cultural patterns. However, similar to ethnography, the research begins with a broad query. Based on what the investigator knows through the action of conducting the research, subquestions and specific inquiries are developed that further inform the overarching query related to the meaning of experience for the individuals participating in the study.

Grounded Theory

Grounded theory is a method in naturalistic research that is used primarily to generate theory.[9] The researcher begins with a broad query in a particular topic area and then collects relevant information about the topic. As the action processes of data collection continue, each piece of information is reviewed, compared, and contrasted with other information. From this constant comparison process, commonalities and dissimilarities among categories of information become clear, and principles and ultimately a theory that explains observations are inductively developed. Thus, queries that will be answered through grounded theory do not relate to specific domains but to the structure of how the researcher wants to organize the findings (Box 7-4).

As you can see, each query indicates that the research aim is to reveal theoretical principles about the phenomenon under study. Grounded theory can also be used to modify existing theory or to expand on or uncover differences from what is already known. In the two queries in Box 7-5, grounded theory is structured to address current theory from a new and inductive perspective.

Developing Naturalistic Research Queries

Ethnography, phenomenology, and grounded theory reflect distinct approaches in naturalistic inquiry. Queries developed within each methodology and design reflect a different purpose and a preferred way of knowing and are shaped by the particular resources available to the investigator. Nevertheless, underlying each of these approaches is an essential iterative process of query-subquestion-reformulation that is central to the structuring of the research enterprise in naturalistic inquiry.

INTEGRATING RESEARCH APPROACHES

Another important category of research is referred to as *integrated designs*. Table 7-3 includes this category in summarizing experimental and naturalistic question/query formulation. Integrated designs

TABLE 7-3

Form and Function of Question/Query Formulation Across Research Traditions

	Experimental-Type	Naturalistic Inquiry	Integrated Design
Form	Focused question	Broad query	Both, or either
Function	Define variables, population, and level of inquiry	Identify phenomena of interest and context	Both, or either

combine different research traditions and approaches and, by their nature, may be complex. As such, these designs may rely on the formulation of a query, a question, or both and may order the formulation of these in diverse ways to accomplish the overall research purpose.

Consider the following examples to highlight the differences in approach among the experimental-type and naturalistic research traditions and an integrated design.

You want to study caregiving of older frail adults. Your purpose is to understand how caregiving affects the psychological stance of family members. You pose a specific question, such as, "What is the relationship between the cognitive status of impaired individuals and perceived mental health in caregivers of spouses with the diagnosis of dementia?" Can you guess what type of question this is? If you guessed Level 2 in the experimental-type tradition, you are correct. This question narrows the area of concern of relationships between cognitive status of the individual with dementia and a specific caregiver outcome—perceived mental health.

The investigator in this example has isolated constructs based on a particular theoretical framework (e.g., a stress process model), a deductive thinking process, and an orientation to knowing about phenomena, which favor experimental-type design. The constructs posed in the research question may have been identified from reading the research literature, from practice experience, or from federal funding initiatives that isolate self-efficacy and management as important constructs by which to understand caregiver experiences. The question lends itself to a design that involves interviewing a substantial number of caregivers to examine the stated relationships. The way the question is posed assumes that the investigator has the necessary fiscal resources and personnel to implement the research action processes that will answer the question.

In contrast, let us assume your purpose is to understand the everyday experience of caregiving and caregivers' appraisals of their actions using an epistemological framework based in naturalistic tradition.

In this case you will develop a research query that is initially posed as a broad statement. For example, "How do caregivers experience the act of caring for their spouses with dementia in the home?" This query identifies "caregiving spouses in the home" as the field of query and the "personal and lived experience of caring" as the particular phenomenon of interest. In such a study, relevant constructs will emerge based on uncovering and revealing the meaning of caregiving from the caregivers. Also, given the focus on spousal caregivers, the researcher will want to look at prior and current feelings toward marital relationships.

The initial formulation of the problem as "caregiver experience" assumes that the investigator in this example does not know the range of such experiences for spousal caregivers. The investigator proceeds inductively, based on the framework that there are multiple caregiver experiences and realities that need to be discovered and understood in order to derive a comprehensive view of spousal caregiving. It is from understanding different realities of spousal caregivers that meaningful concepts, constructs, and relationships will emerge in the course of the study. In this case the monetary and personnel resources available to the investigator will determine the scope of the field that is investigated and the time engaged in field observation and the interview process.

An integrated study may pose both a concise question and a query, and the studies may be conducted sequentially or simultaneously.

As shown, integrated designs can be complex. Therefore it is important for the investigator to clearly articulate the specific questions and queries that are posed jointly and to delineate how each contributes to the other.

The initial question, "What is the level of spouse caregiver upset with specific aspects of dementia?" may be complemented by a related query such as, "How do spousal caregivers experience disruptive behaviors such as wandering or repetitive vocalization?" The investigator would then set up a structured interview to obtain numerical ratings on different standardized scales that address the constructs of "upset," the frequency of types of behavior, and perhaps related scales such as burden. The interview may also integrate more open-ended questioning or other methodologies to evaluate the lived experience of a disruptive behavior. The value of such a combined approach is that it yields a more nuanced and multifaceted understanding of the phenomenon of interest.

SUMMARY

There are many ways to frame a research problem. Each approach to problem formulation and query or question development differs within the two traditions of research design. In experimental-type design the question drives each subsequent research step. Refinement of a research question occurs before any further action processes can be implemented. Conciseness and refinement are critical to the conduct of the study and are the hallmarks of what makes the research question meaningful and appropriate. Experimental-type questions are definitive, structured, and derived deductively before the researcher engages in specified actions.

In naturalistic inquiry the query establishes the initial boundaries for the study but is reformulated in the actual process of collecting and analyzing data. The researcher fully expects and prepares for new queries and subquestions to emerge in the course of conducting the study. That is, refinement of query and question emerges from the action of conducting the research. The development of specific questions occurs inductively and emerges from the interaction of the investigator within the field or with the phenomenon of the study. Thus an initial research question and query have different levels of meaning and implications for the conduct of studies in experimental-type design and naturalistic research. Research queries and subquestions are dynamic, ever changing, and derived inductively.

Integrated studies use the strengths of both experimental-type and naturalistic traditions to pose questions and queries that can reveal, describe, relate, or predict.

EXERCISES

1. To test your understanding of the differences between levels of questioning in experimental-type designs, select a problem area in which you are interested. Frame the problem in terms of Level 1, Level 2, and Level 3 questions.
2. Using the problem area you selected, formulate a broad query to pursue within a naturalistic design.
3. Review your different problem statements and specific queries or questions. Identify the different assumptions that each makes about level of knowledge, preferred way of knowing, and required resources to conduct the study. Use the table below to assist you.
4. Select three research articles in the literature and identify each research question or query. After you have identified them, characterize the nature of each using the table below.

Comparison of Studies According to Level of Knowledge, Preferred Way of Knowing, and Resources

Question/ Query	Assumed Level of Knowledge	Preferred Way of Knowing	Required Resources
1.			
2.			
3.			

REFERENCES

1. Brink PJ, Wood MJ: *Basic steps in planning nursing research: from question to proposal,* ed 3, Boston, 1998, Jones & Bartlett.
2. Gitlin LN, Levine R, Geiger C: Adaptive device use in the home by older adults with mixed disabilities, *Arch Phys Med Rehabil* 74:149-152, 1993.
3. Gitlow L: *Attitudes of occupational therapy faculty towards inclusion,* Minneapolis, Minn, 1997, Paper presented at the Society for Disability Studies.
4. McMurtry SL, McClelland RE: Trends in student-faculty rations and the use of non-tenured faculty in MSW programs, *J SW Educ* 33(3):293-306, 1997.
5. Chandler JM et al: The fear of falling syndrome, *Top Geriatr Rehabil* 11(3):55-63, 1996.

6. Neuman WL: *Social research methods: qualitative and quantitative approaches,* ed 3, Boston, 1997, Allyn Bacon.

7. Agar M: *Speaking of ethnography,* Newbury Park, Calif, 1986, Sage.

8. Farber M: *The aims of phenomenology: the motives, methods, and impact of Husserl's thought,* New York, 1966, Harper & Row.

9. Glaser B, Strauss A: *Grounded theory: strategies for qualitative research,* New York, 1967, Aldine.

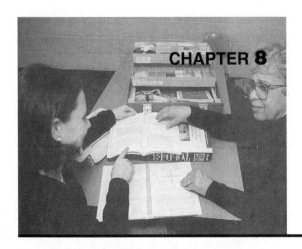

CHAPTER **8**

Language and Thinking Processes

KEY TERMS

Bias
Conceptual definition
Context specificity
Control
Dependent variable
Design
Emic
Etic
External validity
Independent variable
Instrumentation
Internal validity
Intervening variable
Manipulation
Operational definition
Rigor
Statistical conclusion validity
Variable

Flexibility
Language
Emic and Etic Perspectives
Gathering Information and Analysis
Naturalistic Design Summary
Integrated and Mixed-Method Approaches
Summary

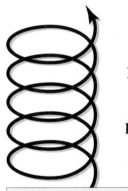

Language
and
thinking
processes

Philosophical Foundations

CHAPTER OUTLINE

W̲e now are ready to explore the language and thinking of researchers who use the range of designs relevant to health and human service inquiry. As discussed in previous chapters, significant philosophical differences exist between experimental-type and naturalistic research traditions. Experimental-type designs are characterized by thinking and action processes based in deductive logic and a positivist paradigm in which the researcher seeks to identify a single reality through systematized observation. This reality is understood by reducing it to its parts, observing and measuring the parts, and then examining the relationship among these parts. Ultimately the purpose of research in the experimental-type tradition is to predict what will occur in one part of the universe by knowing and observing another part.

Unlike experimental-type design, the naturalistic tradition is characterized by multiple ontological and epistemological foundations. However, naturalistic designs share common elements that are reflected in their languages and thinking processes. Researchers in the naturalistic tradition base their thinking in inductive and abductive logic and seek to understand phenomena within the context in which they are embedded. Thus the notion of multiple realities and the attempt to characterize holistically the complexity of human experience are two elements that pervade naturalistic approaches.

Mixed-method designs draw on and integrate the language and thinking of both traditions.

Now we turn to the philosophical foundations, language, and criteria for scientific rigor for experimental-type and naturalistic traditions. *Rigor* is a term used in research that refers to procedures that enhance and are used to judge the integrity of the research design. As you read this chapter, compare and contrast the two traditions and consider the application and integration of both.

EXPERIMENTAL-TYPE LANGUAGE AND THINKING PROCESSES

Within the experimental-type research tradition, there is consensus about the adequacy and scientific rigor of action processes. Thus, all designs in the experimental-type tradition share a common language and a unified perspective as to what constitutes an adequate *design*. Although there are many definitions of research design across the range of approaches, all types of experimental-type research share the same fundamental elements and a single, agreed-on meaning (Box 8-1).

BOX 8-1
CHARACTERISTICS OF EXPERIMENTAL-TYPE RESEARCH

- Based in one epistemology
- Historically accepted as the "scientific method" for discovering "fact"
- Evaluated and described by a unified and an agreed-on vocabulary that is well established

---

In experimental-type research, design is the plan or blueprint that specifies and structures the action processes of collecting, analyzing, and reporting data to answer a research question. As Kerlinger states in his classic definition, design is "the plan, structure, and strategy of investigation conceived so as to obtain answers to research questions and to control variance."[1] "Plan" refers to the blueprint for action or the specific procedures used to obtain empirical evidence. "Structure" represents a more complex concept and refers to a model of the relationships among the variables of a study. That is, the design is structured in such a way as to enable an examination of a hypothesized relationship among variables. This relationship is articulated in the research question. The main purpose of the design is to structure the study so that the researcher can answer the research question.

In the experimental-type tradition, the purpose of the design is to control variances or restrict or control extraneous influences on the study. By exerting such control, the researcher can state with a degree of statistical assuredness that study outcomes are a consequence of either the manipulation of the independent variable (e.g., true-experimental design) or the consequence of that which was observed and analyzed (e.g., nonexperimental design). In other words, the design provides a degree of certainty that an investigator's observations are not haphazard or random but reflect what is considered to be a true and objective reality. The researcher is thus concerned with developing the most optimal design that eliminates or controls what researchers refer to as disturbances, variances, extraneous factors, or situational contaminants. The design controls these disturbances or situational contaminants through the implementation of systematic procedures and data collection efforts, as discussed in subsequent chapters. The purpose of imposing control and restrictions on observations of natural phenomena is to ensure that the relationships specified in the research question(s) can be identified, understood, and ultimately predicted.

The element of design is what separates research from both the everyday types of observations and the thinking and action processes in which each of us engages. Design instructs the investigator to "do this" or "don't do that." It provides a mechanism of control to ensure that data are collected objectively, in a uniform manner, with minimal investigator involvement or bias. The important points to remember are that the investigator remains separate from and uninvolved with the phenomena under study (e.g., to control one important potential source of disturbance or situational contaminant) and that procedures and systematic data collection provide mechanisms to control and eliminate bias.

Sequence of Experimental-Type Research

Design is pivotal in the sequence of thoughts and actions of experimental-type researchers (Figure 8-1). It stems from the thinking processes of formulating a problem statement, a theory-specific research question that emerges from scholarly literature, and hypotheses or expected outcomes. Design dictates the nature of the action processes of data collection, the conditions under which observations will be made, and, most important, the type of data analyses and reporting that will be possible.

Do you recall our previous discussion on the essentials of research? In that discussion we illustrated how a problem statement indicates the purpose of the research and the broad topic the investigator wants to address. In experimental-type inquiry the literature review guides the selection of theoretical principles and concepts of the study and provides the rationale for a research project. This rationale is based on the nature of research previously conducted and the level of theory development for the phenomena under investigation. The experimental-type researcher must develop a literature review in which the specific theory, scope of the study, research questions, concepts to be measured, nature of the relationship among concepts, and measures that will be used in the study are discussed and supported. Thus the researcher develops a design that builds on both the ideas that have

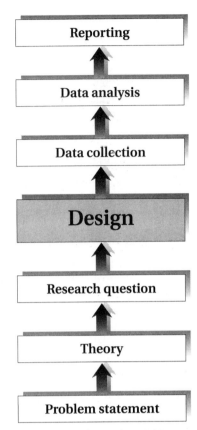

Figure 8-1   Sequence of experimental-type research.

been formulated and the actions that have been conducted in ways that conform to the rules of scientific rigor.

The choice of design not only is shaped by the literature and level of theory development, but also is dependent on the specific question asked. There is nothing inherently good or bad about a design. Every research study design has its particular strengths and weaknesses. The adequacy of a design is based on how well the design answers the research question that is posed.

Structure of Experimental-Type Research

Experimental-type research has a well-developed language that sets clear rules and expectations for the adequacy of design and research procedures. As you see in Table 8-1, nine key terms structure experimental-type research designs. Let us examine the meaning of each.

TABLE 8-1

Key Terms in Structuring Experimental-Type Research

Term	Definition
Concept	Symbolically represents observation and experience
Construct	Represents a model of relationships among two or more concepts
Conceptual definition	Concept expressed in words
Operational definition	How the concept will be measured
Variable	Operational definition of a concept assigned numerical values
Independent variable	Presumed cause of the dependent variable
Intervening variable	Phenomenon that has an effect on study variables
Dependent variable	Phenomenon that is affected by the independent variable or is the presumed effect or outcome
Hypothesis	Testable statement that indicates what the researcher expects to find

Concepts

A concept is defined as the words or ideas that symbolically represent observations and experiences. Concepts are not directly observable; rather, what they describe is observed or experienced. Concepts are "(1) tentative, (2) based on agreement, and (3) useful only to the degree that they capture or isolate something significant and definable."[2] For example, the terms "grooming" and "work" are both concepts that describe specific observable or experienced activities in which people engage on a regular basis. Other concepts, such as "personal hygiene" or "sadness," have various definitions, each of which can lead to the development of different assessment instruments to measure the same underlying concept.

Constructs

As discussed in Chapter 6, constructs are defined as "theoretical creations based on observations but which cannot be observed directly or indirectly."[3] A construct can only be inferred and may represent a larger category with two or more concepts or constructs.

The construct of "function" may be inferred from observing concepts such as grooming, personal hygiene, and work. However, the construct of function is not observable unless it is broken down into its component parts or concepts.

Definitions

The two basic types of definition relevant to research design are conceptual definitions and operational definitions. A *conceptual definition,* or lexical definition, stipulates the meaning of a concept or construct with other concepts or constructs. An *operational definition* stipulates the meaning through specifying how the concept is observed or experienced. Operational definitions "define things by what they do."

The construct of "self-care" may be conceptually defined as the activities that are necessary to care for one's bodily functions, whereas it is operationally defined as observations of an individual engaged in bathing, dressing, and grooming.

Variables

A *variable* is a concept or construct to which numerical values are assigned. By definition, a variable must have more than one value even if the investigator is interested in only one condition.

If an investigator is interested in evaluating the adequacy of self-care routines of persons with disabilities who are employed, both self-care routine and employment are variables. Self-care routine may have multiple values of relevance to the investigator, such as the level of dependence, safety and efficiency of performance, and difficulty. The investigator needs to determine which of the potential values that may be attributed to self-care would be of most interest in the inquiry. Likewise, employment status can have multiple values (e.g., employed vs. not employed, number of hours working outside the home), and the investigator needs to determine, based on the study's purpose, how best to operationalize this variable.

There are three basic types of variables: independent, intervening, and dependent. An *independent variable* "is the presumed cause of the dependent variable, the presumed effect."[4] Thus a *dependent variable* (also referred to as "outcome" and "criterion") refers to the phenomenon that the investigator seeks to understand, explain, or predict. The independent variable almost always precedes the dependent variable and may have a potential influence on it. The dependent variable is also referred to as the "predictor variable." An *intervening variable* (also called a "confounding" or an "extraneous" variable) is a phenomenon that has an effect on the study variables but that may or may not be the object of the study.

> In the study of adequacy of self-care routines of employed individuals with disabilities, employment status represents the independent variable, whereas level of difficulty performing self-care routine represents the dependent variable. Intervening variables in this study may include any other variable that potentially influences either the independent or the dependent variable, such as family support, type and degree of disability, motivational status, and functional ability.

Investigators treat intervening variables differently depending on the research question. For example, an investigator may only be interested in examining the relationship between the independent and dependent variables and may thus statistically control or account for an intervening variable. The investigator would then examine the relationship after statistically "removing" the effect of one or more potential intervening variables. On the other hand, the investigator may want to examine the effect of an intervening variable on the relationship between the independent and dependent variables. For this question the researcher would employ statistical techniques to determine the interrelationships.

Hypotheses

A hypothesis is defined as a testable statement that indicates what the researcher expects to find, based on theory and level of knowledge in the literature. A hypothesis is stated in such a way that it will either be verified or falsified by the research process. The researcher can develop either a directional or a nondirectional hypothesis (see Chapter 7). In a directional hypothesis, the researcher indicates whether she or he expects to find a positive relationship or an inverse relationship between two or more variables. A positive relationship is one in which both variables increase and decrease together to a greater or lesser degree.

> In a positive relationship the researcher may hypothesize that the employed individual with a disability has greater self-esteem than the unemployed individual with a disability. Thus the hypothesis tests the positive movement of both variables.

In an inverse relationship the variables are associated in opposite directions (i.e., as one increases, the other decreases). An inverse relationship may involve a hypothesis similar to the following:

> An individual with a disability who remains employed will demonstrate less difficulty in performing self-care routines than an individual who is unemployed.

In this statement, the expectation is that as the variable "employment" increases, difficulty in self-care will decrease.

Now that we have defined nine key terms that are essential to experimental-type designs, let us review the way they are actually used in research. Experimental-type research questions narrow the scope of the inquiry to specific concepts, constructs, or both. These concepts are then defined through the literature and are operationalized into variables that will be investigated descriptively, relationally, or predictively. The hypothesis establishes an equation or structure by which independent and dependent variables are examined and tested.

Plan of Design

The plan of an experimental-type design requires a set of thinking processes in which the researcher considers five core issues: bias, manipulation, control, validity, and reliability.

Bias

Bias is defined as the potential unintended or unavoidable effect on study outcomes. When bias is present and unaccounted for, the investigator may not

> **BOX 8-2**
> **POSSIBLE SOURCES OF BIAS IN A STUDY**
>
> ■ Selection of inappropriate instrumentation
> ■ Sample selection process that favors a particular unintended group
> ■ Improper training of interviewers
> ■ Deviation from the plan and from structure of the design

be able to fully understand whether the study findings are accurate or reflect sources of bias and thus may misinterpret the results. Many factors can cause bias in a study (Box 8-2). We already discussed one source of bias, the "intervening variable."

Another source is *instrumentation.* This involves the ways in which data are obtained in experimental-type approaches. The two major sources of bias from instrumentation are inappropriate data collection procedures and inadequate questions.

> Assume you are a counselor working in a community mental health center. Your supervisor, the agency administrator, is conducting a survey of worker satisfaction. To obtain information from employees, the supervisor decides to interview people. Knowing that this person is your superior, how likely are you to provide responses to job satisfaction questions, particularly knowing that your performance evaluation is next month?

In the situation portrayed above the procedures for data collection are problematic and introduce bias into the study.

> Using this same example, now consider how questions are asked to obtain the data. Suppose this question is asked: "Don't you agree that this is a great place to work?" Certainly this question is poorly phrased; it implies a socially and politically correct response and in essence urges the responder to agree. Now consider this question: "Don't you think that the physical environment and the climate are excellent here?" In this case the question is confusing and ambiguous. What does "the climate" refer to? Does it signify the weather? The emotional climate? The social climate? In this case the responder is prompted or guided to produce a socially desirable response. It is also not clear what is being asked.

Interview questions that elicit a socially correct response and questions that are vague, unclear, or ambiguous introduce a source of bias into the study design.

Sampling is another major source of bias.

> Suppose that only the supervisor's social friends were selected as the targeted sample to participate in the survey and are viewed as representing the agency population. Such a sample would not represent the overall level of job satisfaction for all employees. In this example the characteristics of the sample serve as potential bias or influence the outcomes of the study.

Improper or uneven training of data collectors and interviewer "drift," in which an interviewer strays from the interview protocol from fatigue or over-familiarity, can all bias the study outcomes as well.

> In the same study of employee satisfaction, if multiple persons collected information about job satisfaction, but each asked the survey questions differently or in a nonuniform manner, interviewer procedures will serve as a strong bias.

Experimental-type designs are characterized by having detailed and elaborate plans and procedures that are established before conducting the study. Thus, any deviation from the original plan for data collection and analysis may be a potential source of bias. The violation of standard procedures is an important point at which bias may be introduced into an experimental-type study.

> Suppose that the agency director decided to collect data regarding the level of job satisfaction of agency employees on Monday. Monday was selected because all employees were normally available. However, the data collection was accomplished on Tuesday because Monday was a holiday. On Tuesday, all home-based service providers were in the field and therefore were not surveyed for their degree of job satisfaction. This deviation in the plan could have significantly affected the study outcome, since a large segment of the agency employee population would have been omitted from the study.

An essential part of planning a design is to introduce systematic procedures to minimize or eliminate as many sources of bias as possible. As you read subsequent chapters, think about the potential sources of bias. Also, as you conduct your own studies or read and analyze published studies, consider findings and conclusions in light of potential bias.

Manipulation

Manipulation is defined as the action process of maneuvering the independent variable so that the effect of its presence, absence, or degree on the dependent variable can be observed. To the extent possible, experimental-type researchers attempt to isolate the independent and dependent variables and then manipulate or change the condition of the independent variable so that the cause-and-effect relationship between the variables can be examined.

Research studies that examine the effects of different types of interventions on the well-being of caregivers of persons with Alzheimer's disease illustrate the concept of manipulation. To determine which types of interventions (e.g., skills training, social support, group counseling, education) promote positive outcomes, the most effective research plan would be to use a randomized, two-group design. In this type of design, caregivers would be evaluated with regard to well-being at baseline or before introducing an intervention. Study participants would then be randomly assigned (assigned on a chance-determined basis; see Chapter 11) to different intervention conditions and tested again after completing the interventions. Then caregivers are asked to switch groups and participate in the intervention group that they had not experienced. They would then be tested again to evaluate change in the dependent variable, "well-being." The interventions represent the independent variables being manipulated (received, not received). By manipulating the intervention timing and sequence, an investigator is able to examine the effect of each intervention and combinations on caregiver well-being.[5]

Control

Control is defined as the set of action processes that direct or manipulate factors to achieve an outcome. Control plays a critical role in experimental-type design. By controlling not only the independent variable but also other aspects of the research context, such as how study participants are assigned to groups, the relationship among the study variables can be observed. In experimental-type design, procedures to establish control are implemented to minimize the influences of extraneous variables on the outcome or dependent variable.

Two basic methods of control are typically introduced: random group assignment and control group. By randomly assigning subjects to one group or the other, the investigator attempts to develop equivalence, or eliminate subject bias, caused by inherent differences that may occur in the two groups.

In evaluating the outcome of interventions on caregivers' well-being, assume you do not use random assignment. Instead, you assign the first 10 volunteers to the first group, who receive the intervention involving group counseling, and the next 10 volunteers to the second group, who do not receive counseling. It is possible that the first 10 subjects know each other and agreed to participate in the study first because they were highly motivated to seek help and each person encouraged the other to join. In contrast, suppose the last 10 subjects were somewhat less motivated to participate. Familiarity with other subjects and a high motivation to seek help (two factors inherent in the subjects assigned to the first group) may influence caregiver responses to the outcome measure of "well-being." By not using random assignment, the investigator may risk developing groups that initially differ from each other. In turn, this initial difference may make it difficult to discern what effect, if any, the independent variable has on the outcome variable.

Another method to enhance control is the use of a control group. A control group is one in which the experimental or comparative condition is absent.

In caregiver intervention research, the experimental treatment is typically compared to a group who does not receive any intervention, sometimes referred to as a "usual care" group, or a group who receives only what they usually would, independent of the study. Occasionally, the experimental treatment group is compared to an "attention" control group, or a group who receives some form of attention to control for its occurrence in the treatment group. By comparing caregiver scores in an attention control group to those in an intervention group, the investigator is able to determine whether changes in the dependent variable resulted from (1) the passage of time, (2) the attention factor inherent in a behavioral intervention (or intervention involving interaction with a health or human service professional), or (3) the particular content of each group.

Validity

Validity is a concept that has numerous applications in experimental-type research. However, the concept as it applies to design refers to the extent to which your study answers the research questions and your findings are accurate or reflect the underlying purpose of the study. Although many classifications of validity have been developed, we discuss four fundamental types of validity, based on Campbell and Stanley's classic work.[6] These are internal validity, external validity, statistical conclusion validity, and construct validity.

Internal Validity. The ability of the research design to answer the research question accurately is known as *internal validity.* If a design has internal validity, the investigator can state with a degree of confidence that the reported outcomes are the consequence of the relationship between the independent variable and dependent variable and not the result of extraneous factors. Campbell and Stanley[6] identify seven major factors that pose a threat to the researcher's ability to determine whether the observable outcome is a function of the study or the result of external and unintended forces (Box 8-3).

To illustrate these threats to validity, consider a hypothetical example.

Suppose you are conducting a study to determine the extent to which an acquired immunodeficiency syndrome (AIDS) prevention program has reduced behavior that increases the risk of developing AIDS in an adolescent population. This study is designed to answer the following research question: "To what extent is adolescent risk behavior reduced by the experimental preventive intervention?" Before the intervention, you evaluate the extent to which subjects exhibit risk behavior. You conduct a prevention program and retest the participants. The retest shows an amazing reduction in risk behavior, and you claim that your program is a success. In doing so, you are making a claim that a relationship exists

---

> **BOX 8-3**
> **SEVEN THREATS TO INTERNAL VALIDITY**
>
> 1. *History.* Effect of external events on study outcomes
> 2. *Testing.* Effect of being observed or tested on the study outcome
> 3. *Instrumentation.* Extent to which the instrument is accurate in its measurement and extent to which the instrument itself may be responsible for outcomes
> 4. *Maturation.* Effect of the passage of time
> 5. *Regression.* Effect of a statistical phenomenon in which extreme scores tend to regress or cluster around the mean (average) on repeated testing occasions
> 6. *Mortality.* Effect on outcome caused by subject attrition or dropping out of a study before its completion
> 7. *Interactive effects.* Extent to which each of these threats interacts with sample selection to influence the outcome of a study

From Campbell DT, Stanley JC: *Experimental and quasi-experimental design,* Chicago, 1963, Rand McNally.

between your program (the independent variable) and risk behavior (the dependent variable). Furthermore, you are claiming that there is a causal relationship between the variables; that is, you claim that your program causes the reduction in behavior that increases the risk of developing AIDS.

Consider how each of the seven threats to internal validity affects your research outcomes.

First, let us assume you have just learned that a celebrity has held a news conference in which he announced that he has tested positive for the human immunodeficiency virus (HIV). This announcement has come immediately after you first administered your test to your subjects but before the final testing occasion. It is possible that this historical event, rather than the independent variable, was the factor responsible for reducing risk behavior in your subjects.

However, assume that your subjects already knew about the celebrity before beginning the study. Now consider the threat of testing to the validity of your claims. As a sensitive researcher, you have decided to measure risk behavior by observing a discussion group about sexual behaviors among adolescents. Each time you hear a risk behavior, you score it as such without informing your subjects. In the first testing situation, the adolescents appear to discuss their sexual decision making openly. However, you note that they are aware of group norms and of being observed, and that they stay well within the boundaries tacitly set by the group when discussing their personal behavior and views. In the second test, you note a significant reduction in reported risk behaviors or in risky decision making.

Although the prevention program may be responsible for the reduction in risk behavior, there are alternative explanations. In the first testing situation the adolescents may have revealed what was normative and acceptable in the group rather than accurately representing their risk potential. In the second test the adolescents who underwent the intervention may have restricted their conversation to what they learned was desirable rather than revealing their own behavior.

Another alternative for the observed reduction in risk behavior may be the result of the testing situation itself. Participants who are aware of what is being observed and recorded may answer more cautiously. In other words, the testing procedures may pose yet another threat to the internal validity of the design. The reduction in reported risk behaviors may be a function of participants actively changing or adjusting their behaviors or thoughts on the topic as a consequence of participating in a group discussion with peers. The test itself or mode of data collection may have influenced a change in behavior independent of the effect of participating in the intervention. Therefore, it is difficult to determine whether observed change is a consequence of the test, a consequence of the intervention, or both.

This example also illustrates the threat to validity posed by instrumentation. In this example the instrumentation may not be measuring what was intended. Instead of measuring risk behavior, the instrumentation may be a more accurate indicator of group norms related to sexual decision making.

Another way in which instrumentation poses a threat to a study is through changes that may occur within interviewers over time or with the instrument itself. For example, if you are collecting data regarding weight or blood pressure, any deviation in the calibration of a scale or blood pressure cuff from one testing occasion to the next will pose a significant threat to the validity of the data that are obtained.

Further, interviewer fatigue or any change in the way interviewers pose questions may cause a deviation in responses that will affect how the investigator interprets the findings.

To illustrate the threat posed by maturation, assume that the AIDS prevention program is being conducted over a 1-year period. It is possible that the participants have matured in their thinking and have become more responsible in their decision making as a function of time rather than as a result of the prevention program.

The threat of regression frequently occurs when subjects with extreme scores are selected to participate in a study.

Assume that adolescents who are sexually active participate in the study and therefore tend to report extremely risky behaviors. Those who are high scorers at the beginning of the program tend to report lower scores at the end.

This change in scores, however, may be a consequence of a statistical principle known as "statistical regression toward the mean," in which extreme scores tend to move toward the mean on repeated testing.

Fifty participants began the AIDS prevention program, but only 10 remained by the final testing period. It is possible that as a result of "experimental mortality" (attrition of participants before a study's conclusion), those who remained in the study may be more committed to reducing risk behavior than those who dropped out.

Thus, experimental mortality poses a threat to the interpretation of study findings. Numerous interactive effects could also confound the accuracy of the findings.

Consider that the selected sample for the study was a population of adolescents on probation. This group was highly motivated to report a change in their risk behavior (a sampling bias) and was also sensitive to being tested because of their judiciary status. The interactive effect of the sample bias and the testing condition may wreak havoc on claims that the outcome was a result of the prevention program.

External Validity. *External validity* refers to the capacity to generalize findings and develop inferences from the sample to the study population stipulated in the research question. External validity answers the question of "generalizability."

> Remember our research question: "To what extent is adolescent risk behavior reduced by the experimental preventive intervention?" In this question the population is all adolescents. Now, assume that the investigator obtained a sample by asking for volunteers from a large group of adolescents between ages 12 and 18 years who were on probation in Philadelphia. The potential to generalize the findings from the sample to all adolescents on probation is limited by several important factors. First, the sample was a volunteer sample, making them potentially different from adolescents who did not volunteer. Second, the experiences of adolescents who live in large cities may not necessarily represent the experiences of adolescents in other geographical locations. Third, because the sample was voluntary, the researcher cannot know in what ways the sample may differ from the study population, which includes those who refused participation or did not have the opportunity to volunteer. Fourth, in selecting a volunteer urban sample on probation, the investigator limits generalizability to that select sample and will not be able to infer the experiences of the research sample to all adolescents, such as those who are not on probation, who live in rural communities, or who may be sexually active and at risk.

These factors represent some of the threats to external validity that may occur in a study. Although randomization decreases some of the threats to external validity, even when a sample is randomly selected, threats remain.[7] The two threats in Box 8-4 result

BOX 8-4
POTENTIAL THREATS TO EXTERNAL VALIDITY

1. *Reactivity.* Extent to which the subjects are responding to the condition of being part of a study and thus do not represent the population from whom they are selected
2. *Realism.* Extent to which the experimental conditions simulate actual life situations to which the population is exposed

from the experimental condition, not from the limitations of sample selection. Consider your own behavior when being watched in a simulated situation. Certainly you act differently than you would under similar but unobserved and nonsimulated conditions.

The internal validity and external validity of a study are interrelated. As an investigator attempts to increase the internal validity of a study, the ability to make broad generalizations and inferences to a larger population decreases. That is, as more controls are implemented and extraneous factors are eliminated from a study design, the population to whom findings can be generalized becomes more limited. Thus, although investigators try to enhance the internal validity of a study to ensure that valid and accurate conclusions can be drawn, these efforts may limit the degree of external validity of the findings. It is a balancing act, but the investigator must err on the side of ensuring that the study has internal validity first, then external validity. If a study lacks internal validity, there would be no purpose in generalizing to a larger population. As you read further in this text, look for ways to balance internal validity and the scope of generalization that may be possible.

Statistical Conclusion Validity. *Statistical conclusion validity* refers to the power of your study to draw statistical conclusions. One aim of experimental-type research is to find relationships among variables and ultimately to predict the nature and direction of these relationships. Support for relationships is contained in the action process of statistical analysis. However, selection of statistical techniques is based on many considerations. Even though the expectation of making errors in determining relationships is built into the theory and practice of statistical analysis, the accuracy and potential of the statistics to support or predict a relationship among variables must be considered as a potential threat to the validity of a design.

> Assume you want to ensure that you do not overestimate the effects of your AIDS prevention program on risk behavior. You select a statistic that will be less likely to find a false relationship when there is none. However, this decision increases the possibility that you may not find a significant relationship when, in fact, one exists. Thus, your statistical testing may lead you to believe that no relationship exists

when there is one or, conversely, to believe that there is a relationship when there is none.

Construct Validity. Construct validity addresses the fit between the constructs that are the focus of the study and the way in which these constructs are operationalized. As stated earlier, constructs are abstract representations of what humans observe and experience. The method used to define and measure constructs accurately is in large part a matter of opinion and consensus. It is possible for several factors related to construct validity to confound a study. First, a researcher may define a construct inappropriately.

Although smiling may be one indication of happiness, if a researcher measured level of happiness exclusively by observing the frequency of smiling behavior, the full construct of "happiness" would not be captured.

Poor or incomplete operational definitions can result from incomplete conceptual definitions or from inadequate translation of the construct into an observable one.

Second, when a cause-and-effect relationship between two constructs is determined, it may be difficult to define each construct exclusively (referring to both independent and dependent variables) and to isolate the effects of one on the other.

You are an occupational therapist who is attempting to test a feeding program for persons with Alzheimer's disease. You design a program in which you choose certain foods and techniques to improve independent feeding. To ensure that your design can reveal cause and effect, you randomly select your sample and randomly assign them to the experimental group (who receives the program) and the control group (who does not receive the program). You measure feeding behavior by two methods: observation of independent feeding and volume of food consumed independently. You implement your feeding program with the experimental group and test all participants after the program to determine whether the experimental group scored higher on your measures of feeding than the group who did not receive the intervention. You conclude that your program was successful in improving independent

feeding, because the experimental group performed significantly better than the group without the intervention.

However, you begin to consider other confounding influences that cannot be separated from your two constructs—independent feeding and the experimental program. The attention of the experimenter may have influenced the improvement in the experimental group, because eating is a social behavior and may change under different social conditions. Also, food preferences may have influenced the response of the groups to their respective conditions. Interactive effects of being observed and participating in an experiment (referred to as the "attention factor" or "Hawthorne effect"[8]) may also limit your capacity to isolate a causal relationship between the constructs.

Reliability

Reliability refers to the stability of a research design. In experimental-type design, rigorous research is shown to be well planned and properly executed when, if repeated under the same circumstances, the design would yield the same results. Investigators frequently replicate or repeat a study in the same population or in different groups to determine the extent to which the findings of one study are accurate in a broader scope. To replicate a study, the procedures, measures, and data analysis techniques must be consistent, well articulated, and appropriate to the research question. Reliability is threatened when a researcher is not consistent and changes a design in midstream, does not articulate procedures in sufficient detail for replication, or does not fully plan a sound design.

Experimental-Type Design Summary

Design is a pivotal concept in the experimental-type research process that indicates both the structure and the plan of the action processes. Experimental-type designs are developed to eliminate bias and the intrusion of unwanted factors that could confound findings and make them less credible. Five primary considerations in the plan of a design are bias, control, manipulation, validity, and reliability. Four types of validity threaten study outcomes: internal, external, statistical conclusion, and construct.

Experimental-type research is designed to minimize the threats posed by extraneous factors and bias through maximizing control over the research action process. In Chapter 9 we discuss how each type of design in the experimental-type tradition addresses these considerations in structuring and planning a design and using action processes to increase control.

NATURALISTIC LANGUAGE AND THINKING PROCESSES

Let us now turn our attention to the attributes of naturalistic inquiry and the implications for design with these traditions. There are eight elements that are common to designs in the naturalistic tradition and that are listed in Box 8-5.

Purpose

Designs within the tradition of naturalistic research vary in purpose from developing descriptive knowledge to evolving full-fledged theories about observed or experienced phenomena. As discussed in earlier chapters, naturalistic designs tend to be preferred when no adequate theory exists to explain a human phenomenon or when the investigator believes that existing theory and explanations are not accurate, true, or complete. The structure of naturalistic designs is exploratory, enabling new insights and understandings to be revealed without the imposition of preconceived concepts, constructs, and principles.

Although the specific purpose of a study may differ, all naturalistic designs seek to describe, understand, or interpret daily life experiences and structures within the contexts in which they occur. Naturalistic inquiry has emerged through five phases of development to its current form of action-oriented social criticism, in which grand narratives are replaced by more local, small-scale theories fitted to specific problems and specific situations.[9] Thus the importance of naturalistic inquiry is now widely recognized because of its usefulness in examining and revealing phenomena that can help guide health and human service practitioners to address specific problems that emerge in the clinical context.

In *Tally's Corner,*[10] Liebow is interested in understanding the nature of a street-corner culture to which he does not belong. Although there has been extensive research on the population he has chosen to examine, these investigations have not characterized the group from the perspective of its members. Naturalistic method, in this case, ethnography, is a viable way to reveal the complexity and richness of the culture. Liebow gains valuable insights because his informants speak for themselves and describe their life experiences.

Context Specificity

As in *Tally's Corner,* to discover "new truth" rather than impose an existing frame of reference, the investigator proceeding from a naturalistic tradition must travel to the setting where the human phenomena occur or must seek information from the perspective of individuals who experience the phenomena of interest. Because of the revelatory nature of naturalistic research, this form of investigatory action is conducted in a natural context or seeks explanations of the natural context from those who experience it. Naturalistic research is therefore context specific, and the "knowing" derived from this context is embedded in the context and does not extend beyond it. The designs in the tradition of naturalistic inquiry share this basic attribute of *context specificity* and development of knowledge that is grounded in or linked to the data that emerge from a particular field.

Complexity and Pluralistic Perspective of Reality

As a result of its underlying epistemology and its inductive and abductive approaches to knowing, naturalistic research assumes a pluralistic perspective of reality that characterizes complexity.

With inductive reasoning, principles emerge from seemingly unrelated information. One of its hallmarks is that the information can be organized differently by each individual who thinks about it. The end result

---

BOX 8-5
EIGHT ELEMENTS OF NATURALISTIC DESIGN

1. Purpose of research
2. Context of research
3. Pluralistic perspective of reality
4. Concern with transferability
5. Flexibility
6. Concern with language
7. Emic and etic perspectives
8. Interactive and analytical process

of induction is the development of a complex set of relationships among smaller pieces of information (not the reduction of principles to their parts, as in deductive reasoning). It is therefore possible that the same information may have different meanings or that there may be pluralistic interpretations by different individuals. Adding abduction to this equation ensures that the information will be revisited and reanalyzed at several points, thereby sharpening and rendering the accuracy of the interpretation more credible and trustworthy.

In the classic study by Maruyama[11] on prison violence, the nature of violence was investigated in two separate institutional settings. The findings from each prison, although yielding some similarities, indicated cultural differences between the two prisons in the reported causes of violence and the inmates' interpretation of the meaning of that violence. The naturalistic design was able to reveal the pluralistic nature of prison violence while shedding light on the basic elements common to both settings.

Transferability of Findings

The findings from naturalistic design are specific to the research context. It is not the desired outcome of naturalistic design to generalize findings from a small sample and apply this generalization to a larger group of persons with similar characteristics. You may ask, "Why bother doing a naturalistic study if you cannot use the research beyond the actual scope of the study?" The answer lies in one of the primary purposes of naturalistic research, generating theory. Naturalistic researchers use their methods and findings to generate theory and to reveal the unique meanings of human experience in human environments. Because the investigator assumes that current knowledge does not adequately explain the phenomenon under investigation, the outcome of naturalistic design is the emergence of explanations, principles, concepts, and theories. Liebow illustrates this point well when he states:

> There is no attempt here to describe any Negro men other than those with whom I was in direct immediate association. To what extent this descriptive and interpretive material is applicable to Negro street corner men elsewhere in the city or in other

cities or to lower class men generally in this society or any other society is a matter of further and later study. This is not to suggest that we are dealing with unique or even distinctive persons and relationships. Indeed, the weight of the evidence is the other direction.[10]

In this passage, even though the researcher is highlighting the contextual limitations of the knowledge, he is also indicating that the principles revealed in his study may have relevance to other arenas. Further, he suggests that additional research is the appropriate means to ascertain the degree of fit, or what Guba[12] calls the "transferability of findings," to other similar populations and contexts.

Because phenomena are context bound and, according to naturalistic principles, cannot be understood apart from the context in which they occur, naturalistic inquiry is not concerned with the issue of generalizability or external validity as articulated in experimental-type inquiry. Rather, naturalistic inquiry is concerned with understanding the richness and depth in one context and with the capacity to retain unique meanings that are lost when generalization is a goal.[9] The development of "thick"[13] and in-depth descriptions and interpretations of different contexts leads to the ability to transfer meanings in one context to another context. In so doing, the researcher is able to compare and contrast contexts and their elements to gain new insights as to the specific context itself.

Flexibility

The experimental-type research design provides the basic structure and plan for the thinking and action processes of the research endeavor. The design must be followed as initially developed. In naturalistic research, however, the opposite is the case; design is a fluid, flexible concept. Design labels such as "ethnography," "life history," and "grounded theory" suggest a particular purpose of the inquiry and orientation of the investigator. However, these labels do not refer to the specification of step-by-step procedures, a blueprint for action, or a predetermined structure to the data gathering and analytical efforts.

Rather, a characteristic of naturalistic design is flexibility.[14] An important and expected feature of a naturalistic study is that the procedures and plans for conducting it will change as the research proceeds.

The investigator may use the results of preliminary findings as guidance for planning or altering subsequent action processes. Not only do procedures change, but also the nature of the research query, the scope of the study, and the manner by which information is obtained are constantly reformulated and realigned to fit the emerging truths as they are discovered and obtained in the inquiry. This flexibility is illustrated more fully in Chapters 17 and 20.

Language

A major shared concern in naturalistic inquiry is understanding language and meanings. This concern with language is not only relevant to the ethnographer, who studies a cultural context in which the language used is different from that of the investigator. Even within the same cultural or language context, people use and understand language differently. For some naturalistic investigators, language, symbols, and ways of expression provide the data through which the investigator comes to understand and derive meaning within each context.[15] Investigators proceeding from a postmodern philosophical foundation are particularly concerned with language itself. In contrast to previous philosophies that attribute meaning to symbols, postmodern thinkers suggest that language as a set of symbols does not necessarily have any of the underlying reality that the symbols describe.[16]

Depending on the philosophical approach, the investigator concerned with language may engage in a rigorous and active analytical process to "translate" the meaning and structure of the context of the studied population into meanings and language structures represented in the investigator's world. In this type of inquiry the investigator must be careful to represent the meanings and intent of expression accurately in this translation of the analytical and reporting process. As mentioned, however, not all investigators concerned with language believe that naturalistic inquiry can reveal meaning. Postmodern inquiry aims to "deconstruct" language, or unravel language to illustrate its arbitrary structure and identify its political and purposive usage. For example, a postmodern investigator might examine the text of legislation designed to protect women against domestic violence to uncover the metaphors that help retain men's dominance and political power over women.

Throughout the full range of philosophical approaches that underpin the naturalistic tradition, the description and analysis of language is a primary concern.

Emic and Etic Perspectives

Design structures vary as to their emic or etic orientation. An *emic* perspective refers to the insider's or informant's way of understanding and interpreting experience. This perspective is phenomenological in that experience is understood as only that which is perceived and expressed by informants. Data gathering and analytical actions are designed to enable the investigator to bring forth and report the voices of individuals as they speak and interpret their unique perceptions of their reality. The concern with the emic perspective is often the motivator for naturalistic inquiry. For example, in her classic work,[17] Krefting explained why she decided to study head injury from an ethnographic perspective, highlighting the preference for an emic viewpoint shared by designs in this tradition, as follows:

> Until recently, the investigation of health problems was dominated by the outsider perspective, in which important questions of etiology and treatment are identified by the professions. Studies based on this perspective assume that professionals are the authorities on what wellness is and that they alone know what questions ought be asked to investigate methods to promote and maintain wellness while preventing and treating illness.. . .Ethnographic studies of the experience of illness and disability. . .consider what these experiences look like from an insider's perspective.17

An *etic* orientation reflects the structural aspects or those that are external to a group; that is, the etic perspective is held by those who do not belong to the group being investigated but who select an analytical and epistemic lens through which to examine information. Unlike the emic perspective, in which those who experience are considered to be most knowledgeable, the etic perspective assumes that those who do not experience a phenomenon can come to know it through (1) structuring an investigation, (2) selecting a theoretical foundation that expands beyond the group being examined, and (3) through that lens, conducting the interpretation of data.[18] Many investigators integrate an emic with an etic perspective. Typically, investigators will start by using an emic perspective, or a focus on the voices of individuals. Further along the process, other pieces of information are collected and analyzed to place individual articulation and expression within a social structural or systemic framework. Although she started with an emic consideration, Krefting used a range of data collection strategies to integrate her understandings with an etic viewpoint, as follows:

> While gathering data, I was able to review theory and check it for pertinence. There was, then, a constant movement back and forth between the concrete data and the social science concepts that helped explain them.[17]

Some designs, such as phenomenology and life history, favor only an emic orientation. Frank describes her preference for an emic perspective and the purpose of her life history approach as follows:

> The life history of Diane DeVries represents a collaborative effort, between the subject and researcher, to produce a holistic, qualitative account that would bear on theoretical issues, but that primarily and essentially would convey a sense of the personal experience of severe congenital disability. The life history, conceived in this way, emerged from a humanistic interest in presenting the voices of people often unheard, yet whose lives were otherwise studied, and acted upon, based on data that are decontextualized and fragmented from the standpoint of the individual.[19]

Because the investigator enters the inquiry having bracketed, suspended, or let go of any preconceived concepts, the naturalistic researcher defers to the informant or experiencer as the "knower." This abrogation of power by the investigator to the investigated is characteristic of naturalistic designs, to a greater or lesser degree.

An extreme example of relinquishing control over the research process is illustrated by Maruyama's classic work.[11] In the prison study, not only did the inmates function as the informants, but they also planned and conducted the research in its entirety.

Where the investigator stands regarding an emic or etic perspective shapes the overall design that is chosen, as well as the specific data collection and analytical action processes that emerge within the context of the inquiry.

Gathering Information and Analysis

Analysis in naturalistic designs relies heavily on qualitative data and is an ongoing process throughout data-gathering activities. Thus, in the naturalistic tradition, data gathering and analysis are interdependent processes. As one collects information or data, the investigator engages in an active analytical process. In turn, the ongoing analytical activity frames the scope and direction of further data collection efforts. This interactive, iterative, and dynamic process is characteristic of designs within the tradition of naturalistic inquiry and is explored more fully later in this text.

Naturalistic Design Summary

The purpose of naturalistic inquiry and the nature of the concept of design in this tradition are vastly different from experimental-type research. The language and thinking processes that characterize naturalistic design are based on the notion that knowing is pluralistic and that knowledge derives from understanding multiple experiences. Thus the thinking process is inductive and abductive; the action processes are dynamic and changing; and these processes are carried out within the actual or theoretical context where the phenomena of interest occur or are experienced. The outcome of these thinking and action processes is the generation of theory, principles, or concepts that explain human experience in human environments and capture its complexity and uniqueness.

Within any naturalistic design, the investigator can implement the 10 essentials in various ways. Designs vary from informant-driven and no structure to researcher-driven and more structure.

The nature of qualitative inquiry has evolved in its forms, scope, and purposes.[9] Naturalistic inquiry is continuing to evolve in its standards, vocabulary, and criteria for design adequacy, and it is becoming a well-respected tradition in its own right as it is increasingly used to answer questions about health and human service practice.

INTEGRATED AND MIXED-METHOD APPROACHES

As discussed in previous chapters of this book, studies which integrate experimental-type and naturalistic traditions have increased despite skepticism about philosophical inconsistencies. The mixed-method approach for advancing knowledge has recently been referred to as the "third tradition"[20] with a foundation in pragmatism.

Mixing methods is a systematic way to address the limitations of each approach, and we therefore support its use whenever possible. As discussed, however, both experimental-type and naturalistic traditions conform to diverse sets of rules, languages, and strategies for rigor. As such, the investigator who proceeds with an integrated approach must heed the important tenets of both traditions as well as the emerging tenets of a third tradition. Because of its nascence and limited epistemological underpinning, we do not yet view a mixed-method approach as a solid tradition in itself. Rather, at this point in its development, we view it as an attempt to integrate experimental-type and naturalistic approaches within a defined and purposive context and incorporating language and thinking processes from each of the two traditions.

SUMMARY

Experimental-type and naturalistic traditions have distinct language and thinking processes. Experimental-type researchers approach their studies with intact theory and a set of procedures. Procedures are developed and followed to eliminate the potential for factors other than those studied to be responsible for the findings. Dissimilarly, naturalistic language and thinking processes are flexible, fluid, and changing. As the investigator proceeds throughout the research design, the aim of capturing complexity from the perspective of the individuals or phenomena studied is actualized through systematic but dynamic interaction between collecting and analyzing information.

REFERENCES

1. Kerlinger FN: *Foundations of behavioral research,* ed 2, New York, 1973, Holt, Rinehart, & Winston.

EXERCISES

1. Select a research article from a journal that uses an experimental-type design. Identify the independent variable or variables, the dependent variable or variables, and any intervening variables that may be confounding the study.
2. Identify the conceptual definitions and the operational definitions in the article that you selected.
3. Using the same article, determine (a) threats to validity of the study, (b) how the investigator minimized bias and enhanced control and validity, and (c) ethical issues that shaped the design.
4. Select a research article that uses naturalistic inquiry. Identify and provide evidence of the eight elements of the researcher's thinking process:
   a. Purpose of research
   b. Context of research
   c. Pluralistic perspective of reality
   d. Concern with transferability
   e. Flexibility
   f. Concern with language
   g. Emic and etic perspectives
   h. Interactive and analytical process
5. Using the same article, determine some of the ethical issues that shaped the investigator's behavior in the inquiry.

---

2. Wilson J: *Thinking with concepts,* Cambridge, Mass, 1966, Cambridge University Press.
3. Babbie E: *The basic of social research,* ed 6, Belmont, Calif, 2005, Wadsworth.
5. Gitlin LN, Winter L, Corcoran M et al: Effects of the home environmental skill-building program on the caregiver-care recipient dyad: six-month outcomes from the Philadelphia REACH Initiative, *The Gerontologist* 43(4), 532-546, 2003.
6. Campbell DT, Stanley JC: *Experimental and quasi-experimental design,* Chicago, 1963, Rand McNally.
7. Neuman WL: *Social research methods: qualitative and quantitative approaches,* ed 3, Boston, 1997, Allyn Bacon.
8. Babbie E: *The basics of social research,* ed 6, Belmont, Calif, 2005, Wadsworth.
9. Denzin NK, Lincoln YS: *Handbook of qualitative research,* ed 2, Thousand Oaks, Calif, 2000, Sage.
10. Liebow E: *Tally's corner,* Boston, 1967, Little Brown.
11. Maruyama M: Endogenous research: the prison project. In Reason P, Rowan J, editors: *Human inquiry: a sourcebook for new paradigm research,* New York, 1981, Wiley & Sons.
12. Guba EG: Criteria for assessing the trustworthiness of naturalistic inquiries, *Educ Commun Technol J* 29:75-92, 1981.
13. Geertz C: Thick description: toward an interpretative theory of culture. In *The interpretation of cultures: selected essays,* New York, 1973, Basic Books.

14. Anastas JW, MacDonald ML: *Research design for social work and the human services*, New York, 1994, Lexington.

15. Hodge R, Kress G: *Social semiotics,* Ithaca, NY, 1988, Cornell University Press.

16. Silverman D: *Doing qualitative research: a practical handbook*, ed 2, Thousand Oaks, Calif, 2004, Sage.

17. Krefting L: Reintegration into the community after head injury: the results of an ethnographic study, *Occup Ther J Res* 9:67-83, 1989.

18. Headland TN, Pike KL, Harris M: *Emics and etics: the insider/outsider debate,* Newbury Park, Calif, 1990, Sage.

19. Frank G: Life history model of adaptation to disability: the case of a congenital amputee, *Soc Sci Med* 19:639-645, 1984.

20. Tashakkori A, Teddlie C: *Handbook of mixed methods social and behavioral research*, Thousand Oaks, Calif, 2002, Sage.

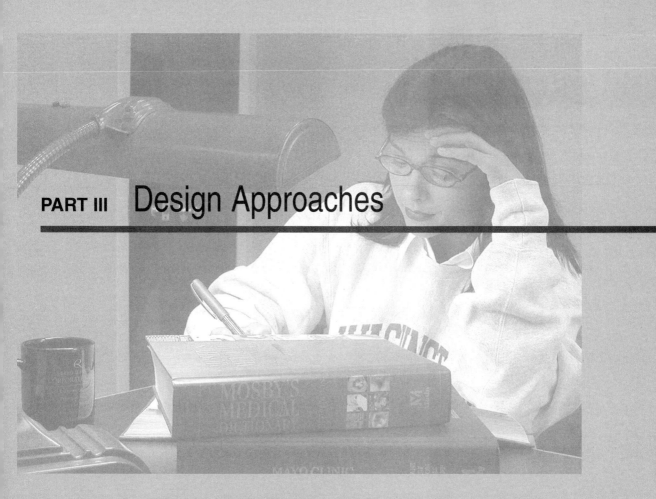

PART III   Design Approaches

Now that we have delved into the thinking processes of research, we are ready to examine its structure. The *structure* of research refers to the design elements used by researchers to answer queries and questions. In Part III, we present diverse approaches to design that are used to conduct research in experimental-type, naturalistic, and integrated inquiries.

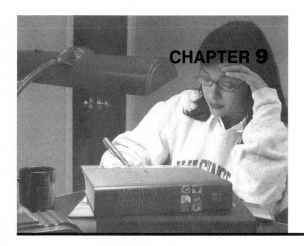

CHAPTER 9

Experimental-Type Designs

KEY TERMS

Counterbalance designs
Effect size
Factorial designs
Manipulation
Meta-analysis
Nonexperimental designs
Pre-experimental designs
Quasi-experimental designs
Randomization
Solomon four-group designs
True-experimental designs

Pretest-Posttest Design
Static Group Comparison
Pre-Experimental Design Summary
Nonexperimental Designs
  Survey Designs
  Passive Observation Designs
  Ex Post Facto Designs
  Nonexperimental Design Summary
Experimental-Type Meta-Analysis
Criteria for Selecting Appropriate and Adequate Designs
Summary

CHAPTER OUTLINE

True-Experimental Designs
  Randomization
  Control Group
  Manipulation
True-Experimental Design Variations
  Posttest-Only Designs
  Solomon Four-Group Designs
  Factorial Designs
  Counterbalance Designs
True-Experimental Design Summary
Quasi-Experimental Designs
  Nonequivalent Control Group Designs
  Interrupted Time Series Designs
  Combined Design
  Quasi-Experimental Design Summary
Pre-Experimental Designs
  One-Shot Case Study

Using the language introduced in Chapter 8, we are ready to examine the characteristics of designs in the experimental-type research tradition. Experimental designs have traditionally been classified as true-experimental, quasi-experimental, pre-experimental, and nonexperimental. The true experiment is the criterion by which all other methodological approaches are judged. Most people think that the only real research or science is the experimental method. Of all the experimental-type designs, the true-experimental design offers the greatest degree of control and internal validity. It is this design and its variations that are used to reveal causal relationships between independent and dependent variables. Also, this design is often upheld as the highest level of scientific evidence, particularly in evidence-based practice model research and ratings that are applied to studies

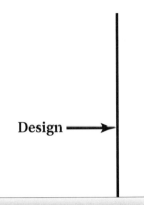

Design ⟶

Philosophical Foundations

for the development of clinical guidelines (see Chapter 24).

Although the true-experimental design is continually upheld as the most "objective" and "true" scientific approach, we believe it is important to recognize that every design in the experimental-type tradition has merit and value. The merit and value of a design are based on how well the design answers the research question that is being posed and the level of rigor that the investigator brings to the plan and conduct of the inquiry. This view of research differs from the perspective of the many experimental-type researchers who present the true experiment as the only design of choice and suggest that other designs are deficient or limited.[1,2]

We believe that a design in the experimental-type tradition should be chosen because it fits the question, level of theory development, and setting or environment in which the research will be conducted. True experimentation is the best design to use to predict causal relationships, but it may be inappropriate for other forms of inquiry in health and human service settings. In other words, not all research questions seek to predict causal relationships between independent and dependent variables. Moreover, in some cases, using a true-experimental design may present critical ethical concerns such that other design strategies may be more appropriate.

TRUE-EXPERIMENTAL DESIGNS

To express the structural relationships of true-experimental designs, we use Campbell and Stanley's classic, widely adopted notation system to diagram a design: X is used for the independent variable, O for the dependent variable, and R for random sample selection,[3] as follows:

R	O	X	O
R	O		O

We also find it helpful to use the symbol r to refer to random group assignment. It is often difficult and frequently inappropriate or unethical for health and human service professionals to select a sample from a larger, predefined population based on random selection (R); rather, typically in health and human service research, subjects enter studies on a volunteer basis. Such a sample is one of convenience in which subjects are then randomly assigned to either the experimental or the control group. The addition of r denotes this important structural distinction.

True-experimental designs are perhaps best known by beginning researchers and laypersons. True-experimental design refers to the classic two-group design in which subjects are randomly selected and randomly assigned (R) to either an experimental or control group condition. Before the experimental condition, all subjects are pretested or observed on a dependent measure (O). In the experimental group the independent variable or experimental condition is imposed (X), and it is withheld in the control group. After the experimental condition, all

You are interested in enhancing shoulder range of motion in persons with stroke. The dependent variable would be a measure of shoulder range of motion, the independent variable or experimental condition a particular physical therapy protocol that is introduced, and the control condition a control group who receives usual care. Subjects in a rehabilitation facility who meet specific criteria for study participation would be pretested on the measure of shoulder range of motion, randomly assigned to receive the experimental condition or usual care, and then retested using the same range of motion measure.

subjects are posttested or observed on the dependent variable *(O)*.

In this design the investigator expects to observe no difference between the experimental and control groups on the dependent measure at pretest. In other words, subjects are chosen randomly from a larger pool of potential subjects and then assigned to a group on a "chance-determined" basis; therefore subjects in both groups are expected to perform similarly. In the example, we would expect that subjects in experimental and control group conditions would have similar shoulder range of motion scores at the first baseline or pretest assessment. On the other hand, the investigator anticipates or hypothesizes that differences will occur between experimental and control group subjects on the posttest scores. However, this expectation is expressed as a null hypothesis, which states that no difference is expected. In a true-experimental design, the investigator always states a null hypothesis that forms the basis for statistical testing. Usually in research reports, however, the alternative hypothesis is stated (i.e., an expected difference). If the investigator's data analytical procedures reveal a significant difference (one that does not occur by chance) between experimental and control group scores at posttest, the investigator can fail to accept the null hypothesis with a reasonable degree of certainty. In failing to accept the null hypothesis, the investigator accepts with a certain level of confidence that the independent variable or experimental condition *(X)* caused the outcome observed at posttest time in the experimental group. In other words, the investigator infers that the difference at posttest time is not the result of chance but is caused by participation in the experimental condition.

Three major characteristics of the true-experimental design allow this causal claim to be made (Box 9-1).

BOX 9-1
THREE CHARACTERISTICS OF TRUE-EXPERIMENTAL DESIGN

- Randomization
- Control group
- Manipulation of an independent variable

Randomization

Randomization occurs at the sample selection phase and/or at the group assignment phase. If random sample selection is accomplished, the design notation appears as presented earlier *(R)*. If randomization occurs only at the group assignment phase, we represent the design as such *(r):*

$$\begin{array}{cccc} r & O & X & O \\ \hline r & O & & O \end{array}$$

This variation has implications for external validity. A true-experimental design that does not use random sample selection is limited in the extent to which conclusions can be generalized to the population from whom the sample is selected. Because subjects are not drawn by chance from a larger identified pool, the generalizability or external validity of findings is limited. However, such a design variation is common in experimental research and can still be used to reveal causal relationships within the sample itself.

Although random sample selection is often not possible to achieve, random assignment of subjects to group conditions based on chance is essential in true experimentation. It enhances the probability that subjects in experimental and control groups will be theoretically equivalent on all major dependent variables at the pretest occasion. Randomization, in principle, equalizes subjects or provides a high degree of assurance that subjects in both experimental and control groups will be comparable at pretest or the initial, baseline measure. How is this possible? By randomizing, people are assigned by chance, and as such, the researcher does not introduce any systematic order to the selection and assignment of the sample. Thus, any influence on one group theoretically will similarly affect the other group as well. In the absence of any other differences that could influence outcome, an observed change in the experimental group at posttest then can be attributed with a reasonable degree of certainty to the experimental condition.

Randomization is a powerful technique that increases control and eliminates bias by neutralizing the effects of extraneous influences on the outcome of a study. For example, the threats to internal validity by historical events and maturation are theoretically eliminated. Based on probability theory, such influences should affect subjects equally in both the experimental and the control group. Without randomization of subjects, you will not have a true-experimental design.

Control Group

We now extend the concept of control introduced in Chapter 8 to refer to the inclusion of a control group in a study. The control group allows the investigator to see what the sample will be without the influence of the experimental condition or independent variable. A control group theoretically performs or remains the same relative to the independent variable at pretest and posttest, since the control group has not had the chance of being exposed to the experimental (or planned change) condition. Therefore the control group represents the characteristics of the experimental group before being changed by participation in the experimental condition.

The control group is also a mechanism that allows the investigator to examine what has been referred to as the "attention factor," "Hawthorne effect," or "halo effect."[4] These three terms all refer to the phenomenon of the subject experiencing change as a result of simply participating in a research project. For example, being the recipient of personal attention from an interviewer during pretesting and posttesting may influence how a subject feels and responds to interview questions. A change in scores in the experimental group may then occur, independent of the effect of the experimental condition. Without a control group, investigators are not able to observe the presence or absence of this phenomenon and are unable to judge the extent to which differences on posttest scores of the experimental group reflect experimental effect, not additional attention.

Interestingly, this attention phenomenon was discovered in the process of conducting research. In 1934 a group of investigators were examining productivity in the Hawthorne automobile plant in Chicago. The research involved interviewing workers. To improve productivity, the investigators recommended that the lighting of the facility be brightened. The researchers noted week after week that productivity increased after each subsequent increase in illumination. To confirm the success of their amazing findings, the researchers then dimmed the light. To their surprise, productivity continued to increase even under this circumstance. In reexamining the research process, they concluded that it was the additional attention given to the workers through the ongoing interview process and their inclusion in the research itself that caused an increased work effort.[5]

Manipulation

In the true-experimental design, the independent variable is manipulated either by having it present (in the experimental group) or absent (in the control group). *Manipulation* is the ability to provide and withhold the independent variable that is unique to the true experiment.

According to Campbell and Stanley,[3] true experimentation theoretically controls for each of the seven major threats to internal validity (see Chapter 8). However, when such a true-experimental design is implemented in the health care or human service environment, certain influences may remain as internal threats, thereby decreasing the potential for the investigator to support a cause-and-effect relationship. For example, the selection of a data collection instrument with a learning effect based on repeated testing could pose a significant threat to a study, regardless of how well the experiment is structured. It is also possible for experimental "mortality" to affect outcome, particularly if the groups become nonequivalent as a result of attrition from the experiment. The health or human service environment is complex and does not offer the same degree of control as a laboratory setting. Therefore, in applying the true-experimental design to the health or human service environment, the researcher must carefully examine the particular threats to internal validity and how each can be resolved.

TRUE-EXPERIMENTAL DESIGN VARIATIONS

Many design variations of the true experiment have been developed to enhance its internal validity. For example, to assess the effect of the attention factor, a researcher may develop a three-group design. In this structure, subjects are randomly assigned to (1) an experimental condition, (2) an attention control group who receives an activity designed to equalize the attention that subjects receive in the experimental group, or (3) a silent control group who receives no attention other than that obtained naturally during data collection efforts. The term "silent control group" can also refer to the situation in which information is collected on subjects who have no knowledge of their own participation.

> Extracting information from medical records on a group who remains unaware may provide the researcher with an understanding of how subjects in the study compare with those who are not, at least regarding identified demographic and medical characteristics.

Let us examine four basic design variations of the true experiment.

Posttest-Only Designs

Posttest-only designs conform to the norms of experimentation in that they contain the three elements of random assignment, control group, and manipulation. The difference between classic true-experimental design and this variation is the absence of a pretest. The basic design notation for a posttest-only experiment follows:

R	*X*	*O*	*or*	*r*	*X*	*O*
R		*O*		*r*		*O*

In a posttest-only design, groups are considered equivalent before the experimental condition as a result of random assignment. Theoretically, randomization should yield equivalent groups. However, the absence of the pretest makes it impossible to determine whether random assignment successfully achieved equivalence between the experimental and control groups on the major dependent variables of the study. There are a number of variations of this basic design. For example, the researcher may add other posttest occasions or different types of experimental or control groups.

Posttest-only designs are most valuable when pretesting is not possible or appropriate but the research purpose is to seek causal relationships. Also, a posttest-only design might be chosen if the threat to

learning is highly likely with repeated testing using the same measure of the dependent variable.

Solomon Four-Group Designs

More complex experimental structures than those previously discussed, *Solomon four-group designs* combine the true-experiment and posttest-only designs into one design structure. The strength of this design is that it provides the opportunity to test the potential influence of the test-retest learning phenomenon by adding the posttest-only two-group design to the true-experimental design. This design is noted as follows:

Group 1: R	*O*	*X*	*O*
Group 2: R	*O*		*O*
Group 3: R		*X*	*O*
Group 4: R			*O*

As shown in this notation, Group 3 does not receive the pretest but participates in the experimental condition. Group 4 also does not receive the pretest but serves as a control group. By comparing the posttest scores of all groups, the investigator can evaluate the effect of testing on scores on the posttest and interaction between the test and the experimental condition. The key benefit of this design is its ability to detect interaction effects. An interaction effect refers to changes that occur in the dependent variable as a consequence of the combined influence or interaction of taking the pretest and participating in the experimental condition.

The following example illustrates the power of the Solomon four-group design and the nature of interaction effects.

> You want to assess the effects of an AIDS informational training program (independent variable) on the sexual risk-taking behaviors (dependent variable) of adolescents. You can pretest groups by asking questions about sexual activities and levels of knowledge regarding behavioral risks of developing acquired immunodeficiency syndrome (AIDS). You can expose one group to the experimental condition, which involves attending an educational forum led by peers. On posttesting you discover that levels of knowledge increased and that risk behaviors decreased in subjects who

received the experimental program. However, you cannot determine the effect of the pretest itself on the outcome. By adding group 3 (experimental condition without pretest), you can determine whether the change in scores is as strong as when the pretest is administered (group 1). If group 2 (control) and group 3 (experimental) show no change but experimental group 1 does, you can be relatively certain that this change is a consequence of an interaction effect of the pretest and the intervention. If there is a change in experimental groups 1 and 3 and some change in control group 2 but none in control group 4, there may be a direct effect of the intervention or experimental condition plus an interaction effect.

This design allows the investigator to determine the strength of the independent effects of the intervention and the strength of the effect of pretesting on outcomes. If the groups who have been pretested show a testing effect, statistical procedures can be used to correct it, if necessary.

As you can see, the Solomon four-group design offers increased control and the possibility of understanding complex outcomes. Because it requires the addition of two groups, however, it is a costly, time-consuming alternative to the true-experimental design and infrequently used in health and human service inquiry.

Factorial Designs

These designs offer even more opportunities for multiple comparisons and complexities in analysis. In *factorial designs* the investigator evaluates the effects of either two or more independent variables (X_1 and X_2) or the effects of an intervention on different factors or levels of a sample or study variables. The interaction of these parts, as well as the direct relationship of one part to another, is examined.

You are interested in examining the effects of an exercise program on older adults. Specifically, you want to determine the extent to which two levels of "health status" (good and poor) influence three "quality of life" areas for participants. In this case the first independent variable that is manipulated assumes two values: participation in an exercise experimental group or participation in a nonexercise control group. The other independent variable that is not manipulated (health) also has two values (good and poor). The dependent variable or outcome measure (quality of life) has three factors (activity level, overall satisfaction, sense of well-being). This study represents a factorial design in which the independent variables have two factors or levels and the dependent variable has three levels. This structure is referred to as a "2 × 2 × 3" factorial design (Figure 9-1). This design allows you to examine the relationship between different levels of health and specific quality-of-life indicators for two different conditions, subjects exercising and subjects participating in a nonexercise control group.

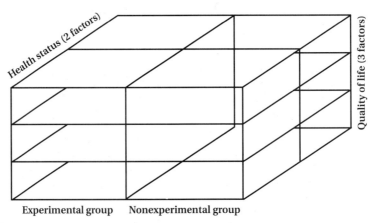

Figure 9-1 Factorial design (2 × 2 × 3) used to investigate quality of life in elder participants in an experimental exercise program.

The factorial design enables you to examine not only direct relationships but interactive relationships as well. You can determine the combined effects of two or more variables that may be quite different from each direct effect. For example, you may want to examine whether the less healthy exerciser benefits more on the activity indicator of quality of life than the less healthy nonexerciser. To evaluate statistically all the possible contrasts in this design, you need to have a large sample size to ensure that each cell or block (see Figure 9-1) contains an adequate number of scores for analysis.

Of course, you can develop more complex factorial designs in which both independent and dependent variables have more than two levels. With more complexity, however, increasingly large sample sizes are necessary to ensure sufficient numbers in each variation to permit analysis.

Counterbalance Designs

When more than one intervention is being tested and when the order of participation is manipulated, *counterbalance designs* are often used. This design allows the investigator to determine the combined effects of two or more interventions and the effect of order on study outcomes. Although there are many variations, the basic design is as follows:

R	O	X_1	O	X_2	O
R	O	X_2	O	X_1	O

Note the subscript numbers on the independent variables. The reversal of the conditions is characteristic of counterbalance designs in which both groups experience both conditions but in different orders. This reversal is called "crossover." In a crossover study, one group is assigned to the experimental group first and to the control condition later; the reverse order is assigned for the other group. Measurements occur before the first set of conditions, before the second set, and after the experiment. Such a study allows you to eliminate the threats to internal validity caused by the interaction of the experimental variable and other aspects of the study.

Suppose you were interested in the psychosocial effects of two different interventions for women whose husbands had been killed in military service in Iraq. You randomly assign your sample to one of two conditions, on-site support group only and peer telephone support, and then reverse their assignment. Testing would occur at three intervals: just before the experiment, after participation in condition one, and after the experiment. By structuring your research with this design, you would be able not only to ascertain the effects of each program on a single group, but also to compare groups over time in each of the conditions.

True-Experimental Design Summary

True-experimental designs must contain three essential characteristics: random assignment, control group, and manipulation. The classic true experiment and its variations all contain these elements and thus are capable of producing knowledge about causal relationships among independent and dependent variables. The four design strategies in the true-experimental classification are appropriate for an experimental-type research question in which the intent is to predict and reveal a cause. Each true-experimental-type design controls the influences of the basic threats to internal validity and theoretically eliminates unwanted or extraneous phenomena that can confound a causal study and invalidate causal claims. The three criteria for using a true-experimental design or its variation are (1) sufficient theory to examine causality, (2) a causal question, and (3) conditions and ethics that permit randomization, use of a control group, and manipulation.

Developing even the most straightforward experimental design, such as the two-group randomized trial, involves many other considerations. It is important to consult with a statistician about the possible approaches to randomization. A statistician can help you determine the best approach to randomizing subjects based on your study design and the basic characteristics of the subjects that you plan to enroll. There are many different ways to randomize to ensure that subjects are assigned to groups by chance. In complex designs or large clinical trials, a statistician is usually responsible for setting up a randomization scheme and placing group assignments in sealed, opaque envelopes so that the investigators or research team members cannot influence the group assignment.

QUASI-EXPERIMENTAL DESIGNS

Although true experiments have been upheld as the ideal or prototype in research, such designs may not be appropriate for many reasons, as we have indicated throughout this book. First, in health and human service research, it may not be possible, appropriate, or ethical to use randomization or to manipulate the introduction and withholding of an experimental intervention. Second, all inquiries do not ask causal questions, and thus the experimental design may not be appropriate. So what can you do when it is not possible or appropriate to use randomization, manipulation, or a control group?

Other design options do not contain the three elements of true experimentation typically used by health and human service researchers to generate valuable knowledge. Even though the language of the experimental-type tradition implies that these designs are "missing something," we suggest that these designs are not "inferior," but rather that they produce different interpretations and uses than true experimentation.

The decision to use *quasi-experimental designs* should be based on the level of theory, type of research question asked, and constraints of the research environment. Cook and Campbell, who wrote the seminal work on quasi-experimentation, define these designs as:

> . . .experiments that have treatments, outcome measures, and experimental units, but do not use random assignment to create comparison from which treatment-caused change is inferred. Instead, the comparisons depend on nonequivalent groups that differ from each other in many ways other than the presence of the treatment whose effects are being tested.[6]

The key to the efficacious use of quasi-experimental designs lies in the claims made by the researcher about the findings. Because random assignment is absent in quasi-experimentation,

---

BOX 9-2
QUASI-EXPERIMENTAL DESIGNS

■ Nonequivalent control group
■ Interrupted time series

---

the researcher can (1) make causal claims while acknowledging the alternative explanations for these claims and design limitations or (2) avoid making causal inferences when they are unjustified by the design.

Designs in the quasi-experimental category have two of the three true-experimental elements: control group and manipulation. Two basic design types fit the criteria for quasi-experimentation (Box 9-2).

Nonequivalent Control Group Designs

There are at least two comparison groups in nonequivalent control group designs, but subjects are not randomly assigned to these groups. The basic design is structured as a pretest and posttest comparison group, as in the following notation:

O	*X*	*O*
O		*O*

It is also possible to add comparison groups or to alter the testing sequence.

You want to test the effectiveness of an innovative mental health program designed to alleviate depression, but it is not possible to use randomization. You arrange for a community mental health center to use the experimental intervention for 1 month. You find another community mental health center in which the population is comparable and assign the comparison condition (conventional intervention) to that group. As with true-experimental design, you pretest and posttest all subjects, then compare group scores. If the group scores for the experimental condition are significantly different, there is strong support for the value of the innovative program. Once again, however, because of the multiple threats to internal validity, most likely you will not use this design to support cause but to explain the comparative changes in each of the study groups. That is, you can indicate that the changes after the intervention in the experimental group were significantly greater than the changes in the comparison group.

Interrupted Time Series Designs

Interrupted time series designs involve repeated measurement of the dependent variable both before and after the introduction of the independent variable. There is no control or comparison group in this design. The multiple measures before the independent variable control for the threat to internal validity based on maturation and other time-related changes. A typical time series design is depicted as follows:

$$O_1 \quad O_2 \quad O_3 \quad X \quad O_4 \quad O_5 \quad O_6$$

Although the number of observations may vary, it is suggested that no less than three occur before and three occur after the independent variable is introduced. The investigator is particularly interested in evaluating the change in scores between the observation that occurs immediately before the introduction of the intervention (O_3) and the observation that follows the intervention (O_4). Any sharp change in score compared with the other measures may suggest that the intervention had an effect. The investigator must evaluate changes in scores in terms of the scoring patterns that occurred both before and after intervention. For example, if there is a trend for scores to increase at each testing occasion, even a sharp difference between O_3 and O_4 may not reflect a change because of the introduction of the intervention.

Because of the absence of the control group and randomization, the interrupted time series design cannot strongly support a causal relationship between the independent and dependent variables. In this type of design, however, the series of premeasures theoretically controls threats to internal validity, except for the threat of history. Maturation, testing, instrumentation, regression, and attrition are considered threats that may occur between all measures and thus are detectable and controlled by repeated measurements. In this design, however, it is extremely important to choose a form of measurement in which there is no learning effect or threat of testing.

In the health and human service context, researchers often use an interrupted time series design when they may not be able to manipulate the experimental intervention but they have knowledge of its introduction. In other words, the intervention or experimental program may be a naturally occurring event in which it is possible to document performance of the dependent variable before and after the event's occurrence.

A hospital announces a plan to implement a new employee benefits program to enhance job satisfaction. The effects of this program on job satisfaction can be determined by taking a quarterly survey of employees for 1 year before the introduction of the new program. The same survey can be used quarterly after employee participation in the new benefits program. In this way, the hospital will have four data points regarding employee satisfaction before the program's introduction that can be compared with four data points after its implementation. This strategy will allow for such extraneous factors as staff turnover and fluctuations in patient census to be tracked over time to account for their effect on job satisfaction.

The interrupted times series design is extremely useful in answering questions about the nature of change over time.

Combined Design

A combination of nonequivalent groups and interrupted time series is a quasi-experimental design that can be considered appropriate for answering causal questions. In this combination, some of the potential bias attributable to nonequivalent groups is limited by multiple measures, whereas the time series design is strengthened by the addition of a comparison group.

Quasi-Experimental Design Summary

Quasi-experimental designs are characterized by the presence of some type of comparison group and manipulation, but they do not contain random group assignment. Although there is no control group in time series and single-subject designs, control is exercised through multiple observations of the same phenomenon both before and after the introduction of the experimental condition. In nonequivalent group designs the control is built in through the use of one or more comparison groups.

We suggest that quasi-experimentation is most valuable when the investigator is attempting to search for change over time, or when a comparison between groups and the constraints of the health or human service environment are such that random assignment is not appropriate, ethical, or feasible.

PRE-EXPERIMENTAL DESIGNS

In *pre-experimental designs,* two of the three criteria for true experimentation are absent. In pre-experiments, it is possible to describe phenomena or relationships. However, the outcomes of the study do not support claims for a causal relationship because of inadequate control and the potential of bias. Pre-experimental designs can be of value to answer descriptive questions or to generate pilot, exploratory evidence, but the investigator using these designs cannot consider causal explanations. The numerous pre-experimental designs are all variations on three designs (Box 9-3).

One-Shot Case Study

In the one-shot case study, the independent variable is introduced, then the dependent variable is measured in only one group, as follows:

$$X \qquad O$$

Without a pretest or a comparison group, the investigator can answer the question, "How did the group score on the dependent variable after the intervention?" As you can see, a cause-and-effect relationship between the two variables cannot be supported because of the seven threats to internal validity (see Box 8-3).

BOX 9-3
PRE-EXPERIMENTAL DESIGNS

■ One-shot case study
■ Pretest-posttest design
■ Static group comparison

Pretest-Posttest Design

The pretest-posttest design is also valuable in describing what occurs after the introduction of the independent variable, as follows:

$$O \qquad X \qquad O$$

This design can answer questions about change over time in that the pretest is given before the introduction of the independent variable. If subjects are tested before the intervention and after the intervention, a change in scores on the dependent variable can be reported but cannot be attributed to the influence of the independent variable. Threats to internal validity, if one were to attempt to infer cause using this design, include maturation, history, testing, instrumentation, experimental mortality, and interactive effects.

Static Group Comparison

In static group comparison, a comparison group is added to the one-shot case study design, as follows:

$$X \qquad O$$
$$O$$

This design, as in other pre-experimental structures, can answer descriptive questions about phenomena or relationships but is not considered a desirable choice for causal studies.

Suppose researchers want to test an intervention that is designed to reduce depression in young adults. The investigator who uses the static group comparison will select two nonequivalent groups, such as two groups of persons with depression receiving treatment in two different community mental health centers. One group will receive the intervention and one will not. A posttest measuring the level of depression will be administered to both groups and then compared. This design can answer the following question with a fair degree of certainty: "How did the experimental group compare with the comparison group on the measure of depression?" Because random assignment did not occur, it is difficult to infer cause. Furthermore, there is minimal control in that the level of depression in either group was unknown before the introduction of the experimental condition.

Some researchers consider the comparison group score as a pretest measure, since the group who did not receive intervention could approximate the pretest condition of the group receiving the intervention.

Introducing a static comparison group offers more control over extraneous factors than the one-shot case and pretest-posttest designs. However, we caution against its use to make statements on causal relationships between the independent and dependent variables.

Pre-Experimental Design Summary

Pre-experimental designs may be valuable in answering a descriptive question. You may want to consider using a pre-experimental design for the specific purpose of pilot testing an intervention protocol or particular measurement approach. However, the absence of two of the three major conditions for true experimentation makes these designs an inappropriate choice if your pursuit is prediction and causal inference. If you attempt to answer predictive or causal questions with these designs, the basic seven threats to internal validity limit effective checks against bias.

NONEXPERIMENTAL DESIGNS

Nonexperimental designs primarily rely on statistical manipulation of data rather than mechanical manipulation and sequencing. By definition, nonexperimental designs are those in which none of the three criteria for true experimentation exists in the structure of sample selection, exposure to an experimental condition, and data collection. These designs are most useful when testing a concept or construct or set of relationships among constructs that naturally occur. Any manipulation of variables is done *post hoc* through statistical analysis. Three nonexperimental designs are frequently used in health and human service research (Box 9-4).

BOX 9-4
NONEXPERIMENTAL DESIGNS

- Surveys
- Passive observation
- *Ex post facto* designs

Survey Designs

Survey designs are primarily used to measure characteristics of a population. Through survey designs, it is possible to describe population parameters, as well as to predict relationships among these characteristics. Typically, surveys are conducted with large samples. Questions are posed either through mailed questionnaires or through telephone or face-to-face interviews. Perhaps the most well-known survey is the U.S. Census, in which the federal government administers mailed surveys and conducts selected face-to-face interviews to develop a descriptive picture of the characteristics of the U.S. population.

Suppose you are interested in examining and predicting job satisfaction of "social work faculty" who are teaching in "distance education programs." You mail questionnaires to program directors of schools of social work with distance education components and ask the directors to distribute these instruments to faculty who are teaching in distance courses. After receiving 500 faculty surveys containing demographic characteristics and job satisfaction scores, you conduct statistical analysis of the data and are able to develop descriptive and predictive conclusions.

The advantages of survey design are that (1) the investigator can reach a large number of respondents with relatively minimal expenditure and time, (2) numerous variables can be measured by a single instrument, and (3) statistical manipulation during the data analytical phase can permit multiple uses of the data set. Disadvantages may result from the survey structure. For example, the use of mailed questionnaires may yield a low response rate, compromising the external validity of the design. Face-to-face interviews are time-consuming and may pose reliability problems.

Many books and online resources can guide you in designing a survey study by mail, by telephone, or in person. For more detailed discussion of surveys, these resources should be consulted.

Passive Observation Designs

Passive observation designs are used to examine phenomena as they naturally occur and to discern the relationship between two or more variables. Often referred to as "correlational designs," passive observation can be as simple as examining the relationship between two variables (e.g., height and weight), or it can be as complex as predicting scores on one or more variables from knowledge of scores on other variables. As in the survey, variables are not manipulated but are measured and then examined for relationships and patterns of prediction.

> In the survey on job satisfaction of social work faculty, you would be able to examine the relationships among multiple variables and to predict the degree of job satisfaction with respondent scores on four other variables.[7]

Ex Post Facto Designs

Ex post facto designs are considered to be one type of passive observation design. In ex post facto ("after the fact") designs, however, the phenomena of interest have already occurred and cannot be manipulated in any way. Ex post facto designs are frequently used to examine relationships between naturally occurring population parameters and specific variables.

> You are interested in understanding the effects of coronary bypass surgery on morale and resumption of former roles for men and women. Coronary bypass surgery is the event that the researcher cannot manipulate, but it can be examined for its effects after its occurrence. For example, ex post facto survey designs might be used to examine phenomena such as career patterns of graduates of professional curricula, recovery process, and differences in job satisfaction between male and female social workers.

Nonexperimental Design Summary

Nonexperimental designs have a wide range of uses. The value in these designs lies in their ability to examine and quantify naturally occurring phenomena so that statistical analysis can be accomplished. Therefore the investigator does not manipulate the independent variable but rather examines it in relation to one or more variables for descriptive or predictive purposes. These designs have the capacity to include a large number of subjects and to examine events or phenomena that have already occurred. Because random selection, manipulation, and control group are not present in these designs, investigators must use caution when making causal claims from the findings.

As in the quasi-experimental and true-experimental situations, the researcher is still concerned with potential biases that may limit the internal validity of the nonexperimental design. The researcher tries to control the influence of external or extraneous influences on the study variables through the implementation of systematic data collection procedures, the use of reliable and valid instrumentation, and other techniques. The researcher also increases the generalizability of a study or its external validity by using random sample selection procedures when appropriate and feasible, to ensure representation and minimize systematic sampling bias.

EXPERIMENTAL-TYPE META-ANALYSIS

A review of the literature is the core action process in meta-analysis (see Chapter 5).

Meta-analysis is a methodology in the experimental-type tradition that can be understood as a form of survey research. In meta-analysis, however, research reports, rather than real people, are surveyed and become the unit of analysis.[8] In using reports as a form of survey research, first a specific research question must be posed, followed by boundary setting, development of a coding sheet, and implementation of analytical action processes. Box 9-5 outlines the basic steps in the meta-analysis research approach.

The purpose of experimental-type meta-analysis is to summarize, integrate, and interpret an empirical body of research or studies in which the outcomes are quantitative. In meta-analysis the findings of more than one study can be combined and averaged. As with all methodologies, there are certain limitations with a meta-analysis. It is only applicable to one tradition at a time and thus cannot be used with mixed methods. Also, it can be used only with studies using similar constructs and reporting specific statistical analyses (e.g., inferential statistics) that can be meaningfully compared.

> **BOX 9-5**
> **BASIC STEPS IN A META-ANALYSIS**
>
> 1. Specify a topic.
> 2. Specify the type of research finding of importance.
>   a. Treatment outcomes
>   b. Co-variation
> 3. Establish "bounding criteria" (inclusion/exclusion criteria for selecting studies).
> 4. Identify, locate, and retrieve studies that meet study criteria.
> 5. Establish a systematic approach to organizing research records.
>   a. Consider using a computer database program
>   b. Entries include bibliographic information, descriptive study information (e.g., type of sample, intervention and study design)
> 6. Derive numerical value or index representing "effect size" for each study.

The strength of meta-analysis lies in its ability to synthesize a body of research that focuses on a specific topic (e.g., treatment for stroke) and to derive interpretations of the degree of effect of similar treatments. Meta-analysis provides a systematic and structured way of summarizing and analyzing research findings from more than one study in a specified area of inquiry. It can be applied to an area of inquiry with few studies or with many studies.

The key concept in experimental-type meta-analysis is *effect size,* a statistic that codes the magnitude of the effect (or outcome) as a result of being exposed to the independent variable (e.g., treatment, intervention, experimental condition). Different statistics to derive an effect size are used, depending on the type of data and specific research question and hypotheses being tested. The calculation of effect size is beyond the scope of this text, but it is important to understand that experimental-type meta-analysis focuses specifically on statistical outcome of an intervention or experimental condition.[9]

Meta-analysis is important in health and human service research. It enables the researcher to derive a systematic interpretation rather than a critical review of the literature as to the state of knowledge in a particular area. With the increasing popularity of evidence-based practice, as discussed in Chapter 24, meta-analysis provides a methodology through which

to combine and integrate studies to identify "the best intervention."

CRITERIA FOR SELECTING APPROPRIATE AND ADEQUATE DESIGNS

As discussed, some researchers believe that the true-experimental design represents the only structure that is appropriate and adequate. However, each design in the experimental-type tradition has its strengths and limitations. The true experiment is the best design for testing theory, making causal statements, and determining the efficacy of treatments. If causality is not your purpose, however, or if the design structure does not fit the particular environment in which the research is to be conducted, true-experimental design is not an appropriate or adequate choice.

It is often difficult to apply strict experimental conditions to a field setting. For example, although subjects may be randomly assigned to a group, it may not be possible to obtain the initial list of subjects for a random sampling process, or it may be unethical to withhold a type of treatment (or experimental intervention) from a consumer in a service setting. Although clinical drug trials or testing of new technologies often obtain the degree of control necessary for true-experimental conditions, research on the social and psychological dimensions of health and human service work often pose a different set of issues and challenges for the researcher. These challenges make it essential for the investigator to be flexible in the use of design so that a research strategy appropriate to the question and to the level of theory, purpose, and practical constraints can be selected and rigorously applied.

To illustrate the value of each type of research design within the experimental-type tradition, apply the concepts in this chapter to an example that you may encounter in your practice.

> You are employed in a hospital in the rehabilitation unit. You have just read about a new computer intervention that seems to enhance the cognitive recovery of persons with traumatic brain injury. You order the program and recruit a group of patients to use it. To determine the extent to which the program works (which you have defined as "significant

improvement in cognitive function"), you select an instrument to measure cognitive function (operationalizing your concept of cognitive improvement), and then you test a sample of 10 patients with the same instrument after their use of the computer intervention.

This type of inquiry is an *XO* design (pre-experimental) in which the computer program is the independent variable and cognitive performance is the dependent variable. The mean score for your sample was within normal limits, with a normal dispersion of scores around the mean. From this design, you have answered the question, "How did subjects score on a test of cognitive performance after their participation in a computer intervention?" Although these data are valuable to you in describing your sample, you still have not answered the question about whether the program "works." Multiple threats to internal validity interfere with your ability to make a causal inference between variables with any degree of assuredness. You therefore decide to build on this study by adding a pretest.

In the next study, you pretest your new sample, introduce the computer intervention, and then posttest the sample.

This type of study is an *OXO* design (also pre-experimental). Because the subjects have greatly improved from the pretest to the posttest, you conclude that your program has worked. However, can you really come to this conclusion? What about the effects of sampling bias, maturation, and history on your sample? You realize that even though you have stronger evidence for the value of the program, the design that you have selected has answered the question, "To what extent did the subjects change in cognitive function after participating in the experimental condition?"

For your next sample, you add a control group so that your research structure is now a quasi-experimental design.

Your design now appears as follows:

O	*X*	*O*
O		*O*

When the experimental group improves more than the control group, you now are convinced that your program works. However, can you make that claim? What about sampling bias and other interactive effects that might confound your study? From this design, you can answer the question, "Which group made more progress?" This type of design provides fairly strong support for the value of your program, but it cannot be used yet to make causal claims.

For your next project, you add random group assignment to your design so that you are conducting a true experiment.

Your design looks like the following:

r	*O*	*X*	*O*
r	*O*		*O*

Because your experimental group has improved significantly more than the control group, you can now make the claim, with reasonable certainty, that the program works. You have used true experimentation to test the efficacy of the computer intervention in your sample. However, can you advise your colleague to use this intervention for his or her clients? The answer is a resounding "maybe."

Because you did not randomly select your sample, the capacity to generalize your findings beyond your own experiment is limited. We are often faced with the desire to generalize, but practical restraints of conducting practice research will not allow us to select our sample randomly, as discussed later in the text. You might select experimental-type meta-analysis to expand your scope of knowledge beyond a single study if studies have used similar methods about the same constructs in your study.

You are interested in examining the extent to which the cognitive intervention produced client outcomes that were satisfactory to family members after a client's discharge. You may then select a nonexperimental survey design to examine the level of satisfaction. You also may include predictor variables, such as length of time in treatment and degree of family support, to inform future use and success with this intervention.

Each research design has strengths and limitations related to claims about the knowledge generated as well as practical and ethical issues. The key to doing rigorous and valued research with experimental-type designs is to (1) state your question clearly; (2) select a design that can best answer the question given the level of theory development, the practical considerations, and the purpose in conducting the study; and (3) report accurate conclusions.

Now that you are aware of experimental-type designs and techniques for enhancing the strength of these designs, you still may wonder how to select a design to fit your particular study question. Begin by asking yourself five guiding questions (Box 9-6).

What does each of these questions really ask you to consider? Question 1 raises the issues of validity. When a design is selected, the project must be internally consistent, the construct valid, and the research capable of providing the level of answer that the question seeks. Question 2 also addresses validity but issues of control and structure as well. The researcher must consider what extraneous influences could confound the study and what ways maximum control can be built into the design. Question 3 summarizes the previous issues raised by guiding the researcher to be most rigorous in planning control and minimizing bias. Question 4 addresses external validity and sampling. The researcher must develop a design that allows as broad a generalization as possible without threatening internal validity. Question 5 reminds the researcher of practical and ethical concerns that shape the design.

If these questions are answered successfully, the criteria for adequacy of experimental-type designs have been addressed. However, keep in mind that design considerations within the experimental-type tradition are more than just knowing the definitions of design characteristics. Knowledge of these design possibilities is your "set of tools," which you can then apply and modify to fit the specific conditions of the setting in which you are conducting research. Developing a design within the tradition of experimental-type research in the health and human service field is a creative process. You must use your knowledge of the language and thinking processes, the basic elements of design, and the issues of internal and external validity to develop a study that fits the particular environment and question that you are asking.

SUMMARY

Experimental-type research designs range from true-experimental to nonexperimental, and each design varies in its level of control, randomization, and manipulation of variables (Table 9-1). Also, field conditions and other practicalities influence the implementation of any type of design. The basic elements of design structure in the experimental-type tradition have many variations, and new applications of experimental designs are being advanced with the advent of meta-analysis and field-based intervention studies.

BOX 9-6

GUIDING QUESTIONS IN SELECTING A RESEARCH DESIGN

1. Does the design answer the research question? Is there congruence between the research question(s) and hypotheses and the design?
2. Does the design adequately control independent variables? Are other extraneous independent variables present that may confound the study?
3. Does the design maximize control and minimize bias?
4. To what extent does the design enhance the generalizability of results to other subjects, other groups, and other conditions?
5. What are some of the ethical and field limitations of the research question that influence the research design?

TABLE 9-1

Summary of Design Characteristics in Experimental-Type Research

	True-Experimental	Quasi-Experimental	Nonexperimental	Pre-Experimental
Randomization	Yes	No	No	No
Control group	Yes	Maybe	Maybe	No
Manipulation	Yes	Maybe	No	Yes

EXERCISES

1. Select an experimental-type research article and identify the dependent and independent variables. Diagram the design using *XO* notation.
2. Develop research questions and designs using the *XO* notation to illustrate (a) true-experimental design, (b) quasi-experimental design, (c) pre-experimental design, and (d) nonexperimental design.
3. Identify up to three potential ethical and field limitations of each research design developed in exercise 2.

REFERENCES

1. Kerlinger FN: *Foundations of behavioral research,* ed 2, New York, 1973, Holt, Rinehart, & Winston.
2. Currier DP: *Elements of research in physical therapy,* Baltimore, 1984, Williams & Wilkins.
3. Campbell DT, Stanley JC: *Experimental and quasi-experimental designs for research,* Chicago, 1963, Rand McNally.
4. Perrow C: *Complex organizations: a critical essay*, ed 2, New York, 1979, Random House.
5. Roethlisberger FJ, Dickson WJ: *Management and the worker*, Cambridge, Mass, 1947, Harvard University Press.
6. Cook TD, Campbell DT: *Quasi-experimentation: design and analysis for field settings,* Boston, 1979, Houghton Mifflin.
7. Rozier C, Gilkeson G, Hamilton BL: Job satisfaction of occupational therapy faculty, *Am J Occup Ther* 45:160-165, 1991.
8. Lipsey MW, Wilson DB: *Practical meta-analysis*, Thousand Oaks, Calif, 2001, Sage.
9. DerSimonian R, Laird N: Meta-analysis in clinical trials, *Control Clin Trials* 7:177-188, 1986.

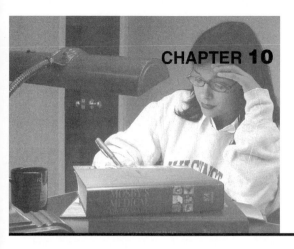

CHAPTER 10

Naturalistic Inquiry Designs

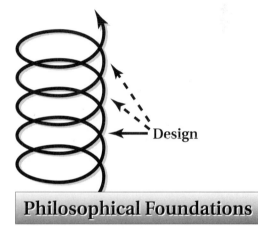

Philosophical Foundations

Using the language and thinking processes you learned in Chapter 8, we are now ready to explore naturalistic inquiry in more detail. Although there are many other approaches in naturalistic inquiry, this chapter highlights 10 specific designs. These designs were selected for inclusion here because of their high relevance to research on health and human service-related concerns. Also, these designs exemplify the wide variation in the naturalistic tradition, the different ways in which complex social phenomena are tackled, and how researchers organize the "10 essentials" of the research process (see Chapter 2).

First, let us reflect a bit on naturalistic inquiry and what we have learned thus far. Do you remember one of the basic principles of naturalist designs? You may recall our discussions in previous chapters that a fundamental principle of all naturalistic designs is that phenomena occur or are embedded in a context, natural setting, or field. As such, research processes are implemented or unfold in an identified context through the course of fieldwork. *Fieldwork* refers to the basic activity that engages all investigators who work in the naturalistic tradition. In conducting fieldwork, the investigator enters an identified setting to experience and understand it without artificially altering or manipulating conditions. The purpose is to observe, understand, and come to know so that theory may be described, explained, and generated. This principle is essential to all naturalistic designs, but the way in which investigators come to know, describe, and explain phenomena differs among designs. That is, although each design shares the basic language and thinking processes discussed in Chapter 8, each design is also based in its own distinct philosophical tradition. As such, these designs differ in purpose, sequence, and investigator involvement (Box 10-1).

This chapter provides the basic framework of 10 designs that are of great methodological value for naturalistic inquiry in health and human ser-

vices: endogenous, participatory action, critical theory, phenomenology, heuristic, ethnography, narrative, life history, grounded theory, and meta-analysis. Table 10-1 summarizes how these naturalistic designs compare in purpose, sequence, and investigator involvement. Remember as you read that the sequence of the 10 essential thinking and action processes is not fixed and therefore cannot be prescribed in each of these 10 naturalistic designs.

ENDOGENOUS RESEARCH

Endogenous research represents the most open-ended approach to research in the naturalistic tradition. This research is "conceptualized, designed, and conducted by researchers who are insiders of the culture, using their own epistemology and their own structure of relevance."[1] The unique feature of this design is the nature of investigator involvement. The investigator relinquishes control of a research plan and its implementation to those who are the subjects of the inquiry. The subjects are primary investigators or co-investigators who work independently or with the investigator to determine the nature of the study and how it is to be shaped. The subjects and investigators make decisions about and participate in the building and testing of information as it emerges.

BOX 10-1
THREE DIFFERENCES IN NATURALISTIC DESIGNS

■ Purpose of the research
■ Sequence and use of the 10 essentials
■ Nature of investigator involvement

TABLE 10-1

Basic Framework of 10 Designs in Naturalistic Inquiry

Design Strategy	Purpose	Sequence	Investigator Involvement
Endogenous	To yield insider perspective through involvement of subject as researcher	Variable	Determined by subjects/informants
Participatory action	To generate knowledge to inform action	Variable	Inclusive team of investigators and participants
Critical theory	To understand experiences for social change	Variable	Investigator directed
Phenomenology	To discover meaning of lived experience	Narrative	Listener/reporter
Heuristic	To reveal personal and lived experience	Variable	Investigator and informant
Ethnography	To understand culture	Prescribed	Investigator directed
Narrative	To understand stories of marginalized individuals	Can be embedded in other designs; analytical strategy	Investigator directed
Life history	To yield biographical experience	Narrative	Investigator directed
Grounded theory	To generate theory	Prescribed	Investigator directed
Meta-analysis	To synthesize body of knowledge	Prescribed	Investigator directed

Endogenous research can be organized in a variety of ways and may include the use of any research strategy and technique in the naturalistic or experimental-type tradition or an integrated design. What makes endogenous research naturalistic is not its investigative structure but rather its paradigmatic framework; that is, the investigator views knowledge as emerging from individuals who know the best way of obtaining that information. *Endogenous* design is consistent with the contemporary notion of "emancipatory research," which is an emerging design category.[2] The endogenous approach rejects the traditional notion of individuals as research subjects. Rather, it views individuals as liberated not only as participants in investigator-facilitated inquiry, but also as leaders in the generation and use of knowledge. The endogenous approach is based on a basic proposition developed by the social psychologist Kurt Lewin, as Argyris and Schon explain:

> Causal inferences about the behavior of human beings are more likely to be valid and enactable when the human beings in question participate in building and testing them. Hence it aims at creating an environment in which participants give and get valid information, make free and informed choices (including the choice to participate), and generate internal commitment to the results of their inquiry.[3]

This design gives "knowing power" exclusively to the persons who are the subjects of the inquiry. Thus the endogenous approach is characterized by the absence of any predefined truths or structures. Because endogenous research is conducted by insiders, no external principles guide the selection of thought and action processes in the study itself. Also, because the researcher's involvement is determined by the individuals who are the subjects of the investigation, the researcher may participate as an equal partner, or not at all, or somewhere between these two levels.

So how exactly does an endogenous design approach work? Let us examine a classic example of endogenous research on prison violence.

Maruyama entered the prison environment as a collaborator and participant observer rather than as the research consultant, an important characteristic of endogenous research.

As a collaborator, Maruyama deferred to the subjects of the investigation to determine the degree of investigator involvement. Two teams, composed of prisoners who had no formal education in research methods, held a series of group meetings and created purposes and plans of action that were important and meaningful to each group. Maruyama describes the research in this way: "A team of endogenous researchers was formed in each of the two prisons. The overall objective of the project was to study interpersonal physical violence (fights) in the prison culture, with as little contamination as possible from academic theories and methodologies. The details of the research were left to be developed by the inmate researchers."[1]

The prisoners chose both experimental-type interview techniques and a form of qualitative data analysis to characterize the violence in the environments in which they were insiders. Maruyama found that the prisoners were able not only to collect extensive and meaningful data, but also to conduct sophisticated conceptual analyses of their data set. The findings from a study "owned" and conducted by insiders may yield very different results from one in which a researcher enters the prison environment as a stranger to ask questions regarding the reasons and nature of violence. From this study, violence was explicated in the language of the inmates, and the findings clearly displayed the cultural nature of violence in each prison. Consider how different the findings may have been if an investigator went to a group of inmates and asked questions about the reasons prison violence occurs. The endogenous methodology not only gave the inmates a voice, but also revealed insights that may never have been uncovered by techniques in which the investigator would have taken an authoritative position in the project.

As you can surmise from this example, the investigator's concerns in the endogenous research design include how to build and work with a team, how to relinquish control over process and outcome, and how to shape the group process to move the research team along in the study of themselves. These concerns rise from the nature of endogenous research and are distinct from other approaches.

PARTICIPATORY ACTION RESEARCH

Participatory action research broadly refers to different types of action research approaches. These varied approaches to action research each reflect a different epistemological assumption and methodological strategy. However, all are "participative, grounded in experience, action-oriented,"[4] and are founded in the principle that those who experience a phenomenon are the most qualified to investigate it. Similar to endogenous research, *participatory action* research involves individuals as first-person, second-person, and third-person[4] participants in designing, conducting, and reporting research. By "first-person research," we mean that individuals who experience the phenomenon of interest systematically reflect on their own lives. "Second-person research" refers to the initiation of an inquiry by a researcher who then branches out to collaborate directly with individuals and communities about a shared problem. In "third-person research" the collaborative nature is still essential, but the direct interaction between researcher and collaborator is not present. Communication takes place through other venues, such as written formats and reports.[4] Consistent with others, we believe that the ideal participatory action inquiry includes all three perspectives and approaches.

The purpose of action research is to generate knowledge to inform responsive action. Researchers using a participatory framework usually work with groups or communities experiencing issues and needs related to health and welfare, disparities in health and access to health care, elimination of oppression and discrimination, equal opportunity, and social justice.

The concept of action research was first developed in the 1940s by Lewin, who blended experimental-type approaches to research with programs that addressed critical social problems. Social problems served as the basis for formulating a research purpose, question, and methodology. Therefore, each research step was connected to or involved with the particular organization, social group, or community that was the focus of inquiry and that was affected in some way by the identified problem or issue. More recently, others have expanded this approach to inquiry. The action research design is now used in planning and enacting solutions to community problems and service dilemmas.[5]

Action research is based on four principles or values (Box 10-2). The principle of democracy means that action research is participatory; that is, all individuals who are stakeholders in a problem or issue and its resolution are included in the research process.

BOX 10-2
FOUR PRINCIPLES OF ACTION RESEARCH

■ Democracy
■ Equity
■ Liberation
■ Life enhancement

Equity ensures that all participants are equally valued in the research process, regardless of previous experience in research. Liberation suggests that action research is a design that is aimed at decreasing oppression, exclusion, and/or discrimination. Life enhancement positions action research as a systematic strategy that promotes growth, development, and fulfillment.

Participatory action research uses thinking and action processes from the experimental-type or naturalistic tradition or an integration of the two. Similar to endogenous design, there is no prescribed or uniform design strategy. Nevertheless, action research is consistent with naturalistic forms of inquiry in that all research occurs within its natural context. Also, most action research relies on action processes that are characteristically interpretive in nature.[6]

Let us examine the sequence in which the 10 research essentials are followed in a participatory action research study. Action research is best characterized as cyclical, beginning with the identification of a problem or dilemma that calls for action, moving to a form of systematic inquiry, and culminating in planning and using the findings of the inquiry. Each step is informed or shaped by the participants of the study. The purpose of the following participatory action study was to establish community programs to enhance the transition of adolescents with special health care needs from high school to work or higher education.[7]

Using the principles of action research and first-, second-, and third-person approaches, the investigators first identified the stakeholders involved in this issue. They included adolescents and their parents, educators, health care providers, employers, and policy makers. To ensure that the research plan reflected the underlying principles of democracy and equity, the investigators convened a group made up of representatives from each of the stakeholder groups. This group became the core participatory researchers. These participatory researchers and the two investigators discussed the research problem and collaboratively negotiated and structured the research method. Focus groups were identified as the primary data collection method, so all team members were trained in this approach. Focus groups of each of the stakeholder groups examined the service needs perceived by each group. Each focus group was facilitated by two members of the participatory team. Data were collected and analyzed by the participatory team. The team reported the findings to planning groups consisting of the same stakeholder groups. A comprehensive service plan was developed, implemented, and evaluated by the participatory action team.[7]

Note that all members of the team were valued and contributed equally to the design, implementation, analysis, and application of the research.

Participatory action research is now used for many purposes, often involving advocacy for underserved groups. The pragmatic foundation combined with its democratic values render action research a useful tool for identifying, empirically supporting, and assessing needed change.

CRITICAL THEORY

Critical theory is not a research method but a "worldview" that suggests both an epistemology and a purpose for conducting research. The debate continues on whether critical theory is a philosophical, political, or sociological school of thought. In essence, critical theory is a response to post-Enlightenment philosophies and positivism in particular. Critical theorists "deconstruct" the notion that there is a unitary truth that can be known by using one way or method.

We believe critical theory is a movement best understood by philosophers. Because critical theory is inspired by diverse schools of thought, including those informed by Marx, Hegel, Kant, Foucault, Derrida, and Kristeva, it is not a unitary approach. Rather, *critical theory* represents a complex set of strategies that are united by the commonality of sociopolitical purpose.[8]

Critical theorists seek to understand human experience as a means to change the world.[9] The common purpose of researchers who approach investigation through critical theory is to come to know about social justice and human experience as a means to promote local change through global social change.

Critical theory was born in the Social Institute at the Frankfurt School in the 1920s. As the Nazi party gained power in Germany, critical theorists moved to Columbia University and developed their notions of power and justice, particularly in response to the hegemony of positivism in the United States. With a focus on social change, critical theorists came to view knowledge as power and the production of knowledge as "socially and historically determined."[10] Derived from this view is an epistemology that upheld pluralism, or a coming to know about phenomena in multiple ways. Furthermore, "knowing" is dynamic, changing, and embedded in the sociopolitical context of the times. According to critical theorists, no one objective reality can be uncovered through systematic investigation. Critical theorists and those who build on their work are frequently concerned with language and symbol as the vehicle through which to uncover multiple meanings and to examine power structures and their interactions.[11]

Critical theory is consistent with fundamental principles that bind naturalistic strategies together in one grand category, such as a view of informant as knower, the dynamic and qualitative nature of knowing, and a complex and pluralistic worldview. Furthermore, critical theorists suggest that research crosses disciplinary boundaries and challenges current knowledge generated by experimental-type methods. Because of the radical view posited by critical theorists, the essential step of literature review in the research process is primarily used as a means to understand the *status quo*. Thus the action process of literature review may occur before the research, but the theory derived is criticized, deconstructed, and taken apart to its core assumptions. The hallmark of critical theory, however, is its purpose of social change and empowerment of marginalized and oppressed groups. Critical theory relies heavily on interview and observation as methods by which data are collected. Strategies of qualitative data analysis are the primary analytical tools used in critical research agendas (as discussed in Chapter 20).

A researcher is interested in understanding the relationship between clients who are substance abusers and formal service providers and the influence of this relationship on the outcome of therapeutic interventions. First, using a critical theory perspective, the researcher would review the literature critically. Of particular importance for the critical theorist would be an examination of the underlying assumptions in the language and textual symbols that reflect a power imbalance based on race, class, and gender differences between client and practitioner. In critical theory this imbalance is presumed to have an effect of oppressing the client while elevating the status, control, and power of the service provider. Second, the researcher would use a range of strategies based in naturalistic inquiry to observe and explore the relationship from the perspectives of both clients and providers. Third, the understandings derived from the research would be used to promote social change, with a particular focus on advancing social justice and equality for clients or oppressed groups.[12]

PHENOMENOLOGY

The specific focus of *phenomenological* research is the explication, narrative presentation, and interpretation of the meaning of lived experiences. Phenomenology differs from other forms of naturalistic inquiry in that phenomenologists believe that meaning can be understood only by those who experience it. In many other forms of naturalistic inquiry, the researcher attributes meaning to experience in the analytical phases of the inquiry. In contrast, however, phenomenologists do not impose an interpretive framework on data but look for it to emerge from the information they obtain from their informants. Phenomenological research is further anchored in the principle that the methods by which we share and communicate experience are limited. "The phenomenon we study is ostensibly the presence of the other, but it can only be the way in which the experience of the other is made available to us."[13]

The primary data collection strategy used in this design is the telling of a biographical story or narrative with emphasis on eliciting experience as it relates to time, body, and physical and virtual space, as well as to other persons. For example, in eliciting experience, the phenomenologist will ask such

questions as, "What is it like to be a patient with breast cancer?" "What was the day like when you learned of your diagnosis?" "What is it like for you to live with breast cancer?" and "What does it mean to you to tell others about your diagnosis?" The elicitation of the ways in which people experience a particular phenomenon differs from other approaches, such as life history. In phenomenology, it is the informant who interjects the primary interpretation and analysis of experience into the interview rather than, as in the life history, the investigator, who imposes an interpretative structure.

How do phenomenologists use literature review? Literature review is framed by the phenomenological principle of the "limits of communication." Thus the literature may be used to illustrate the constraints of our understanding of human experience or to corroborate the communication of the other. It may also support the experiences that emerge from informants.

To help you understand how this approach actually works, suppose that you are conducting a phenomenological research study on the experience of aging. You will seek study participation from a small number of individuals, maybe 10 to 15 persons. Then you would engage in lengthy discourse with each about life experiences and the meanings that each person attributes to his or her lived experience. You may examine the research and clinical literature on aging to ascertain the commonalities of what is being communicated. You may also use the literature to suggest a rationale for using phenomenological methodology, or you may draw on different theoretical perspectives to inform yourself of the context of the experiences that emerge.

In phenomenological research, involvement by the researcher is limited to eliciting life experiences and hearing and reporting the narrative perspective of the informant. Active interpretive involvement during data collection is not typically part of the investigator's role.[14,15]

HEURISTIC RESEARCH

Heuristic research is another important design in the naturalistic tradition. According to Moustakas, heuristic research is an "approach which encourages an individual to discover, and methods which enable him to investigate further by himself."[16]

The *heuristic* design strategy involves complete immersion of the investigator into the phenomenon of interest, including the use of self-reflection of the investigator's personal experiences as primary data. The investigator engages in intensive observation of and listening to individuals who have experienced the phenomenon of interest, recording their individual experiences. The investigator then interprets and reports the meanings of these experiences.

The premise of the heuristic approach is that knowledge emerges from personal experience and is revealed or known to the investigator through his or her own experience of the phenomenon. Thus, investigator involvement in heuristic design is extensive and pervades all areas of inquiry, from the formulation of the query to the collection of data from the investigator as an informant.

Moustakas' classic work provides an excellent example of heuristic research.

When his daughter became ill, Moustakas experienced his own loneliness and realized that health care professionals revealed, by their behavior, that they did not understand the nature of loneliness in persons who were sick. Moustakas therefore engaged in an extensive project where he examined his own loneliness, listened to the stories of hospitalized children, and examined the literature on loneliness to further reveal the meaning of the concept. In this design the literature served as another form of data. It was not used as a source for defining the concept of loneliness before the field was entered.[16]

This example illustrates how heuristic research is conducted by an individual for the purpose of discovery and understanding of the meaning of human experience. The research involves total immersion in the experience of humans, including that of the investigator, as a way of understanding their perspectives. The experiences of the researcher and the information derived from a literature review are considered primary and critical sources of data. Note the sequence and blurring of the 10 essentials in which the literature review is a source of data and is synthesized with other data sources (see Table 2-1).

The name "heuristic" suggests that this form of inquiry serves as a foundation for further inquiry into the human experience that it describes.

ETHNOGRAPHY

Ethnography is a research method primarily derived from the discipline of anthropology, although it is informed by many schools of thought.[17-22] *Ethnography* is a term often used to refer to any type of naturalistic inquiry involving field activity. Although different forms of naturalistic inquiry use fieldwork as a basis for data collection, not all fieldwork represents ethnography.[23]

The intent of ethnography is to understand the underlying patterns of behavior and the meanings of a culture. There are many different definitions of culture. For our purposes, we view "culture" is the set of explicit and tacit rules, symbols, and rituals that guide patterns of human behavior within a group. The ethnographer, as an "outsider" to the cultural scene, seeks to obtain an "insider" perspective. Through extended observation, immersion, and participation in the culture, the ethnographer seeks to discover and understand rules of behavior.[17] Data are collected by interviewing and observing those willing to inform the researcher about behavioral norms and their meanings; participating in the culture; and examining the meaning of cultural objects and symbols. Insiders who willingly engage with the investigator are called "informants." Informants are the investigator's "finger on the pulse of the culture," without whom the investigator would not be able to achieve full understanding. Although the results of ethnography are specific to the culture being studied, some ethnographers attempt to contribute to a broad theory of universal human experience through this important naturalistic methodology.

Ethnography begins by using a range of techniques to gain access to a context or cultural group. Once the investigator enters the field, he or she devotes initial activity to characterizing the context or "social scene"[17] by observing the environment in which the culture operates. Equipped with an understanding of the cultural context, the ethnographer uses participant and nonparticipant observation, interview, and examination of materials, texts, or artifacts to obtain data. Through field notes, voice recordings, and video recordings, qualitative data are logged.[24] Analysis of the data is ongoing and moves from description to explanation, to revealing meaning, to generation of theory. Impressions and findings are verified with the insiders and reported once the findings are determined to represent the culture accurately. Reflexive analysis, or the analysis of the extent to which the researcher influences the results of the study, is an active component of the research process.[23,25] These processes are described in more detail in Chapters 15 and 20.

We classify ethnography as a naturalistic design because of its reliance on qualitative data collection and analysis, the assumption that the researcher is not the knower, and the absence of *a priori* theory, or a theory imposed before entering the field. In this design, investigator involvement is significant and guides the sequence and conduct of the 10 essential thinking and action processes. It is the investigator who makes the decisions regarding the "who, what, when, and where" of each observation and interview experience. The belief that knowledge can be generated about the "other" without the viewpoint of the investigator influencing the study is a different philosophical approach from heuristic and endogenous designs. Furthermore, ethnography is a design that is capable of moving beyond description to reveal complex relationships, patterns, and theory.[8]

Over the past 20 years, contemporary ethnography has emerged and become increasingly integrated in the conduct of health and human service inquiry. Contemporary ethnographic approaches depart from some of the basic assumptions and design elements of classic ethnography. As described by its proponents, Gubrium and Holstein explain: "Where the older ethnography cast its subjects as mere components of social worlds, new ethnography treats them as active interpreters who construct their realities through talk and interaction, stories, and narrative. . . .What is 'new' about this is the sense that participants are ethnographers in their own right."[26]

The new ethnography challenges the basic assumptions held by classic ethnographers, such as investigator objectivity and objective presentation of the social setting.[27] The new concern is how best to represent the participants' own perspectives and their ways of explaining their lives. The focus is on the interpretive practices of people themselves, or how people make sense of their lives as reflected in their own words, stories, and narratives. These concerns are similar to those of the phenomenological and life history approaches. Ethnography is changing in other ways as well. For example, Ulichny[25] discusses a critical ethnography in which ethnographical thinking and action processes are applied to social change. The purposes and action processes of contemporary ethnography are becoming much more diverse, in contrast to classic ethnography. Nevertheless, one key element continues to "bound" all forms of ethnography: the examination of cultural and social groups and underlying patterns and ways of experiencing a social context.

Health and human service investigators increasingly turn to ethnography to obtain an insider's perspective on the meaning of health and social issues as a basis from which to develop meaningful health care and social service interventions or to promote policy and social change. Ethnography has also been used to understand various service environments. One example is the classic ethnography of a nursing home conducted by Savishinsky.[28] Several data collection strategies, including interview and participant observation, were used to describe the culture of the nursing home and the meaning of life in that setting. Through analysis and synthesis of the perspectives of residents and staff, Savishinsky was able to identify ways of changing that environment to improve the quality of life of the residents.

NARRATIVE INQUIRY

The many definitions of and approaches to narrative inquiry all have the common element of "storytelling."[29] The storytelling may be autobiographical, biographical, testimonial, or in another form. Thus, *narrative* is a spoken, written, or visual story[30,31] that can be presented in various discursive formats, serves multiple purposes, and can be approached in diverse analytical and interpretive ways.[8] Narrative inquiry is frequently used to illuminate the voices and experiences of marginalized or excluded populations and individuals, although this is not its only purpose. Because of the complexity and extensive detail, narrative data provide rich description and reveal meanings embedded not only in the content of the story, but also in the words and images (symbols) used to tell the story.[32]

Remember the primacy of language, communication, text, and image in contemporary naturalistic traditions. Narrative has become one of the most popular postmodern methods because it yields a contextually embedded text or set of images that can be subjected to multiple interpretations and discursive analysis. The view of language as a dynamic, embedded human phenomenon drives the analysis of multiple and reciprocal meanings that can be ascertained through examining the symbolic, tacit, deconstructive, and nonneutral nature of the data.[33]

You are interested in influencing state policy so that students with limited financial resources can be recruited and supported to study in health and human service programs at your university. You have decided that one of the most compelling ways to provide evidence of need is to obtain narrative stories from community members who wanted to enter these professions but did not have the opportunity. You select several informants and conduct in-depth interviews with them about their experiences and perspectives. From analyzing the transcripts, you find not only that your informants had to settle for available work, but that embedded in their images, symbols, and stories were unfulfilled lives because of ongoing questions from informants and their families about "what could have been." You then use the narrative findings and the words of your informants to provide a strong and compelling rationale for policy change and financial support for rural recruitment programs.

Narrative has also been used for clinical purposes, such as therapeutic use of autobiography and biography. The power of story in healing has been highlighted in numerous scholarly works.[34-36]

The methods to obtain narrative data are diverse. Interviewing and recording (audio or video) are among the information-gathering strategies used most frequently in health and human services to collect narrative data. Photography,[37] drawing, painting, creative nonfiction, autobiography, and co-constructed narrative[38] are other methods used to tell and present the "story." Selecting the methods for collecting information are first purposive[39] and then practical in

nature. In the previous example, interview provided the forum through which to hear the voices of the informants. But what if you were interested in examining the discursive power in the client-provider relationship? You might turn to video and audio recording, since discursive analysis would be focused on the tacit rules of relationships and social activity. In the recordings, you would then look for how these unspoken rules of communication and behavior were illustrated in the interaction between those observed.

In Chapter 20 we discuss the basic analytical action processes used in the naturalistic tradition. These same strategies are used for narrative analysis.[40] From a data set, inductive analysis is used to reveal the themes, patterns, and meanings that emerge from storytelling.

It is important to keep in mind that many health and human service professionals and those who influence policy, funding, education, and practice have typically been educated to value knowledge that has been generated from experimental-type inquiry.[8] Therefore, investigators who choose narrative strategies for inquiry must be sure to adequately explain its value and purpose and report their narrative in a "clinically convincing" way (Box 10-3).

Although some claim that narrative can generate theory,[34] we do not view this as its primary purpose. Narrative strategies typically employ small numbers of informants in the creation of stories that illuminate underlying processes and meanings of experiences.

BOX 10-3
GUIDELINES IN APPLYING NARRATIVE INQUIRY TO CLINICAL WORK

1. Avoid jargon.
2. Specify the purpose of your inquiry.
3. Detail method and the boundaries of this approach.
4. Make your research credible.
5. Help your audience make the connections between the meaning in the story and professional practice.
6. Highlight what can be learned from this approach that cannot be learned from nomothetic approaches.

From Miller WL, Crabtree BF: Clinical research. In Denzin NK, Lincoln YS: *Handbook of qualitative research,* ed 2, Thousand Oaks, Calif, 2000, Sage.

LIFE HISTORY

Life history, another important design in naturalistic inquiry, uses a narrative strategy. *Life history,* also called "biography of life narrative," is an approach that can stand by itself as a legitimate type of research study, or it can be an integral part of other forms of naturalistic inquiry, such as ethnography. The life history approach is a part of the naturalistic tradition because of its focus on examining the social, cultural, and political context of individual lives. Similar to other designs such as phenomenology, the investigator is primarily concerned with eliciting life experiences and with how individuals themselves interpret and attribute meanings to these experiences.

The aim of life history research is to reveal the nature of the "life process traversed over time."[41] The assumption is that individual lives are unique. These unique life processes are important to examine to understand the context in which people live their lives. Researchers using a life history approach therefore focus on one individual at a time. A study may be composed of just one individual or a few individuals.

There are many diverse purposes for using a life history approach. A life history might be used to explicate the impact of major sociopolitical events on individual lives,[42] the processes of development of disability identity after injury, or the unfolding of self-esteem as women age. Depending on the aim of inquiry, life history researchers sequence the essential action processes and use literature in diverse ways. Investigators who attempt to analyze the value of theory in explaining the complexity of a human life may begin with literature review and use it as an organizing framework. Researchers who seek new theoretical understandings, however, may conduct literature review at different junctures in the research thinking and action processes.

Life history research involves a particular methodological approach in which the sequence of life events is elicited and the meaning of those events examined from the perspective of the informant within a particular sociopolitical and historical context.[42] In eliciting events, the researcher seeks to uncover and characterize marker events, or "turnings," defined as specific occurrences that shape and change the direction of individual lives.[43] Typically, researchers rely heavily on unstructured interviewing techniques. The research may begin with asking an informant to describe the sequence of life events from childhood to adulthood. Based on a time line of events, the investigator may ask questions to elicit the meanings of these events. Participatory and nonparticipatory observation may also be combined with the interview as data collection strategies in order to examine meanings and understand how life is experienced.

Although life history relies mostly on the person who tells his or her story, the investigator shapes the story in part by the types of questions asked. For example, the researcher may ask more detailed questions about a particular life event than is initially offered by the participant. This probing by the researcher structures, in effect, the telling of the story to fit the interests or concerns of the researcher.

Consider how you might use life history to understand the process of developing a disability identity among disability rights activists. First, you would identify an individual or several individuals who are involved in disability rights activities, such as leaders of ADAPT or disabled scholar-activists. For each individual, you would aim to create a narrative or biography through conducting in-depth interviews, to uncover the chronology of life events as well as the symbolic and practical meanings of these events to your informant. Analysis of "turnings" would allow you to examine the types of experience that were most influential in determining the future direction of the informant's life, identity development, and call to action The experience of several individuals who provide narrative would illuminate invaluable insights into the sociocultural world of this group of individuals who have disability and a call to civil action.

Life history studies can be retrospective or prospective. In health and human service research, it is not surprising, in light of practical constraints, that the majority of life history studies are retrospective in their approach; that is, informants are asked to reconstruct their lives and reflect on the meaning of past events. Prospective life histories would rely on the investigator's ability to devote significant time to the observation and analysis of meaning as an individual traveled through chronological time.

GROUNDED THEORY

Grounded theory is defined as "the systematic discovery of theory from the data of social research."[21] It is a more structured and investigator-directed strategy than the previous naturalistic designs that we have thus far discussed.

Developed by Glaser and Strauss,[22] grounded theory represents the integration of a quantitative and qualitative perspective in thinking and action processes. The primary purpose of this design strategy is to evolve a theory or "ground" a theory in the context in which the phenomenon under study occurs. The theory that emerges is intimately linked to each datum of daily life experience that it seeks to explain.

This strategy is similar to other naturalistic designs in its use of an inductive process to derive concepts, constructs, relationships, and principles to understand and explain a phenomenon. However, grounded theory is distinguished from other naturalistic designs by its use of a structured data-gathering and analytical process called the constant comparative method. In this approach, each datum is compared with others to determine similarities and differences. Researchers have developed an elaborate scheme by which to code, analyze, recode, and produce a theory from narratives obtained through a range of data collection strategies.[22,44]

Let us briefly consider how you might use grounded theory.

> You are interested in characterizing single, head-of-household mothers receiving public assistance who have returned to college. After identifying the contextual boundaries of your study, you would interview the women and then, using constant comparison, analyze the narratives. Using this method, you would first read and reread the entire data set to induce categories of data that were repeated throughout the experiences of the women who served as your informants. Then, you would return to the transcripts to analyze each datum, either an experience, articulation, or observation, and compare it with the data in the existing categories to determine similarities and differences between new data and previous information. If it did fit, you would code the datum with an existing code. If it did not fit, a new category or subcategory would be developed and used as a comparison foundation for subsequent data analysis.[45]

The purpose of the constant comparative method is not only to reveal categories but also to explore the diversity of experience within categories, as well as to identify links among categories.

Grounded-theory strategies can also be used to generate and verify theory.[22] A query using a grounded-theory approach begins with broad descriptive interests and then, through data collection and analysis, moves to discover and verify relationships and principles.

NATURALISTIC META-ANALYSIS

Now we turn to another approach, naturalistic meta-analysis that seeks to aggregate small and disparate data sets from which to derive a global synthesis.[46] *Meta-analysis* is a research approach in which multiple independently conducted studies are synthesized and analyzed as a single data set to answer a research question or query. Naturalistic meta-analysis is the application of naturalistic methods to the analysis of many studies. Interestingly, naturalistic meta-analysis is not restricted to the analysis of naturalistic studies. Rather, this approach to meta-analysis is characterized by the philosophical perspective that underpins naturalistic inquiry and the use of inductive methods of analysis applied to multiple studies, literature, and theory.

> If you are interested in understanding the themes in the lives of people living with acquired immunodeficiency syndrome (AIDS), you could aggregate written literature and look for themes throughout narratives, theory, and even experimental-type studies that focus on this population.

There are many purposes of naturalistic meta-analysis.[47] Similar to experimental-type meta-analysis (see Chapter 9), some naturalistic meta-analyses seek to identify and summarize a universe of studies on a particular topic. In anthropology, however, meta-ethnography[48] has been used interpretively to reveal global themes and patterns.[8] The Qual-Quan Evidence Synthesis Group seeks to establish "rigor" standards for naturalistic meta-analysis to contribute to evidence-based practice in health care. This group suggests that meta-analytic approaches are valuable in reviewing diverse perspectives and findings as the basis for deriving single definitions and understandings of complex constructs (e.g., quality, satisfaction).[49]

The thinking and action processes of naturalistic meta-analysis follow the processes that you would use in any naturalistic study. The difference, however, is that your data set comprises studies already conducted and existing sources of literature, theory, and other data sources. Thus, you are aggregating and conducting a secondary analysis of existing knowledge.

If we apply the elements of naturalistic inquiry to existing sources, we begin to see how meta-analysis might be approached from this perspective. First, we need to specify a query or queries that conceptually "bound" a study and provide guidance for seeking sources for analysis. Remember that once the queries are articulated, they can undergo modification as the data sources are initially reviewed and analyzed. In meta-analysis the analogous step to gaining access to the field is deciding which sources to access first. In concert with the thinking and action processes of naturalistic inquiry, data collection and analysis are concurrent and ongoing, and the investigator modifies the inquiry in response to the analysis and emerging findings. Final analysis and reporting to audiences occur once saturation occurs with the data set. Let us consider the investigator who is interested in characterizing the experience of AIDS.

Because there are such diverse findings and accounts of living with AIDS, naturalistic meta-analysis would be an excellent method to choose to determine if any global themes characterize the current knowledge base. But where do you start? You make a decision based on purpose and practicality. You gain access to the literature by entering keywords such as "living with AIDS," "story", and "life history" into a search engine. You search dissertation abstracts for any work done on living with AIDS, regardless of the methodology used. The decision to stop collecting sources is based on saturation and such practical factors as the amount of time and resources that are available to conduct your study.

Naturalistic meta-analysis can be an extremely valuable methodology for health and human service researchers. This approach provides the tools to reveal consensus on competing theories and research, to arrive at single definitions of complex constructs, and to illuminate important themes and patterns across large bodies of literature.

SUMMARY

The 10 design strategies discussed in the chapter differ in their purpose, the sequencing of the essentials of research, and the nature of the investigator's involvement. Naturalistic designs are flexible in the degree to which the investigator participates in the formulation of the design, data collection, and interpretive analysis. Moreover, the sequences of the 10 essential thinking and action processes vary, and boundaries between these processes, such as data collection and analysis, which are clearly delineated in experimental-type designs, may be blurred in naturalistic inquiry.

With this introduction to 10 frequently used designs in the naturalistic tradition, you may want to explore each in greater depth by following up with the references below.

EXERCISES

1. To understand the different purposes of naturalistic designs, identify a broad topic or problem area. Formulate at least four distinct research queries that lead to four different designs discussed in this chapter.
2. Go to a public place and determine how you would conduct a study using classic ethnography to determine public behavior patterns. Determine how you would conduct the study using heuristic research.
3. Plan a study using a naturalistic design to discover the health beliefs of an older Asian population living in an urban community. Plan a study using a naturalistic design with Asian children who are chronically ill and living with their families. How would your strategies differ?
4. Identify an area of your practice in which participatory action research would be useful for defining and guiding necessary change. How would you design your study to ensure that you upheld the four values that underpin all action research?
5. Find, compare, and contrast narrative formats on a single topic. Which presentation do you prefer? Why? Which is most compelling and clinically convincing, and why?
6. Pose a broad query and select four sources of data for your analysis. Look for themes that unify your four sources. After conducting this exercise, identify the strengths and limitations of the approach you have chosen to answer your query.

REFERENCES

1. Maruyama M: Endogenous research: the prison project. In Reason P, Rowan J, editors: *Human inquiry: a sourcebook of new paradigm research,* New York, 1981, Wiley & Sons.

2. Barners C, Mercer JT: *Doing disability research,* Leeds, UK, 1998, Disability Press.

3. Argyris C, Schon DA: Participatory action research and action science compared: a commentary. In Whyte WF, editor: *Participatory action research,* Newbury Park, Calif, 1991, Sage.

4. Reason P, Bradbury H, editors: *Handbook of action research: participative inquiry and practice,* Thousand Oaks, Calif, 2001, Sage.

5. Whyte WF, editor: *Participatory action research,* Newbury Park, Calif, 1991, Sage.

6. Stringer ET: *Action research: a handbook for practitioners,* Thousand Oaks, Calif, 1996, Sage.

7. DePoy E, Gilmer D, Martzial E: Adolescents with disabilities and chronic illness in transition: a community action needs assessment, *Disability Studies Quarterly* 20:34-57, 2000.

8. Denzin NK, Lincoln YS: *Handbook of qualitative research,* ed 2, Thousand Oaks, Calif, 2000, Sage.

9. Rodwell M: *Social work constructivist research,* New York, 1998, Garland.

10. Tierney W: *Culture and ideology in higher education,* New York, 1991, Praeger.

11. Macey D: *Penguin dictionary of critical theory,* 2002, Penguin Books.

12. Nencel L, Pels P: *Constructing knowledge: authority and critique in social science,* Newbury Park, Calif, 1991, Sage.

13. Darroch V, Silvers RJ: *Interpretive human studies: an introduction to phenomenological research,* Washington, DC, 1982, University Press of America.

14. Van Manen M: *Researching lived experience: human science for an action sensitive pedagogy,* Albany, NY, 1990, State University of New York Press.

15. Douglas J, editor: *Understanding everyday life,* London, 1970, Routelage & Kegan Paul.

16. Moustakas C: Heuristic research. In Reason P, Rowan J, editors: *Human inquiry: a sourcebook of new paradigm research,* New York, 1981, Wiley & Sons.

17. Spradley JP: *Participant observation,* New York, 1980, Holt, Rinehart & Winston.

18. Sperber D: *On anthropological knowledge,* Cambridge, Mass, 1987, Cambridge University Press.

19. Levi-Strauss C: *Structural anthropology,* New York, 1960, Basic Books (Translated by C Jacobson and BG Schoepf).

20. Agar M: *Speaking of ethnography,* Newbury Park, Calif, 1986, Sage.

21. Geertz C: *The interpretation of cultures: selected essays,* New York, 1973, Basic Books.

22. Glaser B, Strauss A: *The discovery of grounded theory,* New York, 1967, Aldine.

23. Bogden RC, Biklen SN: *Qualitative research for education,* Boston, 1992, Allyn Bacon.

24. Lofland J, Lofland L: *Analyzing social settings: a guide to qualitative observation and analysis,* ed 2, Belmont, Calif, 1984, Wadsworth.

25. Ulichny P: When critical ethnography and action collide, *Qualitative Inquiry* 3(2):139-168, 1997.

26. Gubrium J, Holstein J: Biographical work and new ethnography. In Josselson R, Lieblich A, editors: *Interpreting experience: the narrative study of lives,* Thousand Oaks, Calif, 1995, Sage.

27. Agar, MH: *The professional stranger:* an informal introduction to ethnography, ed 2, San Diego, 1996, Academic Press.

28. Savishinsky JS: *The ends of time: life and work in a nursing home,* New York, 1991, Bergen & Garvey.

29. Seale C: Resurrective practice and narrative. In Andrews M et al, editors: *Lines of narrative,* London, 2000, Routledge.

30. Center for Narrative Research. http://www.uel.ac.uk/cnr/index.htm

31. Ryan ML: On defining narrative media, *Image Narrative* 6, 2003.

32. Silverman D: *Doing qualitative research: a practical handbook,* ed 2, Thousand Oaks, Calif, 2004, Sage.

33. Abell J, Stokoe E, Billig M: Narrative and the discursive (re)construction of events. In Andrews M et al, editors: *Lines of narrative,* London, 2000, Routledge.

34. Squire C, Centre for Narrative Research, School of Social Sciences, University of East London, 2004.

35. Crossley M: *Introducing narrative psychology: self, trauma and the construction of meaning,* Buckinghamshire, UK, 2000, Open University Press.

36. Labov W, Fanshel D: *Therapeutic discourse: psychotherapy as conversation,* New York, 1977, Academic Press.

37. Bell S: Photo images: Jo Spence's narratives of living with illness, *Health* 6(1):5-30, 2002.

38. Bochner AP, Ellis C: *Ethnographically speaking,* Lanham, Md, 2002, Rowman and Littlefield.

39. Patterson W, editor: *Strategic narrative,* New York, 2002, Lexington.

40. Labov W, Waletsky J: Narrative analysis. In Helm J, editor: *Essays on the verbal and visual arts,* Seattle, 1967, University of Washington Press.

41. Rabin AI et al: *Studying persons and lives,* New York, 1990, Springer-Verlag.

42. Mkhonza S: Life histories as social texts of personal experiences in sociolinguistic studies: a look at the lives of domestic workers in Swaziland. In Josselson R, Lieblich A, editors: *Interpreting experience: the narrative study of lives,* Newbury Park, Calif, 1995, Sage.

43. Frank G: Life history model of adaptation to disability: the case of a congenital amputee, *Soc Sci Med* 19:639-645, 1984.

44. Strauss A, Corbin J: *Basics of qualitative research: techniques and procedures for developing grounded theory,* Thousand Oaks, Calif, 1998, Sage.

45. Butler S: *Homeless women,* Seattle, 1991, University of Washington (unpublished dissertation).

46. Basu A: *How to conduct a meta-analysis,* http://www.pitt.edu/~super1/lecture/lec1171/001.htm.

47. Potts A et al: Qualitative meta-analysis for social justice: the creation of an on-line diversity resources database, Social Information Technology Teacher Education International Conference, 2004, pp 832-836; http://dl.aace.org/14388.

48. Noblitt GW, Hare RD: *Meta-ethnography: synthesizing qualitative studies,* Newbury Park, Calif, 1988, Sage.

49. Qual-Quan Evidence Synthesis Group: http://www.prw.le.ac.uk/research/qualquan/publications.htm.

PART IV Action Processes

Now that you have grasped the vocabulary and general thinking processes across the research traditions, we are ready for action. In Part IV we focus on the way in which researchers implement, or put into action, their design strategies. Each chapter introduces specific research action processes of naturalistic inquiry and experimental-type research. You will learn diverse and varied ways to put into action the following four processes:

1. Bounding your study and obtaining individuals, concepts, or other phenomena to study (Chapters 11 through 14).
2. Collecting information or data using a range of strategies (Chapters 15 to 17).
3. Analyzing and interpreting information or data (Chapters 18 to 20).
4. Reporting and using information and conclusions (Chapters 21 and 22).

As you read about each action process, keep in mind that five factors affect the selection of an action process, as follows:

1. Philosophical or epistemological framework of the research
2. Investigator's specific research purpose
3. Nature of the research question or query
4. Particular type of design
5. Resources available and practical limitations or challenges of the environment in which the research occurs

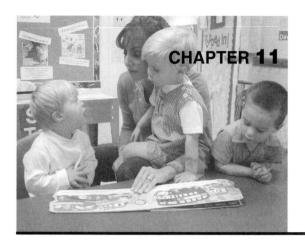

Setting the Boundaries of a Study

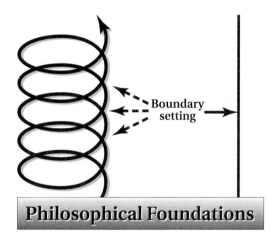

Philosophical Foundations

Assume that you have a research problem and an appropriate design that matches your research purpose and question or query. You are now ready to consider how individuals will be selected for your study and how particular concepts or phenomena will be defined and identified. Selecting research participants and identifying concepts and phenomena represent one of the first action processes that set or establish the boundaries or limitations of a study.

Setting boundaries is inextricably linked to important ethical considerations, such as how people are selected for study participation, how they are informed of study procedures, and how the information they share is managed and treated confidentially. Because of the significance of the ethical component of boundary setting, we examine this in depth in Chapter 12.

WHY SET BOUNDARIES TO A STUDY?

Setting limits or boundaries as to what and who will be in a study is an action that occurs in every type of research design, whether in the experimental-type or the naturalistic tradition. A researcher sets boundaries that limit the scope of the investigation to a specified group of individuals, phenomena, or set of conceptual dimensions. The following example helps show why it is important to set boundaries or limitations.

Consider a study that uses a survey design to describe the health and social service needs of "parents of children with disabilities." It would be impossible to interview every person who falls into this category in the United States. As the researcher, you need to make some decisions as to who you should specifically interview and how. One consideration may be to limit the survey to one or more particular geographical locations. Another way of limiting the study may be to consider only certain types of disabling conditions. Limiting the number of parents of children with disabilities who are selected for study participation is an example of setting a boundary by restricting the characteristics of the persons who will be studied.

Studies are also necessarily limited or bounded by identifying particular data collection strategies and concepts that will be considered.

Assume you are interested in the historical development of the profession of physical therapy. It would not be feasible to examine every historical detail or written document to understand the sociopolitical and health care context of professional growth of physical therapy. In this case, you need to determine criteria for selecting historical documents to examine and identify the key historical events in which professional activity emerged. Deciding which historical documents to examine is an example of limiting your study by specifying the boundaries of the concept and time period that will be explored.

There are numerous ways to limit the scope of a study. As discussed in previous chapters on the thinking processes of research, an investigator actively bounds a study based on five interrelated considerations (Box 11-1).

Your philosophical approach or the particular research tradition you are using to develop your study will set the backdrop from which all action decisions will be made. A deductive, experimental-type study tightly bounds the study to preidentified concepts

---

BOX 11-1
CONSIDERATIONS IN SETTING STUDY BOUNDARIES

1. Researcher's philosophical framework
2. Study purpose
3. Research question
4. Research design
5. Access to the object(s) of inquiry (participants), investigator's time frame, and monetary limitations

---

and a highly specified population. The purpose of the study, the particular research question, and the design will also shape the extent to which concepts, phenomena, and populations are delimited.

For example, an intervention study that tests the effectiveness of a particular home care service in producing a specified outcome must carefully match the intent of the intervention with specific characteristics of the subject group or individuals who will be targeted and recruited for the study. Thus, identifying highly specified criteria as to who is eligible and who is not eligible to participate is a required action process. These criteria are referred to as "inclusion and exclusion criteria," as discussed later.

On the other hand, a broad inquiry designed to investigate the experiences of caring for persons with acquired immunodeficiency syndrome (AIDS) may set few restrictions as to who can participate in the study and thus cast a wide net for participant enrollment.

Finally, your ability to access the population of interest or the phenomenon to be studied is another consideration as to how a study is bounded. Limited resources, such as monetary and time restrictions, will likely yield a study design that is tightly delimited or bounded.

Thus, there are both practical and theoretical considerations in how researchers bound the context of either an experimental-type or a naturalistic form of inquiry. In practical terms, it would be impossible to observe every speech event, personal interaction, or activity in a particular natural setting. You must bound the study by making purposeful selections as to what will be observed and who will be interviewed.[1,2]

In experimental-type designs, *boundary setting* is a process that must occur before entering the field or beginning the study. Boundaries are set in three ways: (1) specifying the concepts that will be operationally defined, (2) establishing inclusion and exclusion criteria that define the population that will be studied, and (3) developing a sampling plan.

This set of action processes is in contrast to naturalistic designs, in which boundary setting occurs throughout the research endeavor. Initial boundaries are set by the investigator through defining the particular domain of interest and the point of access from which to enter that domain.

> This domain may be (1) geographical, as in the selection of an urban community in which to study health behaviors of low-income families; (2) a group of individuals, such as the selection of persons with a particular health condition (e.g., stroke, diabetes, traumatic brain injury), living in an identified community; or (3) a particular experience, such as trauma, dialysis, caregiving, pain, or chronic health problems.

Next, within the context of the defined domain, a selection process then occurs as to who should be interviewed and when, what scenes or events to observe, and which materials or artifacts to review. This selection process occurs or unfolds in the course of performing fieldwork and comprises important boundary-making decisions. Setting boundaries in most forms of naturalistic inquiry is therefore an ongoing process that moves the researcher from a broad stance to a more narrow focus. The actions of data collection, analysis, and further data collection (see Chapters 17 and 18) can be understood as a process of redefining and refining the boundaries of the phenomenon being studied.

IMPLICATIONS OF BOUNDARY SETTING

Bounding a study is a purposeful action process in both research traditions. That is, boundary setting involves making conscious decisions based on a sound rationale that can be documented or articulated to the larger scientific community. The inclusion or exclusion of people, concepts, events, or other phenomena has considerable implications for knowledge development and its translation or use in professional practice. As you make decisions about how to bound

your study and then actively set limits, you must reflect on your actions and understand the implications of each boundary-making decision.

One of the most important consequences of the bounding actions taken by researchers is what can ultimately be concluded (or not) about the phenomenon of interest and the group studied. The ability to generalize from a study sample to the population from which the sample was derived is referred to as *external validity.*

> Suppose you are interested in studying the adaptive mechanisms used by diverse ethnic groups to manage chronic illness. You need to bound your study to one geographical community, in this case an urban low-income community in northeastern United States. Your findings and interpretations will necessarily be limited to this particular group and may not be valid for the full range of ethnic diversity of groups living in rural and southern communities, where the cultural context and access to health care may significantly differ from that of the study participants.

> Assume an investigator is interested in symptom reporting among older men and women. The exclusion of a particular group of individuals, such as Asian or Hispanic elder persons, or other ethnic groups from study participation will limit the researcher's ability to relate or generalize findings from the study to these other groups. This limitation is a consequence of the way in which the researcher sets the boundaries of the study population at the start of the project.

The same principles hold for defining and operationalizing major constructs.

> If a study focuses on mental health outcomes and operationalizes this as "depressive symptoms," the results are specific to this one dimension and how it is measured in the study. The study results cannot be generalized to other aspects of mental health.

The consequences of boundary setting are often described in a proposal or a research report as "limitations" of the study. As you read research articles in professional journals, take a close look at how authors describe their recruitment process, the inclusion and exclusion criteria that they follow to enroll and engage individuals into the study, and how they define and operationalize primary concepts. Also, carefully read how researchers describe the limitations of their study. Finally, look closely at the discussion section of a published article, where the researcher must vigilanty interpret the findings as they relate to specific populations and concepts. Sometimes you will find that researchers overstate their case or stretch their results to include a broader population or set of constructs than was actually studied. They may assert or imply that their findings are not bounded to the studied population and draw conclusions for a broader band of groups or communities than that which was originally included in the study.

The ways in which studies are bounded have particular significance for translating research findings into the professional arena, particularly for evidence-based practice models, as we describe in Chapter 24. For example, in the clinic setting, it is important to know if a particular technique, treatment modality, or teaching approach is effective in producing a desired outcome for a specific client or patient. If you search the literature to identify the evidence for using a particular treatment, you may find that the published studies involve study participants who may or may not match your clients. You must carefully decide how best to interpret and translate such findings for your particular group. The first step in this translational effort is to recognize the ways in which the studies you have identified are bounded. The second step is to evaluate whether specific characteristics of your group would determine whether the results of the studies are applicable (or not).

Another implication of bounding studies relates to building programs of research. Remember that research involves the incremental construction of knowledge. Each study answers a specified question or query and in turn generates the next steps toward understanding a particular phenomenon. The way in which a study is bounded will have implications for building knowledge and for subsequent research steps.

Substantial evidence suggests that case management helps decrease depression in caregivers of persons with dementia. These studies are bounded in the scope of the intervention and the target population. Research steps then may include (but are not limited to) expanding or adding other components to a case management intervention and evaluating the same intervention with another group of caregivers, such as persons caring for individuals who have had stroke.

SPECIFYING WHO PARTICIPATES AND WHO DOES NOT PARTICIPATE

One of the most important ways a researcher sets limits in a study is determining who will be included as well as who will be excluded from participating in the study. The *inclusion and exclusion criteria* developed by an investigator delimit the population (or group) to whom the study results are directly applicable, reflect the underlying purpose of the research endeavor, and reflect the research question or query.

Experimental-type researchers must establish detailed criteria before recruiting individuals into a study. These criteria are highly specified and are used to identify a population and develop a sampling and recruitment plan.

Assume you are planning a study that reflects a Level 2 question (see Chapter 7). You intend to investigate the level of functional ability in a population of older adults with chronic health conditions and the relationship of their functional ability to depression over two points in time—1 month and 12 months after hospitalization for acute illness. First, the purpose of the study limits the inquiry to examining two concepts, "physical function" and "depression." Second, the purpose also limits the study to examining these concepts in one particular population, specifically "Caucasians with an acute health episode." Your inclusion criteria will specify the age, gender, level of physical function, level of cognitive status, and type of disabling conditions of the participants you seek to involve. Your criteria for excluding people may involve certain health conditions, living arrangements, and geographical locations. For example, you may want to include individuals with a hip fracture but not those who also have terminal cancer or heart disease. You will use both types of criteria, those that include and those that exclude, to establish a plan to sample and recruit individuals into your study. (Chapter 13 describes sampling plans in greater detail.) For the purposes of this example, however, you will use a "sample of convenience." Doing so will involve identifying and recruiting any individual who fits your criteria and who has been discharged from one of three area hospitals.

Your next effort is to determine a way of identifying appropriate study subjects and a mechanism to involve them in your study. You want to ensure that your sampling and recruitment procedures are systematically followed so that bias is not introduced into your study; that is, you want to ensure that every person who is truly eligible for your study has an opportunity to be identified and is asked to participate. One recruitment strategy may involve asking discharge coordinators at each participating hospital to identify and screen individuals as they leave the hospital, using your study criteria. You might develop a simple form that can be easily implemented by the discharge coordinator. For each person identified by the coordinator, you seek permission to contact the person and ask his or her willingness to participate in your study.

This set of steps may sound simple. However, suppose the coordinator is busy one week and is unable to screen patients who are being discharged; or assume the coordinator does not refer some patients who fit the study criteria because they are perceived as uncooperative by staff. Both cases may occur in experimental-type field studies and introduce bias to the recruitment process. Selecting individuals for experimental-type study requires constant vigilance by the investigator over the implementation of these recruitment procedures.

In experimental-type designs, there is a high level of specificity in bounding the study. In contrast, usually only broad inclusion and exclusion guidelines are established before engaging in fieldwork in naturalistic designs. However, the structure and extent to which boundaries are established depend on the particular type of naturalistic design. For example, in a phenomenological study the researcher may bound a study only by identifying the type of experience that is of interest to the researcher. The only criterion for participating in the study may be that an individual has experienced the phenomenon of interest. Other factors, such as age, gender, or ethnicity,

may not be specified or used as criteria to include or exclude individuals from the study. Likewise, in a large-scale ethnography, only the context or natural setting may be initially specified or bounded, whereas the participation of individuals in the natural context may not be restricted, at least initially. In a focused life history, however, individuals who meet specific criteria are selected for study participation, and these criteria are articulated before engaging in fieldwork.

Involving humans in health and social service research and establishing participation criteria have important ethical considerations that must be fully understood and carefully thought out by the researcher. When developing a research study and writing a proposal to carry it out (see Chapter 21), whether of the experimental, naturalistic, or mixed-method type, the researcher must address numerous ethical concerns of involving humans, as examined in Chapter 12.

GENERAL GUIDELINES FOR BOUNDING STUDIES

The extent to which a study is bounded depends on your preferred way of knowing, research purpose, question or query, and practical considerations such as monetary and time constraints. It is important to recognize that there is nothing inherently superior about any one boundary-setting approach. The strengths and limitations of a boundary-setting technique depend on its appropriateness and adequacy in how well it fits the context of the particular research problem.

Appropriateness is defined as the extent to which the method of boundary setting fits the overall purpose of the study, as determined by the research problem, purpose, and the structure of the research design. For example, it would be inappropriate to use a random sampling technique when your purpose is to understand how individuals interpret their experience of illness. In this case, the purposeful selection of individuals who can articulate their feelings may provide greater insight than the inclusion of a sample with predetermined characteristics. Purposeful selection to bound the study facilitates understanding, which is the underlying goal of the study.

Adequacy is defined as the extent to which the boundary setting yields sufficient data to answer the research problem. In experimental-type designs, adequacy is determined by sample size and composition. In naturalistic designs, adequacy is determined by the quality and completeness of the information and the understanding that is obtained in the selected domain. "Saturation" in the field, such as reaching a point in the inquiry in which no new information is obtained, is one important cue that the boundary has been met and the investigator has achieved a complete understanding of the identified context.

Thus, appropriateness and adequacy are two criteria that can be applied to boundary-setting decisions.

Subjects, Respondents, Informants, or Participants

Are individuals who are involved in a study the subjects, respondents, informants, or participants?[3] These four terms refer to the individuals who agree to become part of a research study. Each term reflects a different way that an individual participates in a research study and a different type of relationship that is formed between the individual and the investigator.

In experimental-type research, individuals are usually referred to as *subjects,* a term that denotes their passive role and the attempt of the investigator to maintain a removed and objective relationship. In survey research, individuals are often referred to as *respondents* because they are asked to respond to very specific questions. In naturalistic inquiry, individuals are usually referred to as *informants,* a term that reflects the active role of informing the investigator as to the context and its cultural rules. *Participants* can refer to those individuals who enter a collaborative relationship with the investigator, who contribute to decision making about the research process, and who inform the investigator about themselves. This term is often used in endogenous and participatory action research.[4]

Although there are no specific rules to guide the use of these terms, you should select the one that reflects your preferred way of knowing and the role that individuals play in your study design.

SUMMARY

Boundary setting refers to the action process of determining and enacting selection criteria for study participants, study concepts, or study phenomena. Setting boundaries represents one of the first action processes that occurs in experimental-type research. In naturalistic inquiry, boundary setting occurs throughout the data collection and analytical action phases and is an ongoing process.

One crucial way in which studies are bounded is developing inclusion and exclusion criteria for the involvement of human participants. Each tradition handles this action process through different structures and timing sequences.

Given the ethical considerations of working with human subjects in an inquiry, protection from risk is a critical consideration (see Chapter 12).

EXERCISES

1. Identify a research article that tests an experimental intervention. Describe how the authors bound their study with regard to the inclusion and exclusion criteria and recruitment procedures. Identify specific limitations to generalizability of their study given how it was bounded.
2. Identify a research article that reports findings from an ethnographical study. Describe how the authors bound their study. Identify specific boundary scope, strengths, and limitations.

REFERENCES

1. Agar MH: *The professional stranger: an informal introduction to ethnography,* ed 2, San Diego, 1996, Academic Press.
2. Rubin HJ, Rubin IS: *Qualitative interviewing: the art of hearing data,* Thousand Oaks, Calif, 1995, Sage.
3. Subjects, respondents, informants and participants, *Qualitative Health Res* 1:403-406, 1991 (editorial).
4. Reason P, Bradbury H: *Handbook of action research,* Thousand Oaks, Calif, 2001, Sage.

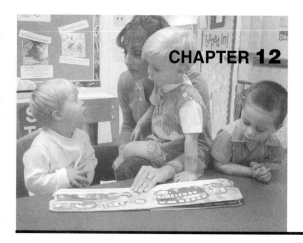

CHAPTER 12

Protecting the Boundaries

KEY TERMS

Assent

Confidentiality

Data and safety monitoring board (DSMB)

Full disclosure

Health Insurance Portability and Accountability Act (HIPAA)

Human subject protection

Informed consent

Institutional review board (IRB)

Voluntary participation

Vulnerable populations

CHAPTER OUTLINE

Health and human service professionals most frequently set boundaries through sampling plans that involve human subjects. Therefore the researcher must follow important ethical considerations and legally binding actions. The basic ethical principle that underlies boundary setting of human subjects in each of the research traditions is that the researcher is obligated to ensure the protection of human subjects.

What do we mean by "the protection of human subjects"? All research in which people are directly involved has potential risks to its participants, even if such risks are minimal or simply involve momentary discomfort with a personal question on a survey. According to federal law,[1] investigators must submit a plan (proposal) for the ethical conduct of any inquiry involving human subjects to a board or group composed of both lay and scientific representatives. This board is mandated to examine proposals with regard to several critical considerations: (1) the level of risk posed to study participants and relationship of risk to potential benefits to society; (2) the adequacy of plan to provide participants with the necessary knowledge about study procedures, risks, and benefits, referred to as "full disclosure"; (3) the plan for ensuring that study participation and all procedures are voluntary; and (4) the plan for ensuring confidentiality.

Large institutions such as hospitals and universities have formal committees, usually called institutional review boards (IRBs). In smaller agencies, review boards may be *ad hoc* committees (with a particular purpose). Regardless of where you are conducting an inquiry, however, you must seek a human subjects review to protect those who are devoting time and effort as participants in your study. Also, if you obtain funding for your research, you will not be allowed to conduct the study until such a review has been conducted and approval obtained. Even if you are conducting a small or pilot-level research study, such as for a research class, you must seek IRB approval. IRBs are the main mechanisms by which protection strategies are reviewed and monitored in the conduct of any type of research study.

PRINCIPLES FOR PROTECTING HUMAN SUBJECTS

Human subject protection is based on three primary principles: full disclosure, confidentiality, and voluntary participation (Box 12-1). All investigators, regardless of the scope or type of research, must follow these principles.

Full Disclosure

Any person who participates in a study, whether participatory action research, single-subject design, or randomized trial, has the absolute right to full disclosure of the purpose and procedures of the study. *Full disclosure* means that the investigator must clearly share with the informant, subject, or research participant the types and content of interviews, length of time of participation, types and length of observations, and other data collection procedures that will occur, as well as the scope and nature of the person's involvement. Full disclosure also means that any risk to a subject, even if the potential is rare or minimal, must be clearly identified and a plan for remediation offered for each risk to every subject.

Identifying and sharing specific study procedures tend to be straightforward in experimental-type research. However, such disclosure can create difficulties for certain forms of naturalistic inquiry. In an experimental-type study, all the procedures are clearly articulated and determined before entering the field. Therefore the researcher can identify in layperson's terms the purpose and scope of the study and the types of data collection efforts that will

---

BOX 12-1
THREE BASIC ETHICAL CONSIDERATIONS FOR INVOLVING HUMANS IN RESEARCH

- Need for full disclosure of study purpose
- Need to ensure confidentiality of all information obtained
- Need to ensure that study participation is voluntary

---

occur. In naturalistic designs, most bounding-type decisions are made in the field and change or evolve over time as knowledge about the context emerges. Researchers who work in this tradition must solve this dilemma in creative, thoughtful, and ongoing ways. In some studies, it may be necessary to introduce a consenting process for each data collection effort.

Discussion in the research literature is ongoing about effective approaches that investigators can use to remain ethical while preserving the integrity of their methodology. All researchers, regardless of tradition, must struggle over the best way to describe the study truthfully without revealing specific aims or hypotheses or introducing biased perspectives that may shape the informant's responses during the study. For example, although it is necessary to state the overall research objective, it is not appropriate to indicate a directional hypothesis that could influence how an informant responds during an interview.

Full disclosure of study intent and procedures is usually provided when initially enrolling participants into a study and when obtaining informed consent. In addition to consent forms, some investigators also provide an informational sheet to participants as a handy reference that outlines the study purpose and the procedures used. In studies that involve multiple testing occasions, the investigator may restate the study aims at each follow-up to ensure that study participants understand the research procedures and what to expect next.

Confidentiality

The investigator must ensure that all information shared by a respondent in the course of a study is kept confidential. *Confidentiality* means that (1) no person other than specified members of the research team can have access to the respondent's information, unless those who have access to the data are identified to the participants before their participation (usually stated in informed consent), and (2) the information provided by a respondent cannot be linked to the person's identity. This second consideration is especially important in studies that focus on political or sensitive topics, such as AIDS research, teenage pregnancy and birth control use, crime, and drug dealing.

An investigator can ensure confidentiality in several ways. The name of the respondent must be removed from the actual information that is obtained. This procedure ensures that the identity of respondents in your study is protected and that the information they provide will not be linked to their names in the future. One typical way to protect a study participant's identity is the assignment of identification numbers. However, this action presents some difficulty for studies that primarily use observation as the principal data collection effort. Also, ensuring confidentiality can be difficult when using audio and video recordings as data collection sources. In these instances the investigator does not usually transcribe names that are recorded. The researcher would more likely establish procedures for coding and storing digital data in locked filing cabinets or offices with restricted access, as well as destroying electronic copies at the conclusion of the study.

Confidentiality of research participants must also be protected when results are reported. In reporting findings from a case study or naturalistic design, the names of individuals and key identifying information are modified so that there is no direct link between the person's identity and the information the person provides. Most experimental-type studies report findings that reflect summative scores or outcomes of an aggregate of individuals, which makes ensuring confidentiality less challenging in this research tradition than in naturalistic inquiry.

Researchers who investigate controversial topics must carefully plan how information will be stored and reported. Studies about HIV, sexual activity, drug trafficking, and substance abuse may obtain information of interest to the legal system. Investigators can refuse to turn over documentation but risk being called into court to testify.

Recent federal regulations such as the *Health Insurance Portability and Accountability Act (HIPAA)* also impose confidentiality rules and restrictions on research activity. HIPAA requires that all health-related information obtained in the course of a study be "deidentified" such that it is not possible to link a person's name to the health information provided. HIPAA also requires that any health information that is shared in the course of a study be documented in the informed consent form that is signed by a participant before entering a study. Furthermore, under HIPAA, researchers are not legally permitted to contact individuals about a study unless that person has given prior permission for such contact to be made. To abide by this regulation, many clinical sites ask patients or clients to sign a form that indicates their willingness to be contacted and informed about a study of potential interest. Researchers are developing similar procedures.

Ensuring confidentiality necessitates that certain office procedures be established. First, written personal identifying information concerning study participants is kept to a minimum. A master list of study participants that includes the assigned identification number (ID#), first and last names, and necessary group designations (e.g., control vs. experimental group) is maintained for tracking purposes on computers and is password protected; hard copies are kept in locked filing cabinets separate from the actual information obtained. In many studies, screening forms and interview cover sheets that include identifying information are used. All this information must be considered strictly confidential and also is kept in locked file cabinets separate from study data. Any information with subject identification that is not needed is shredded.

Second, confidentiality should also be maintained when making telephone contact with study participants or potentially eligible persons. Conversations with or about study participants require common-sense discretion. Attempts to schedule appointments with study participants or telephone conversations discussing issues related to a participant should be conducted in a manner that ensures confidentiality. When talking on the telephone, researchers should keep voices low and should not use last names except as necessary. When possible, they should conduct phone conversations behind closed office doors. If this is not possible, calls can be made when fewer people are in the office or only persons directly involved with the research project are present.

Third, computer files used for tracking study participants can be set up with password protection. Access to such files should be restricted to defined key personnel, and any backup disks must be stored in locked file cabinets.

Fourth, interviewers must be trained and certified in "protection of human subject" procedures before any telephone or face-to-face interviews with study participants. For face-to-face contact, interviewers introduce themselves, explain the study's purpose and procedures, and review the informed consent. Informed consent must be obtained before collecting any study-related information. For telephone interviews, interviewers must obtain verbal *assent,* which is recorded on an institutionally approved form.

Voluntary Participation

When humans are involved in studies, their participation must be strictly voluntary. Individuals have the right to choose to participate or not. Also, an individual who initially agrees to participate in a study has the right to withdraw from the study at any point and the right to refuse to answer a particular question or participate in a particular set of procedures. Thus, the voluntary quality of participation must be protected at three points in a study: initial enrollment, continuation in the study, and right to refuse answering specific questions or a particular study procedure. To ensure *voluntary participation* at each of these points, investigators must develop approaches to recruiting participants that are not coercive and that provide full disclosure of all study procedures.

Although a person may refuse to participate in a study or one of its procedures, it is important for the investigator to understand why refusals occur. Is withdrawal caused by the nature of the procedures, or by excessive demands placed on participants? Is the research team offensive in any way? Is withdrawal based on a change in the health status of the participants or their relocation to another geographical region? Reasons for refusal to participate in a study, withdrawal from a study as a participant, or refusal to answer a particular question may have implications for the

ethical conduct of the study, interpretation of results, and ability to generalize outcomes to other groups, as well as planning future studies. As such, it is important to keep track of and evaluate the reasons why study participants withdraw from a study or refuse participation in a study component. This information enables the investigator to refine ethical plans, evaluate if differences exist between those who participate and those who do not, and prepare for future research.

Refusal to answer a particular question (e.g., "what is your yearly income?") or to engage in a particular study component (e.g., allow observation of home interactions) presents a methodological challenge that the investigator must be prepared to meet. Missing information can be a greater problem in experimental-type research than in naturalistic inquiry because missing data limit the types of statistical analysis that can be used and the inferences that can be derived from the data. For example, a common question on survey studies is level of income as one indicator of socioeconomic status. However, participants may refuse to disclose this information. Missing information can be handled in numerous ways, including using the mean value of the group or using a statistical program to assign a value randomly.

Missing information is less problematic in naturalistic studies. The refusal to answer a question may be an indicator of the salience (or importance) of that particular topic or area, and its "missingness" becomes, in essence, a type of meaning that enters into an interpretive scheme. For the naturalistic inquirer, however, missing an observation, such as an important community event, may be more problematic. Adjustments in collecting information may need to occur to overcome this issue, such as prolonging engagement in a particular context or obtaining information about the event from newspaper reports, community meetings, and personal interviews.

BELMONT REPORT

The ethical issues of conducting research have only recently been a focus of national concern. In 1974 the National Research Act created a commission to delineate the ethical issues and guidelines for the involvement of humans in behavioral and biomedical research in the United States.[1] This act and its subsequent activities arose from revelations of the Nuremberg war crime trials about the devastating human experiments conducted by medical scientists during the Holocaust. Other tragic abuses of human subjects involved in research had occurred in the United States as well. Most notably, the Tuskegee experiments in the 1940s involved poor rural black men diagnosed with syphilis from whom investigators withheld known curative treatment to observe the natural course of the disease process.

The resulting Belmont Commission issued a report in 1979 that outlined three basic ethical principles to guide all research activity in order to protect human subjects.[2] The Belmont Report is a brief document that is required reading by all those involved in human subject research. The first ethical principle is the importance of distinguishing the boundaries between research and practice. This differentiation may be more complex in health and human service research than in other types of science research. However, it is important to distinguish between daily or traditional practice versus systematic efforts to evaluate new approaches and service interventions.

The second principle in the Belmont Report describes three areas that must be addressed: respect for persons, beneficence, and justice. The first area, respect, states that individuals should be treated as autonomous individuals who are capable of personal choice and self-determination. A related mandate is that individuals who are not autonomous or who are vulnerable, such as the person with reduced cognitive capacity, must be protected. The second ethical area, beneficence, specifies that research will "do no harm" and will "maximize" benefits and "minimize possible harm" to individuals. The third ethical area, justice, specifies that people should be treated equitably; that is, research that poses a risk should not be conducted on vulnerable populations.

INSTITUTIONAL REVIEW BOARD

Based on the Belmont Report, the involvement of humans in research must be overseen by a government-mandated board of experts that must be established at each institution engaged in the research process. These boards, referred to as *institutional review boards (IRBs)*, are charged with monitoring the

ethical conduct of research as outlined by the Belmont Report. Most academic settings have an IRB, but only a few health and human service settings have established research committees or IRBs. If you are located in a setting that does not have an established board, you may need to form a partnership with a university or hospital that can review your protocol. Some universities have arrangements with community-based agencies and organizations in which they agree to review protocols for a fee. This linkage is particularly important when seeking funding to support your research effort. All federally funded research studies must be approved by an official IRB. In most institutions, however, any research study—funded or not funded, small scale or large scale—must be reviewed by a committee to examine the nature of human involvement.

Before implementing a study, a researcher must write a brief proposal describing in detail the plans for involving humans. This proposal must be submitted for review to a designated office of research or to an IRB (see Chapter 21).

One of the initial determinations that must be made is whether a particular activity can or cannot be classified as research. This is not as straightforward as it may sound, particularly in clinical settings where some clinical activities cross over to become a form of research.

Assume you are a health professional working in a rehabilitation setting, and (1) you read about a new therapeutic technique in the literature and want to evaluate its benefits for your clients, or (2) you want to examine case records to see if you can identify a set of factors that predict rehabilitation improvement. Are these research studies? Would you need to submit these plans to the IRB for review and their approval?

In the first case, assume your clinical department decides to implement this new technique and track patient outcomes. However, the purpose of this activity is clinical, to improve clinical services, and thus it would not be considered research and would not require IRB approval. Suppose, however, that you want to compare outcomes from this new therapeutic approach systematically to traditional care and assign patients to receive the new or typical treatment, aggregate the data, and report the results formally. In this case the activity would be considered research and fall under the purview of the IRB.

In the second example involving a chart extraction activity, given that you plan to review case records systematically and aggregate the data for reporting purposes, you need IRB approval. Since your methodology involves chart extraction and does not require patient contact or disclosure of patient names, you most likely will receive exempt status (see later discussion); this means your study has minimal risks and thus is exempt from continued reporting requirements. Although you are initially obligated to inform the IRB of any research study, if it is designated as exempt by that board, there will be no legal or ethical requirements for annual IRB reports and updates.

Once the IRB determines that the proposal is research and requires a review, its main goal is to evaluate whether the research protocol will adversely affect study participants and whether the research itself justifies the involvement of humans. Also, the IRB evaluates the procedures that will be used to enroll or engage humans in the study to make certain that participation is voluntary, that confidentiality will be ensured, and that there is full disclosure of study procedures.

Assume you are a rehabilitation clinician and plan to evaluate the relationship between client self-report of functional ability and observation of actual performance. You plan to evaluate the clients you see in the rehabilitation setting. Although this idea does not necessarily present ethical challenges, you must carefully consider how you will introduce the study to your clients. Also, you must establish clear boundaries between your clinical efforts and the information you will gather for research purposes. You must set up procedures to ensure that clients understand three points. First, their participation in the study is strictly voluntary; in other words, it is their decision to participate. You must establish procedures to enroll clients that ensure that they do not feel coerced into participating. Second, a decision not to participate will not affect the type and quality of service intervention they will receive. Third, if clients decide to participate, they can choose to discontinue participation at any point in the study with no consequences to them or their ability to receive other medical and social services for which they are eligible.

The IRB will review all study procedures to make certain that they are ethical and not coercive. You will not be able to begin your study until you have received approval from the IRB.

Three Levels of Review

Most IRBs have three levels of review: full, expedited, and exempt. A full board review involves a formal examination of an investigator's research protocol by members who have been officially appointed by an institution. The composition of board members is mandated to include a consumer representative and a member with scientific expertise in the protocols being reviewed. The board can be composed of as many as 20 individuals or as few as five, depending on how the institution has set up its IRB. A study that involves a vulnerable population must receive a full review. *Vulnerable populations* refer to individuals who may not be able to represent themselves or participate in decision making, or who may be at particular risk when participating in a research study (see later discussion). Examples of vulnerable populations are infants, children, pregnant women, prisoners, mentally incompetent individuals, or persons addicted to substances. Additionally, research studies involving human immunodeficiency virus (HIV) testing, acquired immunodeficiency syndrome (AIDS), investigational drugs, or medical devices also require a full board review. In a full board review, all members read the research protocol, discuss its merits and weaknesses, and vote to either approve (with changes or no changes to recruitment and consent procedures) or disapprove it.

An expedited review involves an evaluation of a research protocol by a subcommittee selected from the full IRB membership. Studies that receive an expedited review do not involve vulnerable populations and do not test invasive techniques, and they represent minimal risk to individual participants. Studies that can have an expedited review include those that collect data from individuals who are 18 years of age or older using noninvasive procedures routinely used in practice, studies that use existing data, and research on group behavior in which the investigator is not manipulating behavior. The previous example of the study in rehabilitation is appropriate for an expedited review.

Exempt status means that a study protocol is exempt from formal review from either the full board or its subcommittee. Although it is necessary to inform the IRB of the intent to conduct the research, the IRB will send a letter of approval of its exempt status and indicate that no future or annual review is necessary. Studies that are exempt from formal review procedures include those involving normal educational practices or the use of educational tests, as well as research involving the collection or study of existing data, documents, and records, provided these sources are publicly available or the information is recorded so that the individuals cannot be identified. An example of the latter situation is a retrospective study involving chart review or hospital census data from the last 10 years of individuals who experienced strokes and their level of functional status at discharge.

In submitting a proposal to an IRB, you must write a brief paragraph addressing each of six considerations (Box 12-2). Although the actual format of a proposal submission to an IRB may differ across institutions, these six points are standard.

INFORMED CONSENT PROCESS

The principles outlined in the Belmont Report are applied to the conduct of research through the

---

> **BOX 12-2**
> **SIX AREAS THAT MUST BE ADDRESSED IN AN IRB PROPOSAL**
>
> 1. Describe the characteristics of the humans who will participate in the study.
> 2. Describe any potential risks and benefits of study participation.
> 3. Describe procedures to ensure confidentiality.
> 4. Describe data collection sources and procedures.
> 5. Describe plans for recruitment and procedures for obtaining informed consent.
> 6. Describe procedures for protecting against or minimizing potential risks.

> **BOX 12-3**
> **TYPICAL ELEMENTS OF INFORMED CONSENT**
>
> ■ Statement of purpose of study in layperson's terms
> ■ Description of study procedures (e.g., number and length of interviews)
> ■ Disclosure of any risks or discomforts from study participation
> ■ Statement describing how confidentiality will be ensured
> ■ HIPAA disclosures
> ■ Statement describing right of refusal and voluntary consent
> ■ Description of benefits of participation
> ■ Signatures of study participant, interviewer, and researcher
> ■ Name of institute and telephone number of investigator

---

informed consent process. *Informed consent* is the process by which potential study participants are informed of the study and its participation requirements. It usually takes the form of an official written document developed by the researcher that informs study participants of the purpose and scope of the study. Although the specific wording and format of informed consent forms vary widely across institutions, they must contain the basic elements listed in Box 12-3.

Important elements of informed consent include a description of the procedures in which you are asking the person to participate and your assurance that participation is voluntary. Also, you need to specify whether participation in the study carries any known risks, and if so, what these risks are and what measures should be taken if they occur. In proposing a study, you need to consider the elements to include in your informed consent and the procedures you will use to introduce it to study participants. A consent form must be read before collecting any information from a person. Usually the participant, the interviewer, and the principal investigator sign the form, and a copy is made for the participant to keep.

A written consent is not required for every type of study. For example, in conducting a mail survey, the act of returning the survey to the investigator is considered an indication of the respondent's consent to participate. Likewise, in a telephone survey, the act of agreeing to answer questions over the telephone is a sign of volunteering or assenting to the study.

Obtaining consent from participants, whether written or assent through verbal acknowledgment, is somewhat straightforward in experimental-type research that involves individuals who are not cognitively impaired. The researcher knows exactly who is eligible to participate in the study and can review informed consent before asking a set of standardized questions. It can be more difficult in naturalistic inquiry, especially when data collection involves observing different events where you cannot predict who will be attending or involved in the setting. Researchers using a naturalistic approach must be creative and thoughtful as to the best and most ethical way of handling consent.

The research of Bluebond-Langer,[3] a medical anthropologist, illustrates the different approaches ethnographers must consider in addressing ethical dilemmas.

Several different procedures were used for obtaining consent in a study of children dying with leukemia and their parents. The study posed several challenges. First, it involved a vulnerable, protected population—children. Second, it involved data collection over time at different sites, in the physician's office, clinical settings, and hospitals. Third, it involved children who were dying and parents who were grieving. Bluebond-Langer first obtained consent from the parents by approaching them during their visits to the clinic. When she observed the same families admitting their children to the hospital, she reintroduced the study. Any parent who appeared uncomfortable or told someone else that he or she would rather not participate was dropped from the study. As the author describes, "I would never take any statement of consent as final, since I felt that the parents needed a way of getting out of the study any time they desired."[3] She also sought assent from the child by asking each for permission to speak with him or her about thoughts and feelings each time she approached him or her. These procedures not only ensured protection of participants but it also led the children and their parents to trust the researcher. She believed that mutual trust and understanding were established very early in the study and were constantly reinforced.

As stated by the Office of Human Subjects Research (OHSR) of the National Institutes of Health, informed consent is best conceptualized as a process:

Informed consent is a process, not just a form. Information must be presented to enable persons to voluntarily decide whether or not to participate as a research subject. It is a fundamental mechanism to ensure respect for persons through provision of thoughtful consent for a voluntary act. The procedures used in obtaining informed consent should be designed to educate the subject population in terms that they can understand. Therefore, informed consent language and its documentation (especially explanation of the study's purpose, duration, experimental procedures, alternatives, risks, and benefits) must be written in "lay language" (i.e., understandable to the people being asked to participate). The written presentation of information is used to document the basis for consent and for the subjects' future reference. The consent document should be revised when deficiencies are noted or when additional information will improve the consent process.

Use of the first person (e.g., "I understand that. . .") can be interpreted as suggestive, may be relied upon as a substitute for sufficient factual information, and can constitute coercive influence over a subject. Use of scientific jargon and legalese is not appropriate. Think of the document primarily as a teaching tool, not as a legal instrument.[4]

To fully understand the significance of informed consent and its pivotal role in the bounding processes of research, access the OHSR website. Also, samples of consent forms from our own research are provided in Appendix A. Although these consents contain the basic elements, each institution requires slightly different wording and approaches.

STUDY APPROVAL AND MONITORING

Once you have submitted a proposal and a sample consent form and obtained IRB review, you will receive a letter indicating that your research protocol has been approved as submitted, conditionally approved, or not approved. Conditional approval indicates that the IRB will provide final approval once specific issues are clarified and elements of the consent are modified. However, an investigator cannot begin a study until final approval is obtained. If your study is not approved, you must carefully consider why and what types of changes are necessary.

In addition to receiving an approval letter, you will also be provided with your original informed consent document with a stamped date at the bottom of the page indicating when IRB approval was granted and the date that approval will expire. You must use only current, dated consent forms. Each year, a report must be submitted to the IRB indicating the number of study participants who have been enrolled, adverse events, and general study progress. Each year, the IRB will restamp a consent form with the current date. The dated consent document ensures that only the current, IRB-approved informed consent documents are presented to study participants. It also serves as a reminder to investigators of the need for continuing review.

Each subsequent year, you will be required to submit a brief annual report updating the IRB as to the number of subjects enrolled and any changes in protocol and level of risk. Additionally, adverse events related to study treatments must be reported to the IRB within 24 hours, then summarized at the annual reporting period.

DEVELOPING AN INFORMED CONSENT DOCUMENT

Guidelines for developing the informed consent document reflect the ethical framework established by the Belmont Report. First, the consent should be written at a sixth-grade to eighth-grade level to ensure that persons with different levels of literacy can fully understand the research process in which they are being asked to participate. Second, familiar words should be used throughout the consent. Scientific jargon, including medical and legal terms, should be avoided. For example, using the term "cholesterol" is preferable to "blood lipids"; and when indicating "random assignment," explain that assignment will be determined "by chance." If a scientific or medical term must be used, be sure to define it. Avoid the use of abbreviations and acronyms.

It is critical that all persons be given the opportunity to participate in the research process. You need to consider different strategies for involving persons with low literacy so that they can understand your study procedures and participate in an informed way. For persons with low cognitive capacity as well, approaches can be used to ensure their understanding of the research process. Different approaches may be necessary to be inclusive for different study populations. For example, you might develop an explanation of your study, with its risks, benefits, and confidentiality procedures, that can be translated into pictures, languages other than English, or Braille if necessary, depending on the target group. The point is that you must consider the characteristics of your target study population and how best to ensure informed participation.

INVOLVING VULNERABLE POPULATIONS

The involvement of vulnerable persons remains a widely discussed and debated issue in research. As noted earlier, vulnerable populations refer to a wide range of persons who may be at risk to research because of not only their intrinsic characteristics, but also their life situation or circumstance. For example, persons may be vulnerable because of a medical condition (e.g., terminal illness), a particular setting (e.g., emergency room of hospital, homeless shelter, prison), a baseline limitation of intellectual function (e.g., developmental disability), a psychosocial stressor (e.g., posttraumatic stress disorder), or an illness that compromises comprehension and decision-making abilities (e.g., dementia).[5]

The concern with involving vulnerable persons is twofold. First, no ethical justification exists for excluding vulnerable populations. In fact, it is unethical to exclude such populations from research in that their exclusion restricts knowledge development in areas that would ultimately benefit that group. Vulnerable populations are typically underrepresented in studies, and it is usually not possible to generalize research findings to the group. A second concern is determining the best way to involve vulnerable populations. Here the investigator must strike a balance between not excluding a particular study group who is vulnerable and avoiding inducement.

Consider how pharmacological studies that use monetary inducements for participation may be particularly attractive to individuals rendered vulnerable because of their life circumstances, such as persons who are homeless or live in prison.[6] Participating in a study based on a hefty monetary inducement, however, may not be in the best interest of these groups.

A related issue is how best to apprise persons with compromised decision-making abilities about the procedures of a study so that they can make an informed decision to participate or not. Remember that an essential principle established in the Belmont Report and overseen by IRBs is that persons must be fully informed before agreeing to participate in a study. For persons with dementia and other populations with impaired comprehension and judgment, how can we be assured that these groups willingly and knowingly agree to participate in a study?

The research community is just beginning to address this important issue and develop tools that can reliably and validly distinguish between persons who can make a judgment regarding their participation and those for whom proxy consent is necessary.[7] For example, persons at the early stages of dementia may be capable of comprehending a typical informed consent written document, whereas persons at the moderate stage may not fully understand what they are committing to in the study. In persons unable to provide their own consent, consent from a legal guardian or family caregiver can be obtained. Even when proxy consent is obtained, however, before administering a test, interview, or any type of procedure, the person with dementia should be provided a brief explanation, and assent should be obtained (e.g., "Hello Mr. Smith, I am going to ask you a few questions; is that okay?").

Although simplifying the language of an informed consent may be helpful for some groups with compromised intellect or decision making, use of pictorial or other visual representations of study procedures may be useful for other populations. Knowing exactly the most effective way to present informed consent can be difficult and only now is becoming the focus of research.

Suppose you want to conduct a study of the quality of life of persons with developmental disabilities living in a group home. You want to include persons living in the group home who have a wide range of capabilities. In this case, your presentation of informed consent may need to be tailored to match persons at different levels of intellectual and cognitive abilities. However, there is no standardized approach to do this, or even to determine how to identify what type of approach a person may need to become fully informed.

Despite the difficulties and challenges of involving vulnerable populations, the scientific community must be committed to develop meaningful approaches that can appropriately involve such populations. Remember that these populations are vulnerable only because of our lack of knowledge and expertise about their involvement in research and their prior exploitation in the research enterprise.

SPECIALIZED OVERSIGHT OF EXPERIMENTAL-TYPE DESIGNS

The true-experimental design, often referred to as a "randomized controlled trial," requires a specialized level of human subject oversight in addition to IRB review. Given that such trials test the efficacy of a new technology, behavioral intervention, device, or therapeutic program, there is heightened concern for the safety of study participants in this type of design strategy. Thus, in addition to the IRB, another level of oversight is required to monitor the safety of study participants in randomized trials.

Assume you plan to test an intervention that involves introducing balance and strength exercises to older adults to reduce fear of falling. A potential harmful outcome of the intervention might be muscle strain, back injury, or possibly a fall as a result of increased movement and activity. Thus the study must be monitored for the occurrence of these possible events. The investigator must track the occurrence of such events and determine whether the event is a direct consequence of the intervention.

To monitor the safety of participants in randomized trials, the investigator is responsible for establishing an independent group of experts as a *data and safety monitoring board (DSMB)*. The extent of involvement of a DSMB in oversight of a study depends on the level of risk associated with the treatment and study procedures. Studies that place participants at high risk require greater monitoring, whereas studies with minimal risk require less oversight.

Regardless of risk level, the primary responsibilities of a DSMB are (1) to review and approve all study procedures; (2) to provide oversight for procedures regarding the safety of human subjects and ethical research practices, including reviewing the investigator's approach to recruitment and the informed consent process; and (3) to determine if and when a study should be terminated because of adverse events that can be attributed to study procedures.

The requirement for DSMB monitoring recently has expanded beyond pharmaceutical research to include behavioral treatments. Some institutions have created a DSMB to serve as a monitoring group for all clinical trials conducted at that setting. In most institutions, however, the investigator is responsible for establishing a committee composed of persons who have expertise in randomized trials and in the specific content of the treatment and who are not involved with members of the research team such that the potential exists for a conflict of interest.

It is important to recognize that even a controlled trial with minimal risk, such as testing a telephone information service to homebound patients, necessitates careful oversight to ensure human subject protection and ethical research practices. The DSMB can be a helpful mechanism for providing feedback and recommendations to the investigative team to enhance study rigor. Search the Internet for DSMBs to see how they function at different institutions. You will find a wide range of approaches, although all cover the essentials of safety monitoring and human subject protection oversight.[8]

SUMMARY

It is your obligation as a researcher to design protection protocols so that all populations, regardless of literacy level or physical or cognitive capacity, can engage in the research process in a fully informed and ethical way. This is both an ethical and a legal obligation of researchers working in any research tradition involving human subjects. Before engaging in any type of research, you must submit a proposal to the IRB for review and approval. If a written consent is necessary, it must contain critical elements describing study procedures, voluntary capacity, risk/benefit ratio, and confidentiality procedures. A current, dated, and stamped consent must be used to enroll study participants. The process of obtaining consent is an essential aspect of bounding one's study.

As in all other thinking and action processes of research, the construction of protection protocols requires careful and thoughtful consideration. Unethical or inappropriate research harms not only study participants, but also the target population, society, and the overall research enterprise.

EXERCISES

1. Contact the office of research and obtain consent templates. Propose a study and develop a corresponding consent form. What aspects of the consent form were particularly challenging to develop? What literacy level is the actual template?

2. Role-play the introduction of a consent to a friend or peer. What types of questions does the person ask about the study and informed consent process? How did the informed consent process flow? Do you think the person understood the purpose of the study and the nature of his or her participation?

3. Identify a published study and develop an informed consent document based on the description of the procedures in the article.

4. Identify a particular vulnerable group that you think is important to study. Design a strategy for informing this group about a study.

REFERENCES

1. National Research Act (Public Law 93-348).
2. National Commission for the Protection of Human Subjects of Biomedical and Behavioral Research: *The Belmont Report: ethical principles and guidelines for the protection of human subjects of research*, Washington, DC, 1979, The Commission.
3. Bluebond-Langner M: *The private worlds of dying children*, Princeton, N.J., 1978, Princeton University Press.
4. Office for Protection from Research Risks: *Tips on informed consent*, 1993, US Department of Health and Human Services; http://www.hhs.gov/ohrp/humansubjects/guidance/ictips.htm.

5. Quest T, Marco CA: Ethics seminars: vulnerable populations in emergency medicine research, *Acad Emerg Med* 10:1294-1298, 2003.

6. Beauchamp TL et al: Pharmaceutical research involving the homeless, *J Med Philos* 27:547-564, 2002.

7. Kim SYH et al: Assessing the competence of persons with Alzheimer's disease in providing informed consent for participation in research, *Am J Psychiatry* 158:712-717, 2001.

8. Ellenberg SS, Fleming TR, DeMets DL: *Data monitoring committees in clinical trials: a practical perspective*, England, 2003, Wiley & Sons.

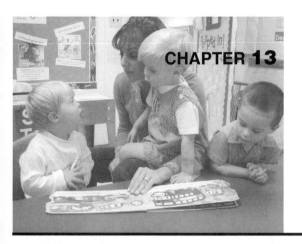

CHAPTER 13

Boundary Setting in Experimental-Type Designs

KEY TERMS

Cluster sampling
Convenience sampling
Effect size
External validity
Nonprobability sampling
Population
Probability sampling
Purposive sampling
Quota sampling
Sample
Sampling
Sampling error
Sampling frame
Simple random sampling
Snowball sampling
Statistical power
Stratified random sampling
Systematic sampling
Target population

Snowball Sampling
Quota Sampling
Comparing Sample to Population
Determining Sample Size
Summary

CHAPTER OUTLINE

Sampling Process
Probability Sampling
   Simple Random Sampling
   Systematic Sampling
   Stratified Random Sampling
   Cluster Sampling
Nonprobability Methods
   Convenience Sampling
   Purposive Sampling

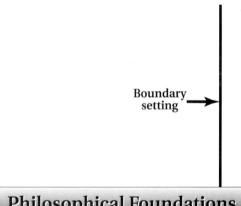

Boundary setting →

Philosophical Foundations

As discussed in Chapter 11, setting boundaries in experimental-type designs is one of the first action processes that occurs. Think about what you have learned thus far about experimental-type designs. What do you think are the characteristics of the process of setting boundaries in this research tradition? If you said the process is primarily deductive, prescribed, and determined before entering the field, you are correct.

Now, think about what would be the primary concern in setting boundaries in experimental-type research. The primary aim of boundary setting is to select a group of study participants or subjects who adequately represent the population that is the target of the study. This is a critical point on which all boundary-setting procedures are based in this research tradition. Now we examine how researchers who use the range of experimental-type designs actually approach the action process of selecting people, groups, or other entities for study participation.

In experimental-type design, the boundary-setting action process is basically deductive. This means that first, the researcher begins with a clear idea of what or whom he or she wants to study. The study group of interest to the investigator is called a *population,* defined as a group of persons, elements, or both that share a set of common characteristics as predefined by the investigator. The researcher must clearly define the characteristics of the population, which includes the individuals or units to be studied. Second, the researcher chooses a set of procedures by which to select a subset or sample from the population who will participate in the study. The individuals or units from the population who actually participate in the study are called a *sample,* which is a subset of the population. The process of selecting a subgroup or sample is called *sampling.*

SAMPLING PROCESS

The main purpose of sampling is to select a subgroup that can accurately represent the population. The intent is to be able to draw accurate conclusions about the population by studying a smaller group of elements (sample). The problem for the experimental-type researcher is how best to select a sample that is representative of an entire population. Accurate representation is critical to allow findings from the study sample to be generalized to the larger group (population) from which the sample is drawn.[1,2]

Sampling designs or procedures have been developed to increase the chances of selecting individuals or elements that will be most representative of the larger population from which they are drawn. The

---

BOX 13-1
FIVE STEPS IN EXPERIMENTAL-TYPE SAMPLING

1. Define population by specifying criteria
   a. Inclusion criteria
   b. Exclusion criteria
2. Develop sampling plan
   a. Probability
   b. Nonprobability
3. Determine sample size
4. Implement sampling procedures
5. Compare critical values of sample to population

---

more representative the sample, the more assured the researcher will be that the findings from the sample also apply to the population. The extent to which findings from a sample apply to the population is called *external validity,* as discussed in Chapter 11. Most researchers conducting experimental-type designs attempt to maximize external validity by using one of the sampling procedures discussed in this chapter.

Investigators follow many different action processes to draw a sample from a population. In this chapter, we discuss five basic steps common to the various experimental-type sampling processes (Box 13-1).

The first step in sampling involves the careful definition of a population. As defined earlier, a population is the complete set of elements that share a common set of characteristics and do not possess any characteristics identified by the researcher as "not to be included." Examples of elements are persons, households, communities, hospitals, and outpatient settings. The "element" is the unit of analysis included in the population, regardless of its type.

In a study of the management practices of hospitals, the investigator would be interested in the hospital as a whole, rather than the people in it. In this case the hospital is the unit of analysis, and the sample is the specified number of hospitals participating in the study. However, in a study of the characteristics of older persons admitted to hospitals in the summer months, each patient, not the hospital as a whole, is the unit of analysis, and the sample is composed of the set of individuals selected for the study.

New investigators often ask how populations are identified and delimited. In experimental-type design, two issues are important to consider: (1) the purpose of the study and (2) the literature support for selecting or excluding population parameters. Thus, it is the investigator who uses previous work and a purposive lens to define or choose the characteristics or parameters of the population that are important to study. Consider the following two examples.

> You are interested in studying the needs of parents caring for children with chronic illness. The first step in selecting your study sample would be to identify the specific characteristics of the larger population you are interested in examining. To identify population characteristics, you will need to identify the purpose of your inquiry and then consult the literature to see how other investigators have conceptualized the important population characteristics that need to be included and excluded.

> You are conducting a needs assessment study as the basis for implementing a hospital-based transition intervention to assist parents of children with cystic fibrosis in their parenting. Because of the hospital policy regarding the age range of children in their cystic fibrosis unit, you decide to include parents caring for children between ages 3 and 8 years who have been diagnosed. Based on the literature, you may also decide to exclude cases in which both parents do not reside together, both are unemployed, or more than one other sibling is in the home. By establishing these inclusion and exclusion criteria, you will have defined a target population from the universe of parents caring for a child with a chronic illness.

In some cases the target population is an "ideal" group only because the investigator cannot access such a population. However, in this chapter we define the *target population* as the group of individuals or elements from which the investigator is able to select a sample. Each element of the target population may possess characteristics other than those specified by the investigator. However, each element must fit three criteria (Box 13-2).

How do investigators using experimental-type designs identify a population? First, the research question guides the investigator. Remember that all

---

BOX 13-2
THREE CRITERIA FOR ELEMENTS OF A TARGET POPULATION

- Must possess all the characteristics that the investigator has identified as "inclusion criteria"
- Must not possess any of the characteristics that the investigator has defined as "exclusion criteria"
- Must be available, at least in theory, for selection into the sample

---

experimental-type questions include the population in whom the variables and their relationships are being studied. Thus the research question contains the basic lexical identification of the population. Second, the researcher uses the literature to clarify and provide support for establishing population parameters.

> If an investigator is interested in studying persons with chronic mental illness, a vast body of literature provides clear descriptions and definitions of this broad category of individuals. An astute investigator may choose a well-accepted source, such as the *Diagnostic and Statistical Manual of Mental Disorders* (DSM-IV),[3] for a definition of chronic mental illness to structure parameters based on this knowledge.

The literature also helps to identify those characteristics that the investigator may want to exclude from the targeted population.

> To isolate and not confound the major population parameter of interest, "chronic mental illness," individuals may be excluded from the target population if they possess a primary physical diagnosis along with a psychiatric diagnosis, or if the mental illness is a secondary consequence of a traumatic head injury.

Consider another example.

> You are interested in understanding the daily routines of persons with quadriplegia. What would be the steps you would follow? First, you would need to define the specific population characteristics of the group you want to study. Some guiding questions you would ask are listed in Box 13-3.

BOX 13-3
GUIDING QUESTIONS IN IDENTIFYING A POPULATION IN A STUDY OF INDIVIDUALS WITH QUADRIPLEGIA

■ Should I include both men and women in the study?
■ Should all persons with quadriplegia be included, regardless of functional level?
■ In what type of setting should the persons included in the study reside (e.g., community, independent living center, institutional setting)?
■ In which geographical location should they live? What ages, ethnic groups, and occupational groups should be included?
■ Should persons with additional diagnoses be excluded?

Reading how other researchers bound their studies is helpful in answering these questions. Your answers will lead to the development of specific criteria by which to include and exclude individuals. Additionally, as indicated earlier, to answer these questions, you will need to consider your purpose in conducting the study. Finally, you will need to refer to the clinical and research literature for definitions of terms such as "quadriplegia" and "functional level."

Defining a population is an important step in sampling and must be carefully and thoughtfully done. Identifying a population can change the nature and findings of a study.

Suppose you are interested in examining the health literacy of veterans who are wounded in Iraq. In your study, you define your population broadly as all soldiers who return home to Veterans Administration (VA) hospitals for treatment of physical injuries sustained in battle. You are surprised when you find an extremely low literacy level. In a similar study, your colleagues study the same population of wounded veterans but exclude those who have visual impairments and who speak English as a second language. The level of health literacy revealed in this study is very high, and thus the finding appears to contradict those from your study.

Including or excluding different population characteristics can change the outcomes of a study. In the example, including English-language competency and excluding potential confounding parameters, such as the inability to see print material, had a major impact on study findings. You must clearly articulate the criteria used for bounding your study. Also, when comparing findings from studies on a similar topic and target population, you must carefully evaluate the differences in boundary setting.

The second major step in boundary setting in experimental-type design involves drawing a sample through the use of a sampling plan. There are two basic categories of sampling plans, probability sampling and nonprobability sampling. Table 13-1 provides an overview of the commonly used sampling plans discussed in this chapter.

PROBABILITY SAMPLING

Probability sampling refers to those plans that are based on probability theory. The two basic principles

TABLE 13-1

Summary of Common Sampling Plans Used in Experimental-Type Research

Probability Sampling	Nonprobability Sampling
Parameters of a population are known	Parameters of a population are not known
Sampling frame is used	No sampling frame is available
Every member/element has same probability of being selected for sample	Probability of selection is not known
METHODS	
Simple random sampling Table of random numbers is used to randomly select sample	*Convenience sampling* Available individuals enter study
Systematic sampling Sampling interval width is determined and individuals are selected	*Purposive sampling* Individuals are deliberately selected for study
Stratified random sampling Subjects are randomly selected from predetermined strata that correlate with variables in study	*Snowball (network) sampling* Informants provide names of others who meet study criteria
Cluster sampling Successive random sampling of units is used to obtain sample	*Quota sampling* Individuals who are unlikely to be represented are included

of probability theory as applied to sampling are as follows: (1) the parameters of the population are known, and (2) every member or element has an equal probability or chance of being selected for the sample.

The important point is that the probability of each element included in the study is known and greater than zero. By knowing the population parameters and the degree of chance that each element may be selected, an investigator can calculate the sampling error. *Sampling error* refers to the difference between the values obtained from the sample and the values that actually exist in the population. It reflects the degree to which the sample is actually representative of the population. The larger the sampling error, the less representative the sample is of the population and the more limited is the external validity of the study. The purpose of probability sampling is to reduce sampling error and to increase the external validity of a study.

To determine sampling error, we can derive a calculation called the "standard error of the mean," which reflects the standard deviation of the sampling distribution and is designated SE_m (see Chapter 19). Many statistical analytical tools used in experimental-type research are based on an assumption of probability: the assumption that a variable will be distributed in a population along a bell-shaped curve. The bell-shaped curve is a graphic depiction of what is expected to occur in a typical group. In other words, it is most probable that the majority of observations will be similar and will cluster around the average. More extreme observations, or those that are farther from the mean, are expected to be less frequent. The distance of a single score from the mean score is called "deviation."

However, the means will most likely vary among the samples, simply as a result of chance error. You will then calculate the standard deviation of each mean. In actuality, however, you will not draw several samples from the population to derive standard error of the mean; a formula can be used with one sample to estimate SE_m. Also, the larger the sample, the smaller is the SE_m. Likewise, the less the variability in a population, the smaller is the SE_m.

Sampling error may be caused by either random error or systematic bias. "Random error" refers to those errors that occur by chance. Not much can be done about random error at the sampling stage of the research process except to calculate the standard error of the mean. On the other hand, "systematic error" or "systematic bias" reflects a basic flaw in the sampling process and is characterized by scores of subjects that systematically differ from the population. Sampling plans based on probability theory are designed to minimize systematic error.

To use probability sampling, the investigator must be able to develop a *sampling frame* from which individuals or elements are then selected. A sampling frame is a listing of every element in the target population. Examples of sampling frames include the white or yellow pages of the telephone book and a complete list of hospitals in a specific region. A sampling frame can range from simple to complex. A simple approach might involve defining the sampling frame as those population members the investigator can easily access. A more complex approach might be the development of a sampling frame to ensure that the investigator can access the total population. This approach can involve extensive time and money.

Assume you want to draw a sample of 50 older adults with cancer from a larger population of older patients with cancer, then evaluate them using a "life satisfaction" measure. Then, you want to draw another sample of 50 older adults, then a third sample, and so forth. If you compute the mean score on life satisfaction for each sample, you will have what is called a "sampling distribution of means."

Theoretically, the distribution of these means should be in a normal shape (bell-shaped curve).

You want to study the needs for adaptive sports equipment in a rural community. There are several ways to proceed with sample selection. The most expansive approach would be to obtain a list of all people who live in the community and then randomly select the appropriate number of people. This approach would allow you to generalize your findings to the total population in the community. However, suppose you decided to use the white pages or phone book as your sampling frame. Your sample will only represent the universe of those who are listed and/or have telephones.

Now let us turn to the four basic sampling procedures that can be used to select individuals or elements from a sampling frame (Box 13-4).

Simple Random Sampling

Simple random sampling (SRS) is the most basic method used to enhance the "representativeness" of a sample. In this case the term "random" does not mean "haphazard." Rather, random means that theoretically, every element in the population has an equal chance of being included in the sample. Theoretically, if elements are chosen by chance, they also have an equal chance to be exposed to all conditions to which all other members in the population are exposed. This random nature of selection therefore precludes the possibility of the sample being selected because of a special trait that is uncommon in the target population or because of exposure to an influence that does not theoretically affect the total population.

Returning to sample selection from the rural community, both sampling approaches involve random selection, one from the roster of residents and one from the telephone book, ensuring that each individual who meets the criteria for inclusion has an equal chance of being selected for the study.

Most researchers who want to attain a large sample size use a table of random numbers to determine which elements should be included in the sample (Box 13-5). The table, only a small portion of which is displayed in Box 13-5, is carefully constructed through computer-generated programs to ensure a random listing of digits that appear with the same frequency. So how does an investigator use this table to select a sample?

You plan to survey all full-time, nonsupervisory nurses in a selected hospital (target population). You will obtain a complete listing of nurses (the sampling frame) who fit the study criteria. You will assign a unique number to each nurse on the list. If there are 150 nurses, the list will run from 001 to 150. Because the numbers contain three digits, you will select the random numbers in sets of three. To use the table, you begin by randomly selecting a starting point and then establishing a plan on how to move through the table. Assume that you decide to start from the third column from the left and one row down (925) and proceed to read down each row. Numbers outside the range of the numbers assigned to the nurses on the list (e.g., numbers greater than 150) are ignored. Therefore the first two numbers, 925 and 623, are outside the range and do not yield a selection. Moving to the top of the fourth row, numbers 143 and 007 reflect number assignments of nurses in the sampling frame. You will proceed through the table as such until the total number of nurses needed for the study have been selected.

Random sampling can be done with or without replacement. By "replacement," we mean that the selection of a unit will always occur from the total sampling frame. Thus, elements selected for the sample will be put back into the sampling frame before the next selection. Using a table of random numbers typically involves replacement because it is possible to select a number more than once. Random sampling without replacement can be as simple as drawing sample member names from a hat that contains all the names listed on a sampling frame.

Let us consider what may happen with smaller numbers in the sampling frame when random sampling without replacement is used. Suppose we have 10 persons in our sampling frame, and we want to select three persons for our sample. Before any subject is selected, the chances are 1 in 10 that an individual will be chosen. However, once the first name is chosen and not replaced in the pool, the next individual has a 1 in 9 chance of being selected. As you can see, the rule of equal chance for selection is violated. However, if we replace the name of the subject who was selected for the subsequent two selections, the chance for sample selection remains 1 in 10. Replacement ensures the same probability of chance of selection for each element throughout the selection process.

Systematic Sampling

SRS can often be time-consuming and difficult to complete when drawing a large sample. *Systematic sampling* offers a more efficient method by which to select elements randomly. After the identification and specification of your population parameters and sampling frame, this sampling approach involves determining a sampling interval width based on the needed sample size, then selecting every Kth element from a sampling frame.

> Suppose you want to survey a sample of 200 health care professionals from a total population of 1000. First, a sampling fraction (the interval width), 200:1000, or 1 in 5, is derived. Second, a random number between 1 and 5 will be selected to determine the first person in the sampling frame. Every fifth person from this starting point will be selected for inclusion in the sample (i.e., 8th, 13th, 18th, and so on). A number from the table of random numbers can also be used to determine the starting point. If the sampling fraction is not a whole number, the decimal is usually rounded upward to the next largest whole number.

When this sampling approach is used, it is critical that the sampling frame itself represents a random listing of names or elements. Also, there must be no hidden biases, purposes, or cyclical arrangements of the elements.

> Now suppose by chance every tenth health professional on your list has just entered the practicing arena. If you used a sampling interval of five and started with the fifth person, you would select only novice practitioners. This would introduce systematic bias in your sample and increase the sampling error.

Stratified Random Sampling

Systematic sampling and SRS treat the target population as a whole. At this point, however, you might be asking how you can ensure that diverse subgroups in your population are represented in the correct proportion in your sample. Stratified random sampling is one way that investigators address the issues of diversity. In *stratified random sampling,* the population is divided into the smaller subgroups, or strata, that the researcher determines to be of importance. Elements are then chosen from each stratum.

Stratified random sampling is a more complex approach than either simple or systematic sampling. Stratified random sampling enhances sample representation and lowers sampling error on a number of predetermined characteristics by increasing the homogeneity and by decreasing the variability in each subgroup. The more homogeneous a population, the fewer the number of elements needed to enhance representation and the lower is the error in generalizing from part to whole. This principle makes common sense; imagine how complicated a sampling plan would be for the population of residents in New York City.

> The Nielsen polls are an example of a complex definition of sampling frames and samples. The researchers clearly specify a multiplicity of characteristics that typify the television-watching population in the United States. Because this population is diverse, it is separated into strata based on characteristics such as geographical location, socioeconomic status, age, and gender. The proportion of each subgroup or stratum in the total population is then determined. Sample subjects are drawn from each stratum in the same proportions represented in the population. For example, if the gender distribution in the population is 59% female and 41% male, then 59% of the subjects will be obtained from the female stratum and 41% from the male stratum. Proportionate stratified sampling is frequently used when it is known that a given characteristic appears disproportionately or unevenly in the population.

If we used SRS or systematic sampling for a diverse population, we might miss the influence on our study question of important characteristics as they exist in the population.

Consider how a health professional researcher may use this technique. Suppose in your population of persons with quadriplegia, only 20% are women. As just noted, the researcher will split the sampling frame into two strata representing each gender. As a result, 20% of the sample from the female group and 80% from the male group will be selected. This selection process will ensure that gender is proportionately represented in the chosen sample. Without stratification, it is likely that the gender balance of the sample would not match the population. Characteristics are chosen for stratification based on the assumption that they will have some effect on the variables under study. In persons with quadriplegia, investigators have posited that gender may be associated with the nature of daily routines. Thus, it would be important to ensure that a comparison between men and women could be made with regard to daily activity.

Suppose in your study of veterans returning from Iraq, you wanted to test the outcome of an Internet support group on veterans' health and emotional well-being. If you did not stratify along literacy, you might miss the effect of reading capacity on participation, comprehension, and outcome of your text-based intervention.

Cluster Sampling

Also referred to as "multistage sampling" or "area sampling," *cluster sampling* is another subject selection plan that involves a successive series of random sampling of units. With cluster sampling the investigator begins with large units, or clusters, in which smaller sampling units are contained. This technique allows the investigator to draw a random sample without a complete listing of each individual or unit.

In testing a rehabilitation intervention for persons with cerebrovascular accident at inpatient rehabilitation settings, the researcher will first list the geographical regions of the United States. Using simple random selection procedures, regions will be selected from this list. Then, in each randomly selected region, the investigator will obtain a complete listing of the freestanding rehabilitation hospitals and make a second random selection among these units, yielding a random sampling of hospitals within a random sample of regions. To obtain the individuals who will participate, the investigator will randomly select participants from a list of individual patients.

Can you see how this approach is efficient in creating a random sample with a large scope of external validity? Because each step of the sampling process was random, the sample of individuals at one hospital center theoretically represents the national population of inpatients who sustained a cerebrovascular accident.

NONPROBABILITY METHODS

In experimental-type design, probability sampling plans are preferred to other methods of obtaining a sample, particularly when the research goal is to generalize from sample to population or, in other words, to increase the external validity of the study. Probability sampling plans provide a degree of assurance that the members selected for the sample will represent those who are not selected. These probability methods are often used in health and human service research for needs assessments, survey designs, and large-scale funded research projects.

However, random methods are often impractical because the researcher must have considerable knowledge about the characteristics and size of the population, access to a sampling frame, access to a large number of elements, and the ability to omit elements from the study for ethical reasons. Therefore, in health and human service research, various forms of nonprobability sampling techniques are frequently and efficaciously used in experimental-type designs.

In *nonprobability sampling*, nonrandom methods are used to obtain a sample. By "nonrandom," we mean that sample members are not chosen on the basis of equal chance to be selected from a larger sampling frame. These methods are used when the parameters of the population are not known or when it is not feasible or ethical to develop a sampling frame. If you are unable to use probability sampling in your research, does that mean that your project is flawed? Not at all; the key to using nonprobability sampling is to attain the greatest degree of representation as possible and to clearly identify to your readers the limitations of your findings.

Suppose you want to study the attitudes of potential students in health professional programs toward working with persons with severe physical disabilities. There are many ways to proceed to obtain a sample, but since you have access to students at your own university who have declared a major or have shown interest in a health professional program, you decide to use this group as your sample. This approach to sampling is a nonrandom process. In your study and report, you would clearly depict your sample process, identify the limits of your work, and indicate that generalization beyond the scope of your sample should not be attempted. Although you might suggest that your findings have applicability to similar populations and contexts, you would clearly state that further research should be done to verify the findings on other populations. However, your work would provide important information for the curriculum of your health professional program as well as contribute to theory to be further tested by others interested in the same phenomenon.

There are four basic nonprobability sampling methods (Box 13-6).

Convenience Sampling

Also referred to as "accidental sampling," "volunteer sampling," and "opportunistic sampling," *convenience sampling* involves the enrollment of available subjects as they enter the study until the desired sample size is reached. The investigator establishes inclusion and exclusion criteria and selects those individuals who fit these factors and volunteer to participate in the study. Sampling health professional students is an example of convenience sampling. Other examples are interviewing individuals in a physician's office and enrolling subjects as they enter an outpatient setting to determine their health service needs.

BOX 13-6
NONPROBABILITY SAMPLING METHODS

- Convenience sampling
- Purposive sampling
- Snowball sampling
- Quota sampling

Purposive Sampling

Also called "judgmental sampling," *purposive sampling* involves the deliberate selection of individuals by the researcher based on predefined criteria. In your study of persons with quadriplegia, you may decide to purposely choose only those who are college educated and able to articulate their daily experiences. In this way, you purposely select individuals to represent insight into the daily routines of a larger group, or you may ask clinical staff which patients with quadriplegia are representative or typical of the patients at their site.

Snowball Sampling

Also called "networking," *snowball sampling* involves asking subjects to provide access to others who may meet study criteria. This type of sampling is often used when researchers do not have direct access to a population.

You are interested in studying the health and human service needs of drug-addicted women with young children. It is not to likely that you would advertise for this sample and expect that people would readily come forward. Rather, you might ask counselors, members of the community where you know the women live, or agency personnel who work with this population to "nominate" informants, who in turn would be also asked to identify additional informants. In this way, you would be able to recruit a sample with techniques in which the women would not feel unsafe or publicly exposed.

Quota Sampling

This technique is often used in market research. The goal of *quota sampling* is to obtain different proportions of subject types who may be underrepresented by using convenience or purposive sampling methods. In quota sampling, parameters of a population and their distribution in the population are known. The researcher then purposively selects a sample that is representative of the population, in that elements are selected to display parameters in the same proportions exhibited in the population. This type of sampling is the nonprobability analog of stratified random sampling in that the investigator identifies the critical population parameters *a priori* and then attempts to obtain elements proportionally with these characteristics.

You are interested in testing the effects of a model day care intervention on the functional level of persons with schizophrenia living in the community. Because schizophrenia represents different types of syndromes, you first determine the proportions of varying types of schizophrenia in your population. You then find that gender and age are distributed differently in each type. To ensure that your nonrandom sample is as representative of your population as possible, you will set up a matrix of diagnoses, ages, and genders and select your sample by filling each cell in the same proportions that are exhibited in your population.

COMPARING SAMPLE TO POPULATION

As we initially stated, the major reason for sampling is to ensure representativeness and the ability to generalize from sample findings to the target population. At this point, you might be asking why probability sampling is even used in light of the numerous nonprobability techniques. The power of probability sampling lies in its capacity to use estimated population parameters from the sample based on statistical theory.

Five basic steps are involved in determining whether findings from the sample are representative of the population, as follows (Box 13-7):

1. State the hypothesis of no difference (null hypothesis) between the population and the sample being compared. This null hypothesis implies that the values obtained in the sample, such as on a depression scale, are the sample values that would have been obtained if depression had been measured in other samples drawn from the same population.

2. Select a level of significance, or the probability that defines how rare or unlikely the sample data must be before the researcher can "fail to accept" the null hypothesis. If the significance level equals 0.05, the researcher is 95% confident that the null hypothesis should not be accepted. Failure to accept the null hypothesis means that, with a degree of certainty, there is a difference between the sample and the population.

3. Compute a statistical value using a formula (see Chapter 19).

4. Compare the computed statistical value with a critical value. Although easily calculated on computers, most statistical texts still have tables of critical values to which the researcher can refer. The critical value indicates how high the computed sample statistic must be at a given level of significance to fail to accept the null hypothesis.

5. Accept or reject the null hypothesis. If the computed sample value is greater than the critical value, the null hypothesis can be rejected, and the researcher will conclude that a significant difference exists between sample and population. In many cases the researcher wants to *accept* the null hypothesis, as when he or she wants to demonstrate that sample values mirror or represent the population from which the sample was selected. In other cases the researcher wants to *reject* a null hypothesis, as when he or she wants to demonstrate that a particular intervention changed the sample significantly from the values represented in the population.

DETERMINING SAMPLE SIZE

Determining the number of participants in the study or the size of the sample is a critical issue that often causes difficulty for new investigators. A common suggestion is to "obtain as many subjects as you can afford." However, a large sample size is not always the best policy and is often unnecessary. The size of your sample can influence the type of data collection techniques, procedures for recruitment, and the costs involved in conducting the study. Also, sample

---

BOX 13-7
STEPS TO COMPARE SAMPLE TO POPULATION

1. State hypothesis.
2. Select level of significance.
3. Compute calculated statistical value.
4. Obtain a critical value.
5. Accept or fail to accept null hypothesis.

size needs to be carefully thought out so that you maximize external validity. Think of the articles that you have read in which claims are made on the basis of testing one group.

If you were a health or human service professional in a school setting, how likely would you be to inform your intervention by a study that reported success in reducing problem drinking behaviors in only *one* urban high school sample?

Although many published research articles discuss the rationale for the size of the sample for a study, you should have a reason for the number you choose. A defense of your sample size is particularly important when you submit a proposal requesting funds to conduct the study. In the proposal you will need to provide justification for the number of subjects that will be included in your study.

Researchers determine the number of elements in a sample once the population and sampling frame have been identified. The determination of sample size may be based on the proportion of units from the population necessary to conduct statistical testing. The number of subjects needed to test a hypothesis is directly related to *statistical power,* which is the probability of identifying a relationship that exists, or the probability of rejecting the null hypothesis when it is false or should be rejected.

Assume you are testing the outcome of a new intervention. Without sufficient power to detect a difference between experimental and control group outcomes, there will be no use in conducting the study. You want to ensure an adequate number of subjects in the study to have the power to determine whether the intervention made a difference in the study outcomes.

There are four considerations in determining the size of your sample (Box 13-8).

As noted, statistical power is the probability that a statistical test will detect a significant difference if one exists. An 80% statistical power level is considered the minimum level of acceptability. If a power analysis is calculated and statistical power is lower

---

BOX 13-8
CONSIDERATIONS IN DETERMINING SAMPLE SIZE

1. Data analytical procedures that will be used
2. Statistical level of significance (usually chosen at 0.05 or 0.01 level)
3. Statistical power (.80 acceptable)
4. Effect size

---

than 80%, the researcher runs the risk of a Type II error (described in Chapter 19) or the inability to detect significance if one exists. If statistical power is too low, it is not wise to conduct the study as planned.

In the 1970s, Cohen[4] advanced the technique of "power analysis." Four factors must be considered in a power analysis: significance level, sample size, effect size, and power. If three of the four factors are known, the fourth can be calculated. Significance level and sample size are straightforward. The investigator sets both these parameters before data collection. Cohen has developed tables indicating power levels for different sample sizes, significance levels, and effect sizes. *Effect size* refers to the strength of differences in the sample values that the investigator expects to find.

Consider a study that tests the benefits of a low-impact aerobic exercise program for elders. Based on empirical evidence from literature reviews and data from small-scale or pilot studies, the investigator hypothesizes that there will be a large effect of the program on muscle strength and a minimal-to-moderate effect on cardiovascular fitness. If the difference between values in experimental and control group subjects is large, only a few subjects will be needed in each group to detect such differences. If the effect size is small, a large sample size will be necessary to detect differences.

The number in the sample is also determined by the number of units in the sampling frame. Practical considerations, such as time and financial support for conducting the research, may also provide guidelines on the number of units to be included in the sample.

SUMMARY

The purpose of boundary setting in experimental-type designs is (1) to complete the study in a timely, cost-effective, and manageable manner and (2) to use the findings about the subset (sample) to inform us about the larger group (population) from whom the sample was selected. A number of probability and nonprobability methods can be used to select a sample from a population. Probability sampling procedures are used to ensure that a sample reflects or is representative of the larger population. Nonprobability methods are used when it is not possible to identify a sampling frame or when random selection is not feasible or desirable. Although this process sounds simple, many decisions must be made along the way. Many print and virtual resources are available that provide in-depth discussion of each procedural step in experimental-type research and the statistical theory of the various sampling plans. Furthermore, you should be aware that an investigator may use variations and combinations of these sampling plans, depending on the nature of the research question and the resources available to the investigator. When probability sampling is used, it is wise to consult a statistical expert to ensure that the sampling plan maximizes representation.

Experimental-type designs increase external validity by achieving "representativeness" of the sample through probability sampling. However, in health and human service research, it is frequently not practical or ethical to use probability sampling techniques. The state of the field is such that most researchers use nonprobability methods to obtain their sample. Even with limited external validity, however, well-planned studies with conclusions consistent with the level of knowledge that the sampling can yield are extremely valuable.

EXERCISES

1. Find a research article that uses probability sampling. Describe the sampling plan.
2. Find a research article that uses nonprobability sampling. Describe the sampling plan, and then compare its usefulness for practice with the article in exercise 1 that uses probability sampling. What conclusions and guidance can you obtain from each, and for what groups?
3. Develop a sampling plan for a study on lifestyles of adults who are hospitalized for chronic heart disease. First, identify population parameters, then suggest how best to obtain a representative sample of that population.
4. Discuss how you may obtain a random sample of children, given the regulation that a child's legal guardian must consent to the child's participation in research.

REFERENCES

1. Babbie E: *Basics of social research,* ed 3, Belmont, Calif, 2005, Wadsworth.
2. Monette DR, Sullivan TJ, DeJong CR: *Applied social research,* ed 6, Belmont, Calif, 2005, Wadsworth.
3. American Psychiatric Association: *Diagnostic and statistical manual of mental disorders,* ed 4 (DSM-IV-TR), Washington, DC, 2000, American Psychiatric Press.
4. Cohen J: *Statistical power analysis for the behavioral sciences,* New York, 1977, Academic Press.

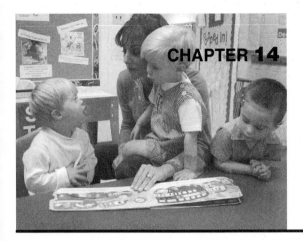

CHAPTER 14

Boundary Setting in Naturalistic Designs

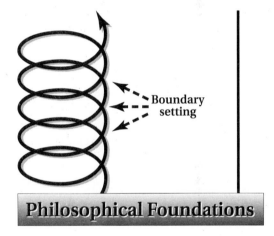

Let us now look at the way in which a researcher engages in the action process of setting boundaries when conducting a study using naturalistic designs. In naturalistic research, setting boundaries is a dynamic, inductive process. It is an action process that is flexible and fluid and that occurs over a prolonged period of engagement in fieldwork.

Because the basic purpose of naturalistic research is exploration, understanding, description, and explanation, the researcher does not often know the specific boundaries of the inquiry or the particular conceptual domains before undertaking the study. Indeed, the very point of the study may be to uncover and

157

establish the specific characteristics that bound or define a group of persons or explicate a particular concept or human experience. Thus, for most naturalistic designs, boundary setting is embedded in the field experience; boundaries emerge and are set based on the process of collecting information and ongoing formative analyses. The final determination of boundaries for a particular concept, or set of constructs, may not actually occur until the formal analysis and reporting phases of the study. Nevertheless, a researcher must start setting boundaries at some point and make decisions as to what to observe, with whom to talk, and how to proceed in the field. Thus, boundary setting in naturalistic inquiry begins broadly and then becomes refined as the research proceeds.

WAYS OF SETTING BOUNDARIES

Researchers working in the traditions of naturalistic inquiry must consider bounding their study along a number of dimensions. These dimensions include the location or physical or virtual setting, the cultural groups, the range and nature of experiences that will be examined, the particular concepts that will be explored, the artifacts that will be examined, and the ways in which individuals are involved.

Geographical Location

Naturalistic studies investigate a wide range of locations, from virtual settings (e.g., Internet chat rooms) to geographical locations and physical settings. Regardless of the setting, there are basic principles for creating location boundaries. Consider the following example of location bounding.

In *Tally's Corner,* Liebow[1] conducted an ethnography to "gain...a clear, first-hand picture of lower class Negro men especially street corner Negroes." Thus the initial boundaries of the research were set broadly to include a subgroup of African American men, those spending time on the street corner. Liebow identified a geographical location in order to enter the field, so his research was initially bounded by the physical location of a neighborhood where the men lived, worked, and "hung out." As the study proceeded, Liebow noted that his data collection took him beyond the initial geographical boundaries to "courtrooms, jails, hospitals, dance halls, beaches, and private houses." Liebow initially set boundaries for entry into the study and then expanded and modified these boundaries as the study proceeded in order to understand the men who congregated on the street corner. This process is characteristic of boundary setting in naturalistic inquiry.

In *Tally's Corner* the geographical location initially formed the boundary because the query sought to understand the lives and experiences of African American men who frequented urban street corners. The identification of a specific locale, geographical region, or area is a customary way of initially bounding a study in the naturalistic traditions. It allows the investigator to enter the field, but the location is only an entry point and may be expanded, as in Liebow's research, to other locales as well.

Choosing a location is a conscious methodological decision, and the investigator may choose to expand or not expand the location. Consider the following example, in which the location remained very bounded throughout the study.

In Gubrium's classic investigation[2] of life at a nursing home, the facility of Murray Manor established the initial boundaries of the study, and Gubrium decided to conduct all his observations in this facility. He consciously chose not to observe prior home life of residents or examine interactions outside the nursing home setting. By focusing or delimiting the study to the world within the nursing home, he achieved a rich or "thick" description of the multiple social worlds of patients and staff. Also, by staying within that one setting, he implicitly makes the interpretive point that it is through the lens of the present status and set of interactions within the nursing home that previous life is reinterpreted and experienced. Thus, similar to the residents themselves, we are forced to relive their history through their current everyday life. By staying within that setting, Gubrium emphasizes its permanence and thus its deep impact on quality of life.

Now we apply the principles from these examples to a virtual location.

Suppose you were interested in identifying the experiences of students with mobility impairments on college campuses in northeastern United States. Rather than spend time on multiple campuses, you choose to enter an online site that mobility-impaired students have created to discuss their experiences.

You therefore choose your initial point of entry into the field as the interactive chat room on the website, setting this virtual location as your initial boundary.

Cultural Groups

Cultural groups are another way in which researchers in the naturalistic tradition may form their study's initial boundary and point of entry. A "culture" may be loosely defined as the customs and tacit knowledge held by individuals who belong to a group, or the culture may be identified by the location in which it exists. Culture can also be defined as the rules, beliefs, and values that guide a person or group of people through a particular experience, such as the "culture of disability" or "culture of caregiving."

Assume you want to study family interactions and the impact of caregiving among Cuban Americans, a cultural group highly concentrated in Florida and in the southern United States. You begin your study in one region of Florida but are uncertain of the impact of "southern" values and culture on interaction patterns. You may want to expand or redefine the boundary of your study to include other geographical locations with Cuban American communities.

As a researcher collects information about a cultural group, he or she may refine the boundaries of the study to obtain a fuller understanding of the group. In the previous example, you could decide to travel to Cuba to understand the cultural underpinnings and historical forces that have shaped your Cuban American study group. A researcher also might use virtual sites to expand cultural boundaries, such as websites devoted to a particular cultural group.

Personal Experience

In studies that focus on the exploration of a particular experience, the phenomenon immediately sets the boundaries for what will be examined; that is, the boundaries of the inquiry lie within the realm of the particular experiences described by the individuals. In phenomenological studies the goal is to understand the experiences of a small set of individuals from their own perspectives. For example, a phenomenologist who wants to describe the experience of a parent who has a child with a terminal illness may choose to interview and observe that parent. The boundary of the study (and thus the understanding derived from it) applies only to the individual's lived experience. As stated earlier, however, the researcher must begin somewhere and make a selection decision as to which individual or individuals to interview who possess the specific characteristic of having a terminally ill child. The selection process may be purposeful in that the researcher makes the judgment as to which parent may be a reasonable "informant" based on the scope or depth of his or her particular experience. Other decisions about how to delimit the study must be made as well. For example, the researcher must decide what other data materials to examine (e.g., parent's diaries, e-mails, favorite book or music selection).

Wiseman,[3] in a phenomenological study of the experience of loneliness, initially identified the domain of concern as the "phenomenon of loneliness among university students." To explore the different meanings of this experience, she selected four students who had high scores on a loneliness trait scale. Her study demonstrated that even though these students had similar scoring patterns on a standardized test, their experiences of loneliness and the meanings attributed to this psychological state varied greatly. Wiseman's study was delimited by the conceptual domain of loneliness. The study purpose shaped other bounding decisions, such as who was selected for study participation.

Similarly, suppose you are interested in the following experience.

To explore the different meanings of the experience of trauma resulting from exposure to war, you might identify soldiers (and/or civilians) from one or more wars with varying levels of exposure to traumatic experiences. Many possible directions are available for you to take. If your purpose is to understand the variability in the experiences of trauma, you would want to maximize the variability of persons and experiences examined. If, however, your intent is to explore a more select or targeted aspect of traumatic experiences (e.g., prisoners of war), you would select individuals accordingly.

The investigator must initially establish the immediate study purpose and bound the personal experience that is to be targeted, at least initially, in order to engage in a feasible research process.

Concepts

As in the previous example, some forms of inquiry explore a particular concept. Thus, it is the particular concept that initially bounds the scope of the study in these types of inquiry. Wiseman's study[3] was limited to the exploration of one concept—loneliness. The study expanded understanding of the dimensions and nature of loneliness by identifying the range of different meanings.

In other types of naturalistic inquiry, the investigator "casts a wide net" and is interested in understanding underlying values or beliefs that guide behaviors.[4] In these forms of inquiry, the concepts of interest may not be immediately identified and may emerge only in the course of the study as a consequence of the analytical process.

Gitlin and colleagues were interested in discovering the meanings attributed to mobility aids and other special assistive devices for persons after their first stroke.[5] The concepts that explicated particular meanings were uncovered from an analysis of interviews with 102 individuals receiving rehabilitation services. Concepts such as social "stigma," "biographic management," and "continuity of self" emerged as important analytical domains that explained the dimensions of meanings associated with device use. Each concept had been defined and developed by other researchers involved in disability studies. Gitlin and associates did not initially bound the study to these conceptual domains; rather,

these concepts emerged as important focal points in the analytical phase of the study.[5]

Some studies, however, begin by setting conceptual boundaries.

A study by DePoy[6] using a Delphi technique (a method in which expert respondents answer questions several times to achieve consensus) sought to define the concept of "mastery" in occupational therapy practice. The investigator wanted to know what is meant by being "good" at clinical practice. In the first part of a two-part study, DePoy used a nonprobability purposive sampling process to select a group of experts who could define mastery. These experts nominated "masters," who were then interviewed to obtain their unique experiences as master clinicians. However, even though a sample of experts provided the initial data, the boundary was the concept of mastery, not the individuals who contributed to its definition. In the second part of the study, DePoy expanded the boundary to the practice arena and examined how mastery was demonstrated by the three masters nominated by the expert respondents. The concept of mastery derived from the first part of the study was examined in the practices of these three informants through an extensive unstructured interview with each informant. DePoy made no claim of external validity but suggested that the model of mastery that was developed (i.e., the domain of the study) should be tested for its relevance to other domains of practice.

The following example further illustrates the process of setting conceptual boundaries in naturalistic research. In his study of the culture of a nursing home, Savishinsky[7] was originally interested in describing the behavioral responses of nursing home residents to pet therapy. He states:

> The approach that I took began with two concepts at the very heart of pet therapy—companionship and domesticity. In the broadest terms, I came to realize that the study had to be a cultural and not just a behavioral one. . . .It had to look at meanings and not simply actions.[7]

As you can see, the initial boundaries of the study—observing actions during pet therapy—became modified and expanded as the study proceeded to the nursing home culture as a whole, including not only behavioral patterns but also meanings embedded within that culture.

INVOLVING RESEARCH PARTICIPANTS

Involving research participants is perhaps the most critical approach to boundary setting in naturalistic inquiry. It is often believed that researchers who engage in naturalistic inquiry simply select any individual, based on convenience or the individual's availability for study participation. This belief is a misconception and a rather simplistic understanding of the actions undertaken by researchers to involve participants. There is nothing haphazard about selecting participants in naturalistic inquiry. The use of a convenience strategy is only one of many important approaches used by researchers working from these multiple traditions. Selecting individuals is a purposeful action process, and the investigator must be acutely aware of the implications of his or her selection decisions. Selection decisions stem from either the investigator's theoretical perspective or the study's purpose and the research query; or selection is informed by judgments or interpretations that emerge in the course of fieldwork.

There are important differences between experimental-type research and naturalistic inquiry in regard to involving humans in research. Knowing these differences provides a basis for a better understanding of the decision-making process used by naturalistic researchers. The concern in identifying subjects in experimental-type research is "representativeness," as discussed in Chapter 13. Basically, the principle of representativeness suggests that the larger the sample size or the more subjects involved in a study, the better are the chances of achieving representation of the target population and detecting group differences or patterns.

In naturalistic inquiry, however, usually the concern is with the selection of individuals who have the potential to illuminate a particular concept, experience, or cultural context. The number of participants in a study is not as important to the naturalistic investigator as the amount of exposure to participants and opportunities to explore phenomena in-depth. The

investigator therefore develops selection strategies that ensure richness of information and complexity of understanding. The concern is not with selecting individuals who represent a population; rather, naturalistic inquiry is typically characterized by a small number of study participants with whom the investigator has repeated exposures and multiple occasions to observe and interview. Decisions as to whom to interview or observe and when to interview in the course of the study are thus based on this principle. Although some researchers label the approaches used in naturalistic inquiry as sampling techniques, we prefer to call them "strategies for involving individuals." Sampling techniques in experimental-type designs are based on the premise of representation and randomization. Therefore, using the term "sampling" in naturalistic inquiry is misleading and does not capture the intent of the decision-making process within these traditions.

The way in which individuals are selected for study participation in naturalistic designs depends on the study's purpose and design. Individuals may be involved differently at distinct points in the fieldwork process. This variability is especially the case for large ethnographical studies or forms of naturalistic inquiry that occur over a long period and that focus on a broad domain of concern. In any case, researchers working from the traditions of naturalistic inquiry use a wide range of strategies for involving participants, and these strategies emerge within the context of carrying out fieldwork. Occasionally, probability or nonprobability sampling techniques may be integrated into naturalistic studies when these approaches are appropriate and fit the structure of the study's purpose and design. These types of strategies have typically been used in large ethnographical studies and after the investigator has identified particular patterns that warrant further explication through the use of these sampling approaches. The ethnographer can use these sampling techniques to determine the representativeness of the particular concept or domain of concern within the cultural group, community, or context. When sampling methods are used in naturalistic designs, we take the position that the design moves to the category of "mixed methods."

Patton[8] and others[9-11] have suggested many distinct strategies that can be used separately or in combination for involving individuals in naturalistic inquiry. The following six strategies are commonly used to identify informants. (Some of these strategies are discussed in Chapter 13 and involve nonprobability methods, such as convenience, purposive, and snowball sampling.) A researcher may begin with one strategy, such as identifying individuals to maximize variation, and then switch to another strategy, such as identifying a disconfirming case to challenge emerging interpretations.

Maximum Variation

Maximum variation is a strategy that involves seeking individuals for study participation who are extremely different along dimensions that are the focus of the study. That is, in using this strategy, the researcher attempts to maximize variation among the broadest range of experiences, information, and perspectives of study participants. Maximizing differences and variability challenges the researcher and attempts to involve a universe of experiences. From the different experiences that are unveiled, the researcher attempts to identify common patterns that cut across variations, as well as to determine the study's boundaries. The challenge for researchers using this approach is uncovering the universe of variations.

> Assume you are interested in understanding and developing a theory of adaptation to life-altering disabling conditions. A grand theory needs to be based on adaptation to many different types of conditions and must involve an examination of individuals from vastly different life circumstances. You will want to maximize variation of disabling conditions and experiences to ensure that a theory of adaptation is comprehensive and captures the broadest possible swath of human experience.

Homogeneous Selection

In contrast to maximum variation, *homogeneous selection* involves choosing individuals with similar experiences. This approach reduces variation and thereby simplifies the number of experiences, characteristics, and conceptual domains that are represented among study participants. This approach is particularly useful in focus group methodology or when group interview techniques are used.

It is important to note that the selection of a homogeneous group does not mean that everyone in that group will express and interpret the experience similarly. The researcher usually discovers wide variation and diversity in expression and interpretation of an identified experience, even among a group initially selected for similarities. DePoy and Gilson[12] refer to this phenomenon as "diversity patina." That is, grouping people by characteristics that are obvious, such as race, class, gender, disability status, and age, may reveal surface differences among groups but barely scratch the surface of the diversity within these groups. Thus, homogeneous selection provides an approach by which to uncover diversity within a particular group of individuals initially selected for their similar characteristic(s), or to uncover what DePoy and Gilson refer to as "diversity depth."

Theory-Based Selection

Theory-based selection involves choosing individuals who exemplify a particular theoretical construct for the purposes of expanding an understanding of the theory. Wiseman's study[3] is an example of a theoretical approach to participant involvement. The individuals selected for this study were those who demonstrated the state of loneliness. Through in-depth interviewing using a phenomenological approach, the investigator was able to elucidate the properties of the theoretical construct. In other words, participants were purposely selected based on a set of experiences that would contribute to a more in-depth examination of the construct "loneliness."

One way the investigator could expand on this study would be to introduce a second phase of data collection. In this second phase the investigator could purposively select individuals who did not experience loneliness. This technique would be an example of using disconfirming cases to elucidate the phenomenon under study, as discussed next.

Confirming and Disconfirming Cases

Confirming cases and *disconfirming cases* are strategies in which the investigator purposely searches for an informant who will either support or challenge an emerging interpretation or theory posited by the investigator. Using disconfirming cases allows the investigator to expand or revise an initial understanding of the phenomena under study by identifying exceptions or deviations. Using data from sources who may provide alternative views and experiences engages the investigator in a process of elaborating and expanding on an understanding that accounts for a fuller range of diverse phenomena than what would have been revealed without this purposive strategy. Based on this expanded understanding, concepts, theories, or interpretations are rethought and developed.

> Assume you are interested in developing a theory of parental caregiving of children with disabilities. You may begin your inquiry with in-depth interviews of parents with a child who is severely disabled. As you develop guiding concepts, you may choose to verify them by interviewing a few parents who have never had a child with a disability. These interviews will offer contrasts. They will confirm or highlight the uniqueness of the experience of families of children with disabilities, or they will reveal similarities to the experience of families without disabled children. If the latter occurred, you would need to rethink your theoretical design because your data would not support a theory that families with a disabled child have experiences that differ from those of families without a disabled child.

Extreme or Deviant Case

In the extreme case, or *deviant case,* the researcher selects a case that represents an extreme example of the phenomenon of interest.

> Suppose you were interested in understanding how body image emerges and develops in girls with congenital amputations. To explore body image, you might select an individual who had a severe congenital amputation resulting in the absence of both arms. By selecting this informant, you would be expecting that every aspect of life for this person was different from a girl with a typical body structure. The extreme case would provide a basis for understanding the development of body image in a girl who does not experience what is typical for most girls.

Typical Case

In contrast to the deviant case, an investigator may choose to select a *typical case.* A typical case is one that typifies a phenomenon or represents the average.

> In your body image study, you might choose to identify girls who typify girls' experiences. Based on the information you gather, your next selection strategy may be to choose an atypical or deviant case.

How Many Study Participants?

There are no specific rules in naturalistic inquiry to assist the researcher in selecting the number of persons needed for interviewing or observation in a study. No procedure for naturalistic inquiry is comparable to a "power analysis" for experimental-type research. Can you guess the reasons for this based on your knowledge thus far of the naturalistic tradition?

Remember that the concern in naturalistic inquiry is *not* with the number of individuals who are enrolled in a study but rather with the types of opportunities and extent of exposure for in-depth observation and interviewing. Some guidelines, however, can be used to determine the number of participants to include in a naturalistic study. If the intent is to examine an experience that has been shared by individuals, a homogeneous strategy should be used to obtain study participants. Given that the naturalistic researcher is minimizing variation, only a small number of individuals (e.g., 5 to 10) will be necessary to include in the study. The small number of participants provides a "representative picture" of the phenomenon or focus of the study. In contrast, if the intent is to examine approaches to family caregiving of patients with dementia and to develop a theoretical understanding of caregiver management techniques, the naturalistic researcher may want to maximize variation in experiences and approaches to derive the broadest understanding of this activity. Thus a larger number of caregivers (e.g., 50 to 100 individuals) may be required, each representing different life circumstances and stages of caregiving.

Note that in naturalistic inquiry the term "representation" does not refer to or imply external validity. Rather, it refers to developing a comprehensive

> **BOX 14-1**
> **FIVE GUIDING PRINCIPLES IN BOUNDARY SETTING**
>
> 1. Inductive process is used.
> 2. Each selection decision informs the next decision.
> 3. Boundaries are adjusted throughout fieldwork.
> 4. A range of strategies is used to select individuals, events, artifacts, and concepts.
> 5. Boundary setting occurs until redundancy or saturation is achieved.

understanding of what may be typical of or common to a group.

PROCESS OF SETTING BOUNDARIES AND SELECTING INFORMANTS

The process of boundary setting in naturalistic research follows several principles (Box 14-1).

Boundary setting begins with the investigator determining an entry point into the inquiry. The actual point of entry into the study is often referred to as *gaining access*.[13] Frequently, an investigator will seek introduction to a group through one of its members. This member acts as a facilitator, or a bridge between the life of the group and the investigator. From that entry point, which could be (but is not limited to) establishing rapport with other group members, examining a concept, or observing a location in which a culture lives, communicates, and performs, the researcher collects information or data to describe the boundaries.

Once a researcher has gained initial access, other issues of access emerge. For example, although the researcher may be initially accepted into a cultural group or community, it may take a prolonged period before participants will share intimate information. Thus, gaining access refers not only to entering the physical or virtual location where the researcher plans to conduct extensive fieldwork, but also gaining entry to the level of information and personal experiences that frame the study's purpose.

Gaining access is not an easy action process. Much literature has been written on this important research action. The approach to gaining entry will differ depending on the context and whether the investigator is a member or stranger of the context.

(Some of these issues are discussed in greater detail in Chapter 17).

> You can think of gaining access as entering a party or new school where you do not know anyone and you are unfamiliar with the rules of behavior and what is acceptable. How would you approach the "scene" or situation? How would you learn about the underlying rules that are governing the partygoers' or students' behaviors? You may choose to stand outside the group and make observations, or you may try to identify someone nearby to introduce yourself and strike up a conversation. How do you think you would feel? Most likely, you would feel unsure of yourself and ask, "What is going on in this 'context' that I am now a part of?" In many respects, this common experience (which we all have had) is similar to gaining access for research purposes.

In the process of discovery and within the context of the field, the naturalistic researcher continually makes boundary decisions as to whom to interview, what to observe, and what to read. There may be an overwhelming number of observational points and potential individuals to interview. Selection decisions are based on the specific questions the researcher poses throughout the research process and the practicalities of the field, such as who is available or willing to be interviewed or observed.

Boundary setting in naturalistic inquiry begins inductively, and as concepts emerge and theory development proceeds, the researcher assumes a more deductive way of selecting observations, individuals, or artifacts to observe and the types of questions or probes to ask. For example, observational points may be chosen to ensure representation of what the researcher observes.

> Assume you want to examine the quality of life of residents with dementia on a separate unit in a nursing home. As part of your study, you might purposely select different times of the day and night to make your observations to ensure representation of time and behaviors. If you have limited resources or access to the context you want to observe, you may need to make less frequent and intense observations and then query participants about how well your observations reflect routine or daily occurrences.

Throughout fieldwork, the researcher is actively determining which sources will be most helpful to gain an understanding of the particular question and to derive a complete perspective of the culture, practices, or experiences of the group or single individual. Thus, once in the field, the investigator uses other techniques and approaches to establish the boundaries of the study. For example, to understand certain practices, an ethnographer may seek a key actor or informant to represent the group. This individual is selected because of his or her strategic position in the group, or because the person may be more expressive or able to articulate what the researcher is interested in knowing.

> Throughout Liebow's study,[1] four key informants continued to provide substantial insights, which Liebow used as the basis of his analysis, although many other men participated. The selection of such informants was purposive and based on the judgment of the investigator.

One could ask whether the same interpretive framework would have emerged had other individuals been selected, and whether Liebow carefully explicates his reason for relying on these four key individuals.

As noted earlier, one strategy in ethnography is to begin broadly. The investigator initially "samples" what is immediately accessible or in view. As fieldwork and interviewing proceed, questions and observational points become increasingly focused and narrowed. The investigator may use a "snowball" or "chain" approach to identify informants, search for extreme or deviant cases, or purposely sample diverse individuals or situations to increase variation.

The process of selecting and adding pieces of information through interview, observation, and review of literature and artifacts, as well as analyzing the data for discovery and description of the boundaries of the phenomenon being examined, is called *domain analysis.*[4] Understanding the domain, or area within the boundaries of a study, is critical in naturalistic inquiry. The intent is to understand, in depth, specific occurrences within the domain of the study. The domain must be clearly understood to ensure that findings or interpretations are meaningful. Although no claim is made about the "representativeness" of a domain in naturalistic inquiry, principles are explicated that that may be relevant to other settings. Therefore, naturalistic boundary setting is unlike boundary setting in experimental-type design, in which the purpose is to maximize representation and external validity. In naturalistic inquiry, selection processes are used to obtain a "thick description" (i.e., detailed or rich data) of a particular domain, allowing the investigator to examine the transferability of principles of one domain to another.[14]

ETHICAL CONSIDERATIONS

There are numerous ethical considerations in making boundary decisions for naturalistic inquiry. Consider the following examples.

> You are observing interactions between therapists and families on an inpatient unit of a hospital; the therapists and family members have granted permission for you to make such observations. Suppose a disoriented and cognitively impaired individual interrupts a therapeutic session you are observing. This interruption is of great interest to you because you want to see how both therapist and family member handle it and then reconnect. However, the person who interrupted the scene has not been approached about your study, and he has not given you permission to make systematic observations of his behavior. What do you do?

> You are observing a community-based program for persons with cognitive disabilities, and you have selected several key informants who attend the program. The inclusion and exclusion of select individuals within the program may be offensive to other participants and may create jealousy or distrust of those selected. Thus, your decision making may have a direct impact on the context you want to observe and may have both positive and negative consequences for those you engage. How should you handle this naturalistic design issue?

Other ethical issues in naturalistic inquiry involve how to exit the field and how to draw appropriate boundaries between the researcher and the individuals studied. Fieldwork is intense, personal, and prolonged, and researchers may have difficulty extricating themselves from the relationships forged. Also, individuals may come to expect certain favors or ways of behaving that are outside the boundary of being an investigator.

> Suppose you are conducting a longitudinal study that involves observations of mothers and their children with disabilities and how parenting decisions are made. Over time, you will naturally become involved in numerous family occasions and will learn about personal and intimate aspects of their daily life.

The boundaries of such relationships in naturalistic research can easily become tenuous, especially in times of duress.

SUMMARY

Boundary setting in naturalistic research is an ongoing and active process. It is part of the process of doing fieldwork and emerges inductively from data collection and analysis. Research is undertaken not only to address a research problem but also to promote further understanding and descriptions of the boundaries of the research. The naturalistic researcher is constantly making decisions and judgments about who should be interviewed and when and what to observe. The investigator uses a range of selection strategies in a study. The selection strategy used to choose an individual to interview, event to observe, or artifact to review is based on the specific focus of the investigator, and this focus usually emerges in the course of fieldwork. These strategies may include probability and nonprobability techniques, as well as others developed specifically for naturalistic inquiry (e.g., typical case, deviant case). Although initially a boundary may be defined globally, the investigator delimits the nature of the group, phenomenon, or concept under investigation through domain analysis and this occurs through ongoing data collection and analysis.

EXERCISES

1. To understand boundary setting in naturalistic inquiry, select a public place, such as a shopping mall, virtual chat room, or restaurant. Spend at least 1 hour observing, then determine patterns of human behavior in the location. As you observe, record how and why you select to focus on specific elements of the location. Reflect on the range of strategies you use. What did each strategy provide in terms of understanding the setting? Reflect on what information and observations you might have missed by your boundary decision making.

2. After leaving the location in exercise 1, write a list of events and behaviors that you believe will be important to observe on another occasion to confirm your emerging understanding.

3. Develop a research plan to examine the experience of being a health professional working at a managed care facility. Identify three strategies for involving study participants, and provide a rationale for using each approach.

REFERENCES

1. Liebow E: *Tally's corner,* Boston, 1967, Little, Brown.
2. Gubrium J: *Living and dying at Murray Manor,* New York, 1975, St. Martin's Press.
3. Wiseman H: The quest for connectedness: loneliness as process in the narratives of lonely university students. In Josselson R, Lieblich A, editors: *Interpreting experience: the narrative study of lives,* Thousand Oaks, Calif, 1995, Sage.
4. Bernard HR: *Social research methods: qualitative and quantitative approaches,* Thousand Oaks, Calif, 2000, Sage.
5. Gitlin L, Luborsky M, Schemm RL: Emerging concerns of older stroke patients about assistive device use, *The Gerontologist* 3(2):169-180, 1998.
6. DePoy E: Mastery in clinical occupational therapy, *Am J Occup Ther* 44:415-420, 1990.
7. Savishinsky JS: *The ends of time,* New York, 1991, Bergen & Garvey.
8. Patton MQ: *Qualitative evaluation and research methods,* ed 3, Thousand Oaks, Calif, 2001, Sage.
9. Kuzel AJ: Sampling in qualitative inquiry. In Crabtree BF, Miller WL: *Doing qualitative research,* ed 2, Thousand Oaks, Calif, 1999, Sage.
10. Gilchrist VJ: Key informant interviews. In Crabtree BF, Miller WL: *Doing qualitative research,* ed 2, Thousand Oaks, Calif, 1999, Sage.
11. Marshall C, Rossman GB: *Designing qualitative research,* Newbury Park, Calif, 1989, Sage.
12. Depoy E, Gilson SF: *Rethinking disability,* Belmont, Calif, 2004, Wadsworth.
13. Spradley J: *Participant observation,* New York, 1980, Holt, Rinehart & Winston.
14. Geertz C: *The interpretation of cultures: selected essays,* New York, 1973, Basic Books.

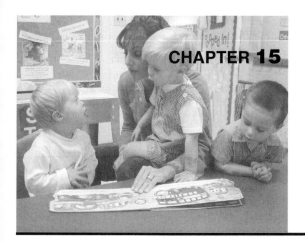

CHAPTER 15

Collecting Information

KEY TERMS

Artifact review
Closed-ended question
Hawthorne effect
Interviews
Materials
Observation
Open-ended question
Probes
Questionnaires
Secondary data analysis
Structured interview
Unobtrusive methodology
Unstructured interview

CHAPTER OUTLINE

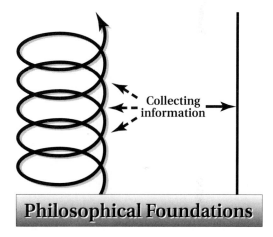

Collecting information

Philosophical Foundations

Y ou now have a better understanding of the methods for involving individuals, events, observations, and artifacts in your study. Now let us explore the different strategies you can use to collect information or data. This chapter provides an overview of the action process of gathering information to answer research questions or queries. A number of strategies are discussed, some of which are used exclusively in experimental-type research or in naturalistic inquiry. Subsequent chapters examine the specific approaches used in each research tradition.

In experimental-type research, data collection is a distinct action phase that represents the crossroads between the thinking processes involved in question formation, development and implementation of design, and the action process of analysis. Strategies for data collection involve actions that are pertinent to the research problem and consistent with the design. In turn, the types of data collected and the methodological approach used to obtain information shape both the type and nature of the analytical process and the understandings and knowledge that can emerge.

In naturalistic inquiry, gathering information stems from the initial query. However, it is embedded in an iterative, abductive approach that involves ongoing analysis, reformulation, and refinement of the initial query.

PRINCIPLES OF INFORMATION COLLECTION

Three basic principles characterize the process of collecting information within the different research traditions (Box 15-1).

First, the aim of collecting information, regardless of how it is conducted, is to obtain data that are both relevant and sufficient to answer a research question or query. Second, the choice of a data collection or information-gathering strategy is based on four major factors: the researcher's paradigmatic framework, the nature of the research problem, the type of design, and the practical limitations or resources available to the investigator (Table 15-1). Third, although the overall data collection strategy reflects the researcher's basic philosophical perspective, a specific procedure, such as observation or interview, may be used by researchers conducting either a naturalistic or an experimental-type study. Many researchers find it useful to collect data and information with more than one procedure or technique in order to be able to answer a question or query more fully. The use of multiple collection techniques is referred to as "triangulation" or "crystallization" and is useful for increasing the accuracy of information.[1] We discuss this technique in subsequent chapters.

TABLE 15-1
Factors Influencing Choice of Strategy for Collecting information

Factor	Specific Issue
Paradigmatic framework	Relationship of investigator to what is being investigated
Research problem	Question or query
Design type	Naturalistic inquiry or experimental-type research
Practical limitations	Time Money Access to research population

In general, the action process of data and information collection uses one or more of the following strategies: (1) watching, listening, and recording; (2) asking; and (3) obtaining and examining materials. Each of these strategies can be structured, semistructured, or open-ended, depending on the nature of the inquiry (Table 15-2). Also, each strategy can be used in combination with another.

WATCHING, LISTENING, AND RECORDING

One important data collection and information-gathering strategy involves systematic observation. The process of *observation* includes three interrelated activities: watching, listening, and recording. The record produced by the investigator comprises the data set. The way in which the researcher watches and listens may range from being structured to unstructured, participatory to nonparticipatory, narrowly to

BOX 15-1
BASIC PRINCIPLES FOR COLLECTING INFORMATION

1. Information needs to be relevant and sufficient to answer the question or query.
2. Selection of collection strategies needs to be purposeful.
3. Use of a single strategy or combination of strategies must enhance validity or trustworthiness.

TABLE 15-2
Summary of Strategies for Collecting Information

Method	Structured	Unstructured
Watching and listening	Checklists Rating scales	Participatory Nonparticipatory
Asking	Closed-ended questions	Open-ended questions Guided questioning
Examining materials	Coding schemes	Open-ended observation

broadly focused, and time limited to ongoing and fully immersed.[2]

In the experimental-type tradition, observation is usually time limited and structured. Criteria to watch, listen, and record are determined *a priori* to gathering data, and the data are recorded as a structured measurement system. For example, checklists may be used that indicate the frequency (or only the presence or absence) of a particular behavior or object under study. Phenomena other than those specified before entering the field are omitted from or remain outside the investigator's record. Rating scales may also be used to record observations; the investigator rates the observed phenomenon on a scale with a predetermined point system (see Chapter 16).

Watching, listening, and recording take on an inductive quality in naturalistic designs, with varying degrees of participation and interaction between the investigator and the phenomena of interest. The investigator broadly defines the boundaries of observation (e.g., a nursing home), then moves to a more focused observational approach (e.g., particular units, staff-resident interactions, language) as the process of collecting and analyzing information from previous observations unfolds.

Let us examine the concept of "intelligence" to illustrate different observational approaches. In experimental-type studies, intelligence testing relies largely on the use of a structured instrument that involves paper-and-pencil or computer-based tests and a tester observing a subject's performance in a laboratory setting. Measurements are obtained on dimensions that have been predefined as composing the construct of intelligence. Typically, a score or set of scores will denote the magnitude of an individual's intelligence. In a naturalistic approach, however, rather than using predefined criteria, the investigator may watch and listen to persons in their natural environments to reveal the meaning of intelligence and the ways it is recognized and responded to in a particular culture. Each approach has its value in addressing specific types of research questions or queries. Structured observation of intelligence is appropriate for the investigator who wants to compare populations or individuals, measure individual or group progress and development, or describe population parameters on a standard indicator of intelligence. On the other hand, naturalistic observation of intelligence is useful to the researcher attempting to develop new understandings of the construct.

ASKING

Health and human service professionals routinely ask a wide range of questions to obtain information for clinical purposes. Similarly, in research, "asking" is a systematic and purposeful aspect of a data collection plan. As in observation, questions can vary in structure and content, from unstructured and *open-ended questions* to structured and *closed-ended questions* or fixed-response queries that use a predetermined response set.

An example of an open-ended question is, "How have you have been feeling this past week?" or "How is it now for you compared to before your stroke?" In contrast, an example of a structured or closed-ended question is, "In this past week, how would you rate your health: excellent, good, adequate, fair, or poor?"

Naturalistic research relies more heavily on open-ended types of asking techniques, whereas experimental-type designs tend to use structured, fixed-response questions. Focused, structured asking is used to obtain data on a specified phenomenon, whereas open-ended asking is used when the research purpose is discovery and exploration.

When asking, you can pose questions through interviews or questionnaires.

Interviews

Interviews are conducted through verbal communication; may occur face-to-face, by telephone, or through virtual communication; and may be either structured or unstructured. Interviews are usually conducted with one individual. Sometimes, however, group interviews are appropriate, such as those conducted with couples, families, and work groups. Group interviews of five or more individuals may involve a focus group methodology in which the interaction of individuals is key to the information the investigator wants to obtain.[3] An audiotape of the group interview is transcribed, and the narrative (along with investigator notes) forms the information base, which is then analyzed.

Structured interviews rely on a written questioning protocol in which maximum researcher control is imposed on the content and sequencing of questions. Each question and its response alternatives are developed and placed in sequential order before an interview is conducted. Interviewers are instructed to ask each question precisely as it is written in the protocol. Most questions are closed-ended or fixed; that is, subjects select one response from a predetermined set of answers. Closed-ended questions vary with regard to the type of response alternatives (Box 15-2). Each response set forms a different type of scale, as discussed later in this chapter.

In a structured interview, the investigator may use a few open-ended questions. However, responses are then examined to derive categories, which are coded and, in effect, changed into a closed-ended response set on a *post hoc* analytical basis; that is, the investigator develops a numerical coding scheme based on the range of responses obtained and assigns a code to each subject. The numerical response is then analyzed.

You are interested in examining the social support of a group of inpatients. Because of comfort, you choose to use a semistructured interviewing approach by asking the inpatients who volunteer to participate in your study to talk about the important people in their lives and the roles that each plays. However, to obtain a score of the level and nature of support for each respondent, you analyze the recorded interview by scoring it according to a preexisting scale of social support.

Unstructured interviews are primarily used in naturalistic research and in exploratory studies with experimental-type designs. The researcher initially presents the topic area of the interview to a respondent, then uses probing questions to obtain the desired level of detailed information. The interview may begin with an explanation of the study purpose and a broad statement or question such as, "Could you

please describe your day as a patient in this hospital?" Other probing questions emerge as a consequence of the information provided from this initial query. *Probes* are statements that are neutral or, to the extent possible, that do not bias the respondent to answer in any particular way. Probes are used to encourage the respondent to provide more information or to elaborate. A probe (e.g., "Tell me more about it," or simply repeating a question) encourages a respondent to discuss an issue or elaborate on an initial response.

Quantitative researchers sometimes use unstructured interviews in pilot studies to uncover domains and response codes for future inclusion in a more structured interview-and-question format.

Questionnaires

Questionnaires are written instruments and may be administered face-to-face, by proxy, through the mail, or over the Internet. Similar to interviews, questionnaires vary as to whether questions are structured or unstructured. (The process of developing questionnaires is examined in Chapter 16 as part of the discussion on measurement in experimental-type research.)

Each way of asking—structured or unstructured—has strengths and limitations that the researcher must understand and weigh to determine the most appropriate approach. There is no "best way" of collecting information. The strengths and limitations of structured (closed-ended) questions must be evaluated in terms of the researcher's purpose (Boxes 15-3 and 15-4). Consider the following example.

As the basis for promoting healthy behaviors among elders residing in a rural community, you are planning to study their activity patterns. You decide to use a structured interview approach in which you list specific physical activities (e.g., walking, running, engaging in various sports) and ask respondents how many hours each week they devote to one or more of these activities. As you suspect, this inquiry documents a low level of activity. In planning your intervention, however, you realize that more information is necessary to determine how to structure the intervention. To obtain the answers to explain why the activity level was low and how to address it, you therefore decide to conduct an unstructured (open-ended) group interview of all community residents meeting your inclusion criteria.

BOX 15-3
STRENGTHS OF STRUCTURED (CLOSED-ENDED) QUESTIONING

1. Honest responses can be obtained.
2. Large cohort can answer questions in short period.
3. Responses can be compared across groups.
4. Statistical analysis can be conducted to describe and compare responses.

BOX 15-4
LIMITATIONS OF STRUCTURED (CLOSED-ENDED) QUESTIONING

1. Researcher is uncertain how respondents interpret or understand the questions.
2. Issues relevant to respondents may not be captured.
3. Respondent answers may reflect socially desirable responses.

Using this example, now consider the advantages of open-ended (unstructured) questions (Box 15-5). Then, identify the limitations of an open-ended approach and see if you can apply these to the example (Box 15-6).

As you can see, both structured asking and unstructured asking have merits and limitations, depending on the research purpose, phenomena to be studied, and study population.

OBTAINING AND EXAMINING MATERIALS

Materials are defined as objects, information, phenomena, or data that already exist. There are numer-

BOX 15-5
STRENGTHS OF OPEN-ENDED (UNSTRUCTURED) QUESTIONS

1. Highly sensitive issue can be explored.
2. Nonverbal behaviors can be captured and analyzed.
3. Issues salient to respondent can be identified.
4. Meaning of questions to respondent can be identified.

BOX 15-6
LIMITATIONS OF OPEN-ENDED (UNSTRUCTURED) QUESTIONS

1. Respondents may not want to address sensitive issues directly.
2. Extensive time is required to conduct interviews and analyze information.
3. Responses across groups cannot be readily compared.

ous reasons to seek out and use existing materials. First, direct observation and interview may not be possible, and thus an investigator may try to answer the research question by seeking a data set that has already been generated in the topic area of interest. Consider the investigator who is conducting inquiries of a sensitive nature, where informants may not want or be able to share their experiences. Seeking information that has already been obtained and organized not only makes sense for the researcher, but saves further discomfort on the part of respondents. Second, the use of existing materials eliminates the attention factor, or the *Hawthorne effect*[4] (change in respondent's answer as a consequence of participating in research process). Third, using existing materials allows the researcher to view phenomena in the past and over time, which may not be possible with a primary data collection strategy that occurs at one point.

As with asking and observing, securing and examining materials in experimental-type design are structured by criteria before the research field is entered. In naturalistic inquiry, the selection of materials to observe or examine emerges as a consequence of the investigative process. Although there are many ways to use existing materials, we organize them here into three distinct approaches: (1) unobtrusive methodology, (2) secondary data analysis, and (3) artifact review.

Unobtrusive Methodology

Unobtrusive methodology involves the observation and examination of documents, objects, and environments that bear on the phenomenon of interest.[5] This methodology is nonreactive; that is, there is minimal or no discernable investigator effect in the research setting.

To estimate the alcohol consumption of a neighborhood, the investigator may search trash cans and count empty alcohol containers. This approach can be used to confirm information obtained from another source. The researcher may have searched trash cans as a way of confirming information obtained during a face-to-face interview on alcohol consumption.

Consider also the investigator who examines text messages posted to a website to ascertain the answer to a research question. Investigators may use many different sources for text-based materials in their analysis (Box 15-7).

Secondary Data Analysis

In *secondary data analysis* the researcher reanalyzes one or more existing data sets.[6] By "data set," we mean information that has been obtained and organized for the purpose of research.

A health care researcher may examine client medical records to obtain data or may combine the data of two studies for subsequent analysis. Also, a social work researcher may examine clinical process recordings as a basis for understanding therapeutic interaction in family therapy.

The purpose of a secondary analysis is to ask different questions of the data from the data set analyzed in the original work. Researchers use several large, national health and social service data sets for secondary data analysis. For example, the census tracts, National Health Interview Surveys, National Health Care Data Set, Medicare and Medicaid data, Annual Housing Survey, and court report recordings

are important sources for secondary analysis in health and human service research.

Artifact Review

Artifact review is a technique primarily used to ascertain the meaning of objects in research contexts. For example, archaeologists examine ruins to learn about ancient cultures. Artifact review in health and human service research may include the examination of personal objects in a patient's hospital room or client's home to determine interests and preferred ways of arranging the environment as a basis for intervention planning.

SUMMARY

Three basic principles guide the action process of obtaining information: (1) collecting relevant and sufficient information for the research question or query; (2) choosing an information-gathering or data-collecting strategy that is consistent with the research question, epistemological foundation, design, and practical constraints of the research effort; and (3) recognizing that methods can be shared across traditions. The three categories of collecting information in all designs are watching, listening, and recording; asking questions; and examining materials.

We are now ready to examine specific data collection strategies in experimental-type design (Chapter 16) and gathering information in naturalistic design (Chapter 17).

BOX 15-7
EXAMPLES OF SOURCES OF WRITTEN DATA

■ Diaries or personal journals
■ Medical records
■ Clinical notes
■ Historical documents
■ Minutes from meetings
■ Letters
■ Newspapers, magazines, and professional journals

EXERCISES

1. You want to study the level of function in individuals with spinal cord injuries immediately after hospitalization. Identify and describe two data collection strategies you may use. Evaluate the strengths and limitations of each.
2. Conduct a brief interview with an older adult. Ask the person to rate his or her health on a five-point scale (excellent, very good, good, fair, poor) and to explain the rating. Compare and contrast the type of information you obtained by asking a structured question and an unstructured question.
3. Select a website for analysis. Ask a question that can be answered through examining the frequency of a particular word or phrase. Then, ask a question that can be answered through inductive analysis. What are the strengths and limitations of each approach when analyzing the same virtual data set?

REFERENCES

1. Denzin, Lincoln: *Handbook of qualitative research,* ed 2, Thousand Oaks, Calif, 2000, Sage.
2. Patton M: *Qualitative evaluation and research methods,* ed 3, Thousand Oaks, Calif, 2001, Sage.
3. Bloor M et al: *Focus groups in social research,* Thousand Oaks, Calif, 2001, Sage.
4. Babbie E: *Basics of social research,* Belmont, Calif, 2005, Wadsworth.
5. Lee RM: *Unobtrusive measures in the social sciences,* Boston, 2000, Open University Press.
6. Stewart DW, Kamins MA: *Secondary research: information sources and methods,* ed 2, Thousand Oaks, Calif, 1992, Sage.

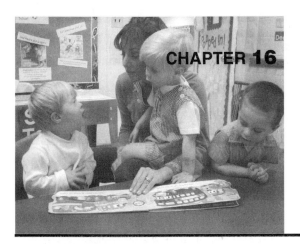

CHAPTER 16

Measurement in Experimental-Type Research

KEY TERMS

Continuous variable
Discrete variable
Guttman scale
Interval
Level of measurement
Likert-type scale
Measurement
Nominal
Ordinal
Proxy
Random error
Ratio
Reliability
Scales
Semantic differential scale
Systematic error
Validity

Confidence in Instruments
   Reliability
   Validity
Considerations in Selecting a Measure
   Purpose of Assessment
   Psychometric Properties
   Population
   Information Sources
   Item Selection
   Response Set
Instrument Construction
Administering the Instrument
Summary

CHAPTER OUTLINE

Measurement Process
Levels of Measurement
   Nominal
   Ordinal
   Interval
   Ratio
   Determining Appropriate Level
Types of Measurement
   Likert-Type Scale
   Guttman Scale
   Semantic Differential Scale

Measurement ⟶

Philosophical Foundations

Think about the nature and scope of experimental-type designs. What would you say is the purpose of data collection using these research designs?

In experimental-type designs, the purpose of data collection is to learn about an "objective reality." In this tradition the investigator is viewed as a separate entity, and every attempt is made to remove the researcher from what is being studied. There is strict adherence to a data collection protocol. A "protocol" refers to a series of procedures and techniques designed to remove the influence of the investigator from the data collection process and ensure a nonbiased and uniform approach to obtaining information. These data are made more "objective" (unbiased, a singular reality known by scientific method) by the assignment of numerical values, which are submitted to statistical procedures to test relationships, hypotheses, and population descriptors. These descriptions are viewed as representing objective reality. Therefore, in experimental-type research, the process of quantifying information or measurement is a primary concern. The investigator must develop instruments that are reliable and valid or have a degree of correspondence to an objective world or truth.

In this chapter we examine the measurement process and issues such as reliability and validity that are critical to the experimental-type research tradition.

MEASUREMENT PROCESS

What is measurement? In research, measurement has a precise meaning. Broadly speaking, *measurement* can be defined as the translation of observations into numerical values or numbers. It is a vital action process in experimental-type research that links the researcher's abstractions or theoretical concepts to concrete variables that can be empirically or objectively examined. In experimental-type research, concepts must be made operational; in other words, they must be put into a format such as a questionnaire or interview schedule that permits structured, controlled observation and measurement. The measurement process involves a number of steps that include both conceptual and operational considerations (Figure 16-1).

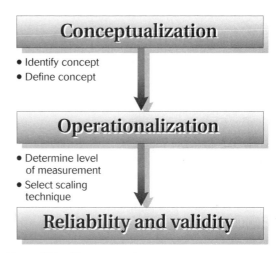

Figure 16-1   Measurement process.

The first step in measurement involves conceptual work by the researcher. The researcher must identify and define what is to be measured. Although this may seem obvious, it is often a difficult initial first step that involves asking, "How will I conceptualize the phenomenon I want to study?" or "How will I define these concepts in words?" Consider such basic concepts as attitude, depression, anxiety, self-mastery, and adaptation. Each has been defined in many different ways in the research literature. Once the researcher identifies a concept, such as "anxiety" or "depression," the literature must be thoroughly reviewed to decide on an appropriate definition.

The second step in measurement involves developing an operational definition of the concept. This operational step involves asking, "What kind of an indicator will I use as a gauge of this concept?" or "How will I classify and quantify what I observe?" A "measure" is an empirical representation of an underlying concept. Because, by definition, a "concept" is never directly observable, the strength of the relationship between an "indicator" and an underlying concept is critical. This relationship is referred to as "validity." In other words, does the measurement measure what it aims to measure? Also, it is important for the indicator to measure consistently the underlying concept. The consistency of a measure is referred to as its "reliability." The greater the reliability and validity, the more desirable is the instrument.

Reliability and validity are two fundamental properties of indicators. Researchers engage in major efforts to evaluate the strength of reliability and validity to determine the desirability and value of a measure, as discussed later.

Information gathering in experimental-type research, an important action process, must begin with identifying key concepts. This step is followed by developing conceptual (lexical) and operational definitions of these concepts. Based on these definitions, specific indicators (scales, questionnaires, rating forms) are specified or developed. These indicators represent the source of information or data that will be collected.

LEVELS OF MEASUREMENT

The first step in developing an indicator involves specifying how a variable will be operationalized. This action process involves determining the numerical level at which the variable will be measured. The *level of measurement* refers to the properties and meaning of the number assigned to an observation. There are four levels of measurement: nominal, ordinal, interval, and ratio. Each level of measurement leads to different types of manipulations. That is, the way in which a variable is measured will have a direct bearing on the type of statistical analysis that can be performed. The decision regarding the level of measurement of a variable is thus a critical component of the measurement process. It is important to understand that the way in which you measure a particular concept dictates the type of analytical approach you will be able to pursue.

> You need to collect information on a person's age. What are some of the ways you could ask about age? You could categorize people as being either young, middle-aged, or old; you could develop categories that reflect specific ranges of ages (18-35, 36-55, 56-65, 66-75, 76+); or you could record actual ages reported or dates of birth and then calculate age in years.

The level of measurement, whether you use age categories or the full range of possible ages mea-

sured in years, will determine the types of analytical approaches you can use, as you will learn here and in Chapter 19.

Several principles are used to determine the level of measurement of a "variable." The first principle is that every variable must have two qualities. The first quality is that a variable must be exhaustive of every possible observation; that is, the variable should be able to classify every observation in terms of one or more of its attributes.

> A simple example is the concept of gender, which most often has been classically defined as either a "male" or "female" attribute. These two categories represent the full range of attributes for the concept of gender.

The second quality of a variable is that the attributes or categories must be mutually exclusive.

> There can be only a male attribute or a female attribute. An attribute cannot be both male and female.[1]

The second principle in determining a variable's level of measurement is that variables can be characterized as being either discrete or continuous. A *discrete variable* is one with a finite number of distinct values. Again, gender is a good example of a discrete variable. Gender, as classically defined, has either a male or a female value. There is no "in-between" category. A *continuous variable,* on the other hand, has an infinite number of values.[1,2] Age (measured in years) and height (measured metrically or in feet and inches) are two examples of continuous variables in that they can be measured along a numerical continuum. It is possible to measure a continuous variable using discrete categories, such as the classification of the age variable as young, middle-aged, or old or the height variable as tall, medium, or short.

Discrete and continuous structures represent the natural characteristics of a variable. These characteristics have a direct bearing on the level of measurement that can be applied. We now examine each level in greater detail.

Nominal

Measuring gender as female or male represents the most basic, simplest, or lowest level of measurement, which is called *nominal*. This level involves classifying observations into mutually exclusive categories. Nominal means "name"; therefore, at this level of measurement, numbers are used, in essence, to name attributes of a variable. This level merely names or labels attributes, and these attributes are not ordered in any particular way.

> Your telephone number, the number on your sports jersey, and your Social Security number are used to identify you as the attribute of the variables "person with a telephone," an "athlete," and a "taxpayer." All are examples of nominal numbers.

Variables at the nominal level are discrete. For example, we may classify individuals according to their political or religious affiliation, gender, or ethnicity. In each of these examples, membership in one category excludes membership in another, but there is no order to the categories. One category is not higher or lower than another. Box 16-1 provides examples of mutually exclusive categories.

For data analysis, the researcher assigns a numerical value to each nominal category. For example, "male" may be assigned a value of 1, whereas "female" may be assigned a value of 2. The assignment of numbers is purely arbitrary, and no mathematical functions or assumptions of magnitude or ranking are implied or can be performed. Many survey analyses, conducted by telephone, mail, or face-to-face, use nominal level questions. The intent of these surveys is to describe the distribution of responses along these discrete categories. This level of measurement therefore is also referred to as

---

BOX 16-1
EXAMPLES OF NOMINAL-TYPE VARIABLES

■ Yes or no
■ Male or female
■ Democrat, Republican, or independent
■ Caucasian, African American, Hispanic, or Asian

"categorical" because the assignment of a nominal number denotes category membership.

> A survey may provide answers to questions such as how many men versus women have low back pain and how many unemployed versus employed people have health care insurance. In these examples the nominally or categorically measured variables are "gender" and "employment." A respondent must (and can) only belong to one gender category and one employment condition.

Ordinal

The next level of measurement is *ordinal*. This level involves the ranking of phenomena. Ordinal means "order" and thus can be remembered as the numerical value that assigns an order to a set of observations. Variables that are discrete and conceptualized as having an inherent order at the theoretical level can be operationalized in a rank-order format. Variables operationalized at the ordinal level have the same properties as nominal categories in that each category is mutually exclusive of the other. In addition, ordinal measures have a fixed order so that the researcher can rank one category higher or lower than another.

> Income may be ranked into categories, such as 1 = poor, 2 = lower income, 3 = middle income, and 4 = upper income. Using this ordinal variable, we can say that middle income is ranked higher than lower income, but we can say nothing about the extent to which the rankings differ.

The assignment of a numerical value is symbolic and arbitrary, as in the case of nominal variables, because the distance or spacing between each category is not numerically equivalent. However, the numbers imply magnitude; that is, one is greater than the other. Because there are no equal intervals between ordinal numbers, mathematical functions such as adding, subtracting, dividing, and multiplying cannot be performed. The researcher can merely state that one category is higher or lower, stronger or weaker, or greater or lesser.

Many scales useful to health and human service researchers are composed of variables measured at the ordinal level. For example, the concept of self-rated health is ranked from 1 = very poor to 5 = excellent. Although the numbers imply a state of being in which 5 is greater than 1, it is not possible to say how much greater the distance is. Also, the difference in magnitude between 5 (excellent) to 4 (very good) may be perceived differently from person to person. Thus, you must be careful not to make any assumptions about the degree of difference between numerical values.

We want to raise a caution here to remind you that ordinal data must denote mutually exclusive phenomena. A common mistake is the inclusion of the extreme points of an interval in more than one category. For example, questionnaires ask us about our age with such categories as 1-10, 10-20, 20-30, and so on. What category do you check if you are 10, 20, or 30 years old? These numbers incorrectly appear in two categories. The investigator should have specified mutually exclusive intervals, such as 1-10, 11-20, 21-30, and so on.

Interval

The next level of measurement shares the characteristics of ordinal and nominal measures but also has the characteristic of equal spacing between categories. This level of measurement indicates how much categories differ. *Interval* measures are continuous variables in which the 0 point is arbitrary. Although interval measures are a higher order than ordinal and nominal measures, the absence of a true 0 point does not allow statements to be made concerning ratios. However, the equidistance between points allows the researcher to say that the difference between scores of 50 and 70 is equivalent to the difference between scores of 20 and 40.

Examples of a true interval level of measurement include Fahrenheit and Celsius temperature scales and intelligence quotient (IQ) scales. In each there is no absolute 0, but there is equal distance between mutually exclusive categories.

In the social and behavioral sciences, there is considerable debate as to whether behavioral scales represent interval levels of measurement. Typically, such scales have a Likert-type response format in

which a study participant responds to one of four to seven categories, such as strongly agree, agree, uncertain, disagree, or strongly disagree. Researchers who accept this type of scaling as an interval measure argue that the distance between "strongly agree" and "agree" is equivalent to the distance between "disagree" and "strongly disagree." Others argue that there is no empirical justification for making this assumption and that the data generated should be considered ordinal. In the actual practice of research, many investigators assume such scales are at the interval level in order to use more sophisticated and powerful statistical procedures that are only possible with interval and ratio data. You should be aware that this issue continues to be controversial among experimental-type researchers.

Ratio

Ratio measures represent the highest level of measurement. Such measures have all the characteristics of the previous levels and, in addition, have an absolute 0 point. Income is an example of a ratio measure. Instead of classifying income into ordinal categories, as in the previous example, it can be described in terms of dollars. Income is a ratio measurement because someone can have an income of 0, and we can say that an income of $40,000 is twice as high as an income of $20,000.

Determining Appropriate Level

Table 16-1 summarizes the characteristics of each level of measurement.

Experimental-type researchers usually strive to measure a variable at its highest possible level. However, the level of measurement also reflects the

---

TABLE 16-1

Characteristics of Experimental-Type Levels of Measurement

	Level of Measurement			
Characteristic	Nominal	Ordinal	Interval	Ratio
Mutually exclusive categories	X	X	X	X
Fixed ordering		X	X	X
Equal spacing			X	X
Absolute 0				X

researcher's concepts. If political affiliation, gender, and ethnicity are the concepts of interest, for example, nominal measurement may be the most appropriate level because magnitude does not typically apply to these concepts.

MEASUREMENT SCALES

Now that we have discussed the properties of numbers, let us examine the different methods by which data are collected and transformed into numbers in experimental-type research.

Scales are tools for the quantitative measurement of the degree to which individuals possess a specific attribute or trait. Box 16-2 lists examples of scales frequently used by health and human service professionals in research.

Scaling techniques measure the extent to which respondents possess an attribute or personal characteristic. Experimental-type researchers use three primary scaling formats: Likert approach to scales, Guttman scales, and semantic differential scales.[10] Each has its merits and disadvantages. The researcher who is developing a scale needs to make basic formatting decisions about response-set structure, whereas the researcher selecting an existing scale must evaluate the format of the measure for his or her project.

Likert-Type Scale

In the *Likert-type scale* the researcher develops a series of items (usually between 10 and 20) worded favorably and unfavorably regarding the underlying construct that is to be assessed. Respondents indicate a level of agreement or disagreement with each statement by selecting one of several response alternatives (usually five to seven). Researchers may combine responses to the questions to obtain a summated score, examine each item separately, or summate scores on specific groups of items to create subindices. In developing a Likert-type format, the researcher must decide how many response categories to allow and whether the categories should be even or odd in number. Even choices force a positive or negative response, whereas odd numbers allow the respondent to select a neutral or middle response.

> The Dyadic Adjustment Scale is an example of a Likert-type scale with several different even-numbered response formats. The first set (22 separate items) has six response categories: always agree, agree a lot, agree a little, disagree a little, disagree a lot, and always agree. The instructions read: "Most persons have disagreements in their relationships. Please indicate the approximate extent of agreement or disagreement between you and your partner for each item on the following list."[3]

> On the other hand, the Family Adaptability and Cohesion Scale (FACES-III), which measures family function, is an example of a scale that allows a neutral response by structuring responses into five ordinal categories: almost never, once in a while, sometimes, frequently, and almost always. The "sometimes" category is the middle response and receives a score of three.[5]

Social science researchers frequently use Likert-type scaling techniques because they provide a closed-ended set of responses while still giving the respondent a reasonable range of latitude. As mentioned, Likert-type scales may be considered ordinal or interval, depending on what is being measured and which analytical procedures are selected. A disadvantage of Likert-type scaling is that there is no way of ensuring that respondents have the same understanding of the magnitude of each response.

Guttman Scale

The *Guttman scale* is referred to as "unidimensional" or "cumulative."[1] The researcher develops

---

BOX 16-2
EXAMPLES OF USEFUL SCALES

- Dyadic Adjustment Scale (measure of marital adjustment)[3]
- Self-Rating Anxiety Scale (measure of clinical anxiety)[4]
- Family Adaptability Cohesion Scale[5]
- State-Trait Anxiety Scale[6]
- Session Evaluation Questionnaire[7]
- CES Depression Scale (CES-D)[8]
- SF-36 (measure of health status)[9]

CES, Center for Epistemological Studies; *SF,* Short Form.

a small number of items that relate to one concept. The items form a homogeneous or unitary set and are cumulative or graduated in intensity of expression. In other words, the items are hierarchically arranged so that endorsement of one item means an endorsement of those items below it, which are expressed at less intensity. Knowledge of the total score is predictive of the individual's responses to each item.

Consider a series of items to measure level of political tolerance.[11] If a person answers "no" to each of the three items in Box 16-3, he or she is most tolerant. On the other hand, a person who answers "yes" to all three questions is the least tolerant. Another person who answers "no" to item 2 will probably answer "no" to item 1.

Thus, in the Guttman approach to scaling, items are arranged according to the degree of agreement or intensity in ascending order, such that each subsequent response along the scale assumes the previous one.

Semantic Differential Scale

The *semantic differential scale* is usually used for psychological measures to assess attitudes and beliefs.[12] The researcher develops a series of rating scales in which the respondent is asked to give a judgment about something along an ordered dimension, usually of seven points. Ratings are "bipolar" in that they specify two opposite ends of a continuum (e.g., good-bad,

happy-sad). The researcher sums the points across the items.

The Session Evaluation Questionnaire is an example of a semantic differential scale.[7] The scale measures two constructs, "depth" and "smoothness," related to clients' perceptions of clinical counseling sessions in which they have participated. The scale also measures two postsession mood constructs, "positivity" and "arousal." The scale includes 24 items, 12 each for the two sections. One item related to the session reads:
    The session was:
        Bad—Good
    One postsession item reads:
        Right now, I feel:
            Happy—Sad
    The respondent is instructed to place an X in the space that most accurately depicts his or her feelings.

Semantic differential scaling is most useful when natural phenomena can be categorized in opposite or contrary positions. However, it limits the range of responses to a linear format.

CONFIDENCE IN INSTRUMENTS

In selecting a scale or other type of measurement, the researcher is concerned about two issues: (1) whether the instrument consistently or reliably measures a variable and (2) whether the instrument represents an adequate or valid measure of the underlying concept of interest.

Reliability

Reliability refers to the extent to which you can rely on the results obtained from an instrument. You will want to be assured that if you were to measure the same variable in the same person in the same situation over and over again, your results would be the same. More formally, *reliability* refers to the degree of consistency with which an instrument measures an attribute. Reliability is an indicator of the ability of an instrument to produce similar scores on repeated testing occasions that occur under similar conditions. The reliability of an instrument is important to consider in ensuring that changes in the variable

---

BOX 16-3
EXAMPLES OF A GUTTMAN SCALE

1. Assume this admitted communist wants to make a speech in your community. Should he be banned from speaking?
2. If some people in your community suggest that a book he wrote favoring government ownership should be taken out of your public library, would you favor removing the book?
3. Suppose he is a clerk in a store. Should he be fired?

Modified from Stouffer SA: *Communism, conformity and civil liberties,* New York, 1955, Doubleday.

under study represent observable variations and not those resulting from the measurement process itself. If an instrument yields different scores each time the same person is tested, the scale will not be able to detect the "objective" value or truth of the phenomenon being examined.

It is easy to understand the concept of reliability when you consider a physiological measure such as a scale for weight. If you weigh an individual on a scale, you can expect to derive the same weight on repeated measures if that subject stepped on and off the scale several times without doing anything to alter weight between measurements. Instruments such as a weight scale or blood pressure cuff must be consistent to assess an accurate value that approximates a "true" physiological value for an individual. Consider an example involving human behavior to see how this principle applies.

> Suppose you are interested in measuring the level of depression in a group of inpatients who are in an experimental intervention program. You want to determine whether depression scores decline after participation in the program. You need to administer a depression scale before beginning the program and after its conclusion. Thus it is important that the depression measure you select is reliable. If the measure is reliable, any change in depression scores that are observed after the intervention will indicate a "true" alteration in level of depression rather than a variation on a scale.

However, there is always some error in measurement. A scale may not always be completely accurate. Suppose you measure a person's weight with shoes, then the next time you measure the person's weight without shoes. As another example, consider a tape measure that is not precisely held at the same place for each measure. This error is "random" in that it occurs by chance, and the nature of the error may vary with each measurement period.

Reliability represents an indication of the degree to which such random error exists in a measurement. A formal representation of *random error* in measurement is expressed by examining the relationship among three components: (1) the "true" score *(T)*, which is unknown; (2) the observed score *(O)*,

which is derived from an instrument or other measurement process; and (3) an error score *(E)*. An observed score is a function of the "true" score and some error. This tripartite relationship can be expressed as follows:

$$O = T + E$$

As you can see in this equation, the smaller the error term (E), the more closely O will approximate T. The standardization of study procedures and instruments serves to reduce this "random error" term. In a questionnaire, for example, a question that is clearly phrased and unambiguous will increase its reliability and decrease random error.

> You want to know whether your client is feeling depressed. You ask, "How do you feel today?" The client answers, "Fine," and then begins to weep. Obviously the client and you do not have the same question in mind, even though you both heard the same words. If you ask the client, "Do you feel depressed today?" you may be more likely to obtain the desired information. Although both questions refer to the same psychological state to you, the second question eliminates room for interpretation by the client. The client understands exactly what you are asking and gives the answer that you seek.

The point just illustrated holds true for measurement as well. Reduction of ambiguity decreases the likelihood of misinterpretation and thus error. Also, the longer the test or the more information collected to represent the underlying concept, the more reliable the instrument will become.

> If your client answers that he or she is not depressed but breaks down in your office and weeps, you may experience some cognitive dissonance. However, if you administer a scale to the client that asks multiple questions, all of which measure aspects of depressive behavior, you may be able to obtain a more accurate picture of your client's mood.

Because all measurement techniques contain some random error (error that occurs by chance) reliability can exist only in degrees. The concept of reliability is thus expressed as a ratio between variation surrounding T (a "true" score) and variation of O (an observed score), as follows:

$$r = \frac{T}{O}$$

Because we can never know the "true" score, reliability represents an approximation to that "objective" reality.

Reliability is expressed as a form of a correlation coefficient that ranges from a low of 0 to a high of 1.00. The difference between the observed coefficient and 1.00 tells you what percentage of the score variance can be attributed to error. For example, if the coefficient is 0.65, then 0.35 reflects the degree of inconsistency of the instrument. On the other hand, 65% of the observed variance is measuring an individual's "true" or actual score.

To assert reliability, experimental-type researchers frequently conduct statistical tests. These tests of reliability focus on three elements: stability, internal consistency, and equivalence (Table 16-2). The choice of a test depends on the nature and intended purpose of the instrument.

Stability

Stability involves the consistency of repeated measures. Test-retest is a reliability test in which the same test is given twice to the same subject under the same circumstances. It is assumed that the individual should score the same on the test and retest. The degree to which the test and retest scores correlate (or are associated) is an indication of the stability of the instrument and its reliability. This measure of reliability is often used with physical measures and paper-and-pencil scales. The use of test-retest techniques is based on the assumptions that the phenomenon to be measured remains the same at two testing times and that any change is the result of random error.

Usually, physiological measures and equipment can be tested for stability in a short period, whereas paper-and-pencil tests are retested in a 2-week to 1-month period. This approach of measuring reliability is not appropriate for instruments in which the phenomenon under study is expected to vary over time. For example, in the measurement of mood or any other transitory characteristic, we anticipate variations in the "true" score at each repeated testing occasion. Thus a test-retest approach is not an appropriate way of indicating stability.

Tests of Internal Consistency

Also referred to as "tests of homogeneity," tests of internal consistency are primarily used with paper-and-pencil instruments. In these tests the issue of consistency is internally examined in relation to a composite score.

In the split-half technique, instrument items are split in half, and a correlational procedure is performed between the two halves. In other words, the scores on one half of the test are compared with the scores on the second half. The higher the correlation or relationship between the two scores, the greater is the reliability. Tests are split in half by comparing odd-numbered with even-numbered responses, by randomly selecting half of the items, or by splitting the instrument in half (e.g., questions 1 through 10 are compared with questions 11 through 20). This technique assumes that a person will consistently respond throughout a measure and therefore demonstrate consistent scores between the halves.

Cronbach's alpha test and the Kuder-Richardson formula are two statistical procedures often used to examine the extent to which all the items in the instrument measure the same construct. The statistic generated is a correlation coefficient between the values of 0 and +1.00 in which a 0.80 correlation is interpreted as adequate reliability. An "80% correlation" basically means that the test is consistent 80% of the time and that error may occur 20% of the time. A score close to +1.00 is most desirable because it indicates minimal error and maximal consistency.

TABLE 16-2

Three Elements in Tests of Reliability

Element	Applicable Tests
Stability	Test-retest
Internal consistency	Split-half technique Cronbach's alpha Kuder-Richardson formula
Equivalence	Inter-rater reliability Alternate forms

Equivalence

There are two tests of equivalence: inter-rater reliability and alternate forms. The inter-rater reliability test involves the comparison of two observers measuring the same event. A test is given to one subject but scored by two or more raters, or the same rater observes and rescores an event on two different occasions. The total number of agreements between raters is compared with the total number of possible agreements and multiplied by 100 to obtain the percentage of agreement. Eighty percent or more is considered to be an indication of a reliable instrument. As in the other tests of reliability, a higher score is more desirable.

Consider the hypothetical data in Table 16-3. There are four potential chances for agreement, but only two occur among the raters. Agreement occurs in the ratio of 2 to 4 (2/4), or 1 to 2 (1/2), so inter-rater reliability is 50%.

The alternate forms test, or "parallel forms" test, involves the comparison of two versions of the same paper-and-pencil instrument. In this case, two equivalent forms of one test are administered to one subject on the same testing occasion. The use of this technique depends on the availability of two equivalent versions of a form.

Validity

An indicator or measure not only must be reliable but must be valid as well. *Validity* addresses the critical issue of the relationship between a concept and its measurement. It asks whether what is being measured is a reflection of the underlying concept. Figure 16-2 diagrams three different degrees of validity and highlights how instrumentation (A_1) only approximates the

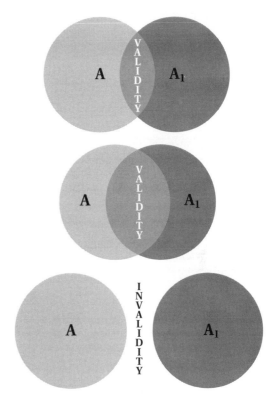

Figure 16-2   Three degrees of validity.

underlying concept (A). The closer an instrument comes to representing the "true" definition of the concept, the more valid the instrument.

Researchers argue whether the Wechsler Adult Intelligence Scale, the traditional indicator of adult intelligence, actually measures what it purports to and whether it is valid for different cultures and populations.[13] Because researchers can only approximate a perfectly valid instrument, validity is a question of degree, as with reliability, and may vary with the intended purpose of the instrument and the specific population for whom it is developed or intended. Thus the Wechsler Adult Intelligence Scale may be a valid measure of intelligence as it has been traditionally defined for white, middle-class Americans, but it is an invalid measure of intelligence for groups such as rural and ethnic minorities and those whose first language is not English.

Unlike reliability, the validation of an instrument occurs in many stages, over time, and with many

TABLE 16-3

Example of Data for Inter-Rater Reliability

Rater 1	Rater 2
30	35
25	25
31	32
33	33

different populations. For example, a scale that assesses problem solving that is validated with college students may need further validation before being used with middle-aged and older persons. A scale that measures cognitive status in an older urban group may not be valid for rural Latino elders. Also, a scale that is valid is necessarily reliable, but the opposite may not be true. In other words, a scale may reliably or consistently measure the same phenomenon on repeated occasions, but it may not actually measure what it is intended to assess. Thus, validation of an instrument is extremely critical to ensure some degree of accuracy in measurement.

Whereas reliability is a measure of the random error of the measurement process itself, validity is a measure of systematic error, or "nonrandom error." *Systematic error* refers to a systematic bias or an error that consistently occurs.

> A weight scale that systematically weighs individuals 5 pounds heavier than an accurate scale is an example of systematic error and an invalid measurement.

A measure that systematically introduces error indicates that it is a poor indicator of the underlying concept it intends to represent. Validity is therefore inversely related to the amount of systematic error present in an instrument; the smaller the degree of systematic error, the greater is the validity of the instrument.

There are three basic types of validity that examine the degree to which an indicator represents its underlying concept: content, criterion, and construct.

Content Validity

Content validity is sometimes referred to as "face validity." It is considered the most basic form by which an instrument is validated. This type of validity addresses the degree to which the indicator reflects the basic content of the phenomenon or domain of interest. Ideally, the steps to obtain content validity include (1) specification of the full domain of a concept through a thorough literature search and (2) adequate representation of domains through the construction of specific items.

If all domains are known, the investigator can sample items that reflect each domain. The problem with content validity is twofold. First, for most concepts of interest to health and human service professionals, there is no agreed-on acceptance of the full range of content for any particular concept. Concepts such as poverty, depression, self-esteem, and physical function have been defined and conceptualized in many ways, but there is no unified understanding of the domains that constitute any of these concepts. Second, there is no agreed-on "objective" method for determining the extent to which a measure has attained an acceptable level of content validity. One way of obtaining some degree of assuredness of content validity is to submit constructed items or drafts of a scale for review by a panel of experts. This review process can be repeated until agreement has been obtained as to the validity of each item. However, this process does not yield a coefficient or other statistical indicator to discern the degree of agreement or the extent to which an instrument is content valid.

Criterion Validity

Criterion validity involves demonstrating a correlation or relationship between the measurement of interest and another instrument or standard that has been shown to be accurate. Central to the validation effort is that scores on a given construct should correlate with conceptually related constructs. Two types of criterion validity are concurrent and predictive.

Concurrent. In concurrent criterion validity, there is a known standardized instrument or other criterion that also measures the underlying concept of interest. It is not unusual for researchers to develop instrumentation to measure concepts, even if prior instrumentation already exists.

> Assume you are interested in developing your own measure of self-esteem. To establish concurrent validity, you will administer your instrument along with an accepted and validated instrument measuring the same concept to the same sample of individuals. The extent of agreement between the two measures, expressed as a correlation coefficient, will tell you whether your scale is accurately measuring the same construct measured by the validated scale.

The problem, however, is that this form of validity can only be used if another criterion exists. Also, the concurrent form is only as good as the validity of the selected criterion.

> You have developed a measure of physical functioning that you believe is more precise than existing measures. You are interested in examining the relationship between your measure and previously evaluated measures, and you expect a strong relationship because they should be measuring the same underlying construct.

Predictive Validity. Predictive validity is used when the purpose of the instrument is to predict or estimate the occurrence of a behavior or event. For example, this type of validity can be used to evaluate whether an instrument designed to assess risk of falls can predict the incidence of falling. Agreement between the instrument and the criterion (a fall, or an established assessment of the risk of falling) is indicated by a correlation coefficient.

Discriminant

To establish validity, it is important to show not only that the instrument is associated with measures of the same concept, but also that it is *not* associated with measures of concepts that are different. In establishing discriminant validity, you first need to hypothesize what measures you expect to be different from your instrument. Then, you examine the level of agreement between the instrument and the criterion, as indicated by a correlation coefficient. In this case, you would want to see a correlation coefficient that is small and not statistically significant.

Construct Validity

Construct validity represents the most complex and comprehensive form of validation. Construct validity is used when an investigator has developed a theoretical rationale underlying the test instrument. The researcher moves through different steps to evolve supporting evidence of the relationship of the test instrument to related and distinct variables. Construct validity is based on not only the direct and full measurement of a concept, but also the theoretical principles related to the concept. Therefore the investigator who attempts construct validity must consider how the measurement of the selected concept relates to other indicators of the same phenomenon.

> The researcher who is developing a measure of depression will base a set of expectations of the measurement outcome on sound theory about the nature of depression. If the instrument is a self-report of depression based in cognitive-behavioral theory, the researcher will hypothesize that certain behaviors and thoughts, such as lethargy, agitation, appetite changes, and melancholia, will frequently be found in subjects who score as "clinically depressed." Thus the relationship of the scale score to other expected relationships will be measured as an indicator of construct validity.

Validating a Scale

There are many complex approaches to construct validity, including different types of factor analysis (see Chapter 19) and confirmatory structural equation modeling.

When validating a scale, it is important to consult with a psychometrician or statistician who is familiar with measurement development. The validation of a scale is ongoing; each form (content, criterion, and construct) builds on the other and occurs progressively or sequentially.

CONSIDERATIONS IN SELECTING A MEASURE

A basic action process in experimental-type research is selecting a measure to use in a study. A vast array of measures is available to health and human service researchers, and the selection of one measure over another should be based on a conscious recognition of the type of information that each measure will yield and its relative strengths and limitations.

Purpose of Assessment

In choosing a measure for your study, you first must match the purpose of your investigation to the intent of a particular instrument. This is the most elemental step in choosing a measure. You must clearly articulate what you want to measure and why.

Suppose you want to assess the physical function of elder individuals who enter your subacute rehabilitation facility after having a stroke. You must decide on the definition, what aspects of physical function you want to measure, and why. Assume you are introducing new clinical treatment guidelines for helping people who have experienced strokes with daily ambulation, and you want to be able to document significant improvements in mobility functioning at discharge. There are many measures of physical function,[14] but not every measure will match your specific purpose and the domain you need to target. You will need to select a measure that includes the ambulation items specific to your treatment focus and that rates physical performance using a response set that is sensitive to detect the type of changes in function that you are hoping will occur. For example, a measure that rates functional difficulty using a three-point scale (1 = no difficulty, 2 = some difficulty, 3 = cannot do at all) may not adequately detect change. However, a measure that scores level of dependence with more response options, such as a seven-point scale (7 = complete independence to 1 = complete dependence), may offer greater specification and opportunity for change before (pre) and after (post) rehabilitation.

The purpose of measuring a particular phenomenon is the initial driving force for selecting an instrument.

Psychometric Properties

Once you have clearly articulated your study's purpose, you can focus on whether a particular instrument conforms to adequate standards of measurement. It is important to use measures that have stable characteristics and that have demonstrated reliability and validity, rather than use a tool you developed yourself or a measure that lacks adequate psychometric properties for the population you intend to study.[15] Given that the validation process occurs over time in multiple studies, it is important to examine what level of validation has been established for the measure you are selecting and for which populations. You can feel somewhat secure in using a new measure if it performs adequately compared with a well-tested measure, even if only convergent validation evidence is available. However, it may be unwise to use a tool for which only content validity has been established.

Population

The choice of a particular measure also largely depends on the study population you plan to recruit and enroll in your study. Diverse personal characteristics (e.g., age, cognitive status, background) may affect your decisions about the measure and the approach you choose to obtain information about the phenomenon of interest.

You want to assess mobility of individuals with severe cognitive impairment undergoing rehabilitation for stroke. Self-report of mobility abilities may not yield reliable ratings. Also, the level of exposure of a particular person or cultural group to the items included in a tool may be important to evaluate. Of this present cohort, a woman in her nineties may not have had prior experience with financial management (a typical question in measures assessing activities of daily living), so questioning her on level of performance in this area may not be particularly valid. The use of a standard measure that includes these items would therefore provide an inconclusive understanding of actual performance and potential capabilities.

Also of concern is whether the measure has a "floor" or "ceiling" effect, such that it is not possible to obtain an adequate rating.

Most measures do not differentiate the types and levels of difficulty that may be present among healthy elder persons who do not experience difficulties or dependencies along traditional items. Thus, there is usually a ceiling effect such that this population scores at the highest level, and a measure may not satisfactorily differentiate among this well elder group.

Likewise, for highly impaired persons who require total assistance in basic areas, traditional measures may not sufficiently assess the components of a particular task that these persons can perform. Thus, there is a floor effect such that this population scores at the lowest level of the scale, with little differentiation possible within this group.

Another population-related consideration is whether to select a measure that is useful for the population at large or a measure that is specific to a particular diversity issue.

Suppose you are interested in studying stress associated with providing care to persons with severe impairment. You will need to decide between a general measure of stress or one that includes items specific to the experience of caregiving. A general measure may be preferred if your purpose is to compare caregiver and noncaregiver stress levels. However, if your purpose is to understand the specific aspects of caregiving that serve as stressors, a condition-specific stress measure would be more useful.

Information Sources

Another consideration in selecting a measure is the source from which evaluative judgments will be obtained. Four basic sources of information are self-report, proxy, direct observation, and chart extraction (e.g., medical records, claims data). Each source has its own strengths and limitations. Your decision of source from which to obtain information will be influenced not only by your purpose but also by your resources (e.g., time, money, expertise).

Self-Report

Self-report involves asking persons to rate themselves using a standard metric. Self-report information can be obtained by a face-to-face or telephone interview or through a mail survey. The use of a self-report approach usually does not require special expertise, although some interviewer training is helpful. This is a quick, relatively simple, and cost-effective approach for obtaining information.

Self-report has some limitations, however, and may not be useful for all study populations.

If you are interested in obtaining functional status information, research has shown that community-living older people tend to overestimate their abilities, underestimate their level of dependence, and may be unaware of unsafe interactions in carrying out daily activities within their living environment.[14] Also, poor sense of personal mastery and feeling depressed may lead to underestimating performance capabilities.

Persons with cognitive impairment also tend to be unreliable sources of information about their health and functioning, often reporting greater functional ability than that reported by their caregivers.

Also, the test-retest reliability of self-report is unclear; certain domains of living may be more amenable to self-report than other domains; and the validity and reliability of obtaining self-report are unclear when using different modalities (e.g., telephone interview vs. home visit).

Nevertheless, increasing evidence supports the important contribution of the self-report perspective to derive a comprehensive understanding of a person's health and well-being. Self-reports on health and function are highly predictive of actual performance, mortality, psychological well-being, and future expenditures for health care.[16]

Proxy

The use of a *proxy,* or informant, is another important source of information, particularly in the clinical setting. This approach involves asking a family member, health professional, or an individual familiar with the targeted person to rate that person on the phenomenon of interest using a standard measure. As in self-report, ratings from a proxy may be obtained through a face-to-face encounter, telephone interview, or mail survey. Proxies play a critical role in obtaining health information, particularly for individuals who may not be able to self-report or evaluate their performance accurately.

At issue, however, is the validity of informant responses and the specific factors that may inflate or otherwise influence proxy ratings. Proxy ratings may be affected by factors such as the relationship of the informant to the person, gender, level of depressive symptoms, or co-residence.[17] Although the specific role of gender, education, age, and relationship is unclear, evidence suggests that co-residency may enhance the accuracy of proxy responses. Nevertheless, families who are providing care to the target group and who are burdened or stressed are more likely to report more impairments relative to the person's self-appraisal.

Proxy responses can be useful, and subjects and proxies tend to agree in most areas.

Direct Observation

Measures that use direct observation of real-time performance tend to be task oriented and highly structured, and they yield numerical ratings. That is, the performance of each step or component of an activity is observed and rated for its successful completion along a number of dimensions, including the time for activity completion and the need for verbal and tactile cueing. Performance-based measures tend to yield more precise judgments as to the particular aspects of an activity that may or may not be able to be performed independently or safely. These measures also offer a more exacting assessment tool to guide intervention and may be especially useful when self-report and proxy are not possible or not good choices.

Nevertheless, direct observation does have several important limitations. First, performance-based measures need to be administered by highly trained raters and thus are often more costly to administer. Second, direct assessment of a specific area of activity may require special setup or stations in a clinic (e.g., use of the cafeteria) or home setting that may not be feasible to implement. Third, this approach can be time-consuming, even though only a few select skill areas may be observed. Fourth, observing an individual simulate an activity in one setting may still not provide an assessment of how an individual performs in another setting. There is little research to date from which to determine whether a simulated context is ecologically valid or if ratings derived in the constructed settings reflect daily performance. Fifth, timed performance-based measures have a wide range of test-retest reliability, particularly for unfamiliar tasks or tasks that do not have discrete start and stop points.

Chart Extraction

Another common source of information, particularly in clinical research, is extraction of recordings from provider notes and charts. This method is an inexpensive, relatively easy approach from which to derive specific types of information, such as health status, number and types of medication, physical function, and psychological well-being. However, professionals may rate phenomena differently, and it is not clear whether ratings in health records reflect the outcome of a standard assessment or whether they are anecdotal and based on casual observations.

Item Selection

Another important consideration in selecting a measure is determining if the items you have included are adequate for the purpose of your study.

Consider the study previously cited on the physical functioning of people who have had strokes, specifically their ability to ambulate after a therapeutic regimen. If you are interested in deriving ratings of "level of dependence" in ambulation and transferring, you will need to ensure that your selected functional measure includes the items that are important to your purpose.

Consider another example. The Child Health Protocol–Adolescent Edition (CHIP-AE) is a global, comprehensive, self-report measure of child health. One of the subsections measures physical endurance and activity by asking questions such as, "When was the last time that you walked a mile?" An adolescent who uses a wheelchair may be in excellent health but is unable to walk. Asking about mobility ability and endurance by restricting its operational definition to walking does not capture health in this case. The health rating for a child using a wheelchair would therefore be misleading because the items are not necessarily relevant to how this child performs.

Response Set

You not only have to consider what items are included in a measure but also whether the response set is suitable for your study purpose.

In your study of functioning in people with strokes, you need to decide whether to obtain information about their level of difficulty in ambulating or their level of dependence.

A measure that asks respondents to rate difficulty level will not yield information about whether they must rely on a helper as well. It is important to identify a measure with the response set that will yield the type and scope of information that reflect your study purpose.

CONSTRUCTING AN INSTRUMENT

Health and human service professionals frequently find that measures must be newly constructed to fit the study or clinical research purpose. The development of a new measure in experimental-type research should always include a plan for testing its reliability and some level of validity (content, at the minimum) to ensure a level of accuracy and rigor to the study findings. This can be a complex and time-consuming enterprise, and investigators often must develop different strategies to address measurement issues. Some investigators combine previously test-ed and well-established measures with a newly constructed measure in order to test their relationships and relative strengths in the study and provide evidence of reliability and validity.

The development of new instrumentation is, in itself, a specialty in the world of experimental-type research. We have introduced the basic components of the measurement process and have provided some principles for ensuring that your items are reliable. However, constructing an instrument and its components is a major research task (Boxes 16-4 and 16-5). Many different sources of error interfere with the reliability and validity of an instrument. It is best to consider consultation.

BOX 16-4
BASIC STEPS IN CONSTRUCTING AN INSTRUMENT

1. Review the literature for relevant instrumentation.
2. Identify the theory from which to develop a new instrument.
3. Specify the concept or construct to be operationalized into an instrument.
4. Conceptually define the full range and content of the concept.
5. Select an instrument format.
6. Translate the concept into specific items or indicators with appropriate response categories.
7. Test the instrument.

BOX 16-5
CONSIDERATIONS IN DEVELOPING AN INSTRUMENT

1. Format or design of the instrument
2. Clarity of the instrument
3. Social desirability of the questions
4. Variation in administration
5. Situational contaminants
6. Response set biases (all "yes" or all "no" responses)

For more detailed information on instrument construction, see the references.

ADMINISTERING THE INSTRUMENT

An instrument in experimental-type research can be administered by self-report using paper-and-pencil, direct observation of the phenomena of interest, face-to-face interview of the subject or a proxy, telephone, or mail. It is important to standardize the administration of an instrument, particularly when more than one person is obtaining information for a study. The influence of the data collector can potentially confound the findings. Consider the following example.

You and another investigator are studying perceived quality of life in a nursing home environment. You both have a set of questions with a closed-ended response set to be answered by the subjects. You begin your interview with a "thank you" statement and then ask the questions, whereas the other interviewer discusses the respondent's poor health status before beginning the interview schedule. In your data analysis, you find that the subjects you interviewed tend to be more satisfied with their lives than those interviewed by the other investigator. Is it possible that the second investigator influenced the subjects by discussing potentially depressing issues before administering the instrumentation?

This scenario highlights the importance of training for data collectors. Training is essential (1) to ensure that data collection procedures are the same for all data collection action processes and (2) to reduce bias that can be introduced by investigator differences. Establishing a strict protocol for administering an interview and training interviewers in that protocol will result in standardization of procedures to ensure "objective measurement."

SUMMARY

Data collection instruments for experimental-type designs vary in structure (open or closed), level of measurement, and objectivity (reliability and validity). The purpose of data collection is to ensure minimal researcher obtrusiveness through the systematic

---

BOX 16-6
ENHANCING CONSISTENCY IN OBTAINING INFROMATION

■ Establish testing procedures and protocols
■ Establish when and how subjects are contacted
■ Establish a script by which to describe the study

---

and consistent application of procedures. The researcher minimizes systematic and random errors through validation and reliability testing, respectively. Other procedures are developed to ensure consistency in obtaining data (Box 16-6).

Reliability and validity represent two critical considerations when a data collection instrument is selected. When experimental-type research is conducted, the researcher's first preference is the selection of instruments that have demonstrated reliability and validity for the specific populations or phenomena the investigator wants to study. In health and human service research, however, as in other substantive or content areas (e.g., diversity, disability, caregiving, gerontology, children, family function), instruments to measure relevant researchable concepts are limited. Because of the lack of reliable and valid instruments, some professional organizations and agencies, such as the Health Resources and Services Administration and National Institutes of Health, have placed a high priority on funding research directed at the development of data collection instruments.

EXERCISES

1. Develop at least five questions on a Likert-type scale to measure job satisfaction among your peers. Ask at least three of your peers to respond to the questions. Ask each to indicate the clarity of the questions. Do you need to revise the questions? Did the questions appear to measure what you intended?
2. Using job satisfaction as your construct, develop a Guttman scale and a semantic differential scale. What are the advantages and disadvantages of each? Ask your peers to respond to these questions, and compare the responses.
3. With a peer, observe a child in a playground and independently attempt to determine the child's age. Record the criteria used to make your judgment. Compare your impressions with those of your peer to determine the extent of interrater reliability.

REFERENCES

1. Kerlinger F: *Foundations of behavioral research,* New York, 1973, Holt, Rinehart & Winston.
2. Miller D: *Handbook of research design and social measurement,* Newbury Park, Calif, 1991, Sage.
3. Spanier GB: Measuring dyadic adjustment: new scales for assessing the quality of marriage and similar dyads, *J Marriage Fam* 38:15-28, 1976.
4. Zung WK: A rating instrument for anxiety disorders, *Psychosomatics* 12:371-379, 1971.
5. Olson DH, Portner J, Lavee Y: FACES-III. In *Family social science,* Minneapolis, 1985, University of Minnesota.
6. Spielberger CD et al: Assessment of anxiety: the State-Trait Anxiety Scale, *Adv Personality* 2:159-187, 1983.
7. Stiles WB, Snow JS: Counseling session impact as seen by novice counselors and their clients, *J Counsel Psychol* 31: 3-12, 1984.
8. Radloff LS: The CES-D scale: a self report depression scale for research in the general population, *Appl Psychol Measure* 1:385-401, 1977.
9. Stewart AL, Ware JE, editors: *Measuring functioning and well-being: the medical outcomes study approach,* Durham, NC, 1992, Duke University Press.
10. DeVellis RF: *Scale development: theory and applications,* Newbury Park, Calif, 2001, Sage.
11. Stouffer SA: *Communism, conformity and civil liberties,* New York, 1955, Doubleday.
12. Osgood CE, Suci GJ, Tannenbaum PH: *The measurement of meaning,* Urbana, 1957, University of Illinois Press.
13. Wechsler D: *The measurement of adult intelligence,* ed 4, New York, 1958, Psychological Corp.
14. Gitlin LN: *Physical function in the elderly: a comprehensive guide to its meaning and measurement,* ProEd Press (in press).
15. Switzer GE et al: Selecting, developing, and evaluating research instruments, *Soc Psychiatry Psychiatr Epidemiol* 34:399-409, 1999.
16. Pacala JT et al: Using self-reported data to predict expenditures of the health care of older people, *J Am Geriatr Soc* 51:609-614, 2003.
17. Neumann PJ, Araki SS, Gutterman EM: The use of proxy respondents in studies of older adults: lessons, challenges, and opportunities, *J Am Geriatr Soc* 48:1646-1654, 2000.

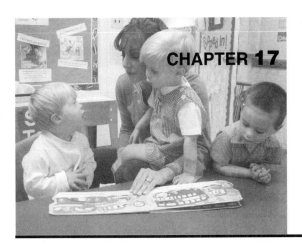

CHAPTER 17

Gathering Information in Naturalistic Inquiry

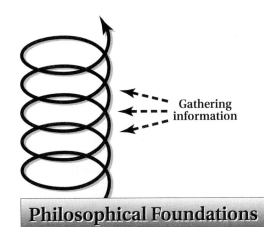

Gathering information

Philosophical Foundations

Gathering information in naturalistic forms of inquiry involves a set of investigative actions that are quite divergent in purpose, approach, and process from experimental-type research. In naturalistic inquiry, knowledge emerges from and is embedded in the unique and shared understandings of human phenomena of interest.

The overall purpose of gathering information in naturalistic inquiry is to uncover multiple and diverse perspectives and underlying patterns that illuminate, describe, relate, and even predict the phenomena under study within the context in which phenomena occur. By "context," we mean the physical, virtual, intellectual, social, economic, cultural, spiritual, and other types of environments in which human experience unfolds. Thus, different from experimental-type approaches, which also aim to predict, the processes of collecting information in naturalistic inquiry serve as discovery and revelation in a contextual field, not verification or falsification of a theory through the specification, collection, and analysis of data in a carefully controlled environment. The investigator gathers sufficient information that leads to description, discovery, understanding, interpretation, meaning, and explanation of the rich mosaic of human experiences.

As you now know, many distinct perspectives compose the rubric of naturalistic inquiry. Thus there is wide variation in the information-gathering approaches of researchers conducting naturalistic inquiry. For example, in semiotics the focus of data collection is on discourse, symbol, and context.[1] In classic ethnography the focus of data collection may be broader than in semiotics and may include verbal exchanges, behavioral patterns, and physical objects.[2]

FOUR INFORMATION-GATHERING PRINCIPLES

Although the process of gathering information differs across the types of naturalistic inquiry, four basic principles provide guidance for action: (1) the nature of involvement of the investigator; (2) the inductive, abductive process of gathering information, analyzing the information, and gathering more information; (3) the time commitment in the actual or virtual field; and (4) the use of multiple data collection strategies.

Investigator Involvement

In experimental-type research, investigators implement a set of procedures designed to remove themselves from informal or nonstandardized interactions with study participants. Naturalistic inquiry, however, is based on *investigator involvement* and active participation (to a greater or lesser degree) with people and other sources of information, such as artifacts, written historical documents or virtual text, and pictorial representations. When working directly with humans, the quality of the data collected often depends on the investigator's ability to develop trust, rapport, and mutual respect with those participating in or being studied. The level and nature of the investigator's involvement with people and other sources of information, however, depend on the specific type of naturalistic study that is pursued (Table 17-1).

In most forms of naturalistic inquiry, but particularly in classic ethnography, life history, grounded theory, and heuristic designs, the process of eliciting stories, personal experiences, and the telling of events is based on a strong relationship or bond that forms between the investigator and the informant. Some researchers characterize this bond as a "collaborative endeavor" or "partnership." In these approaches to inquiry, the primary instrument for gathering trustworthy information from study participants is the investigator. As Tedlock states (in Denzin and Lincoln):

TABLE 17-1

Investigator Involvement in Gathering Information from Study Participants in Naturalistic Designs

Type of Naturalistic Inquiry	Investigator Involvement
Endogenous	Variable; flexible; depends on study team decisions
Participatory action	Variable; flexible; depends on study team decisions
Phenomenological	Active listener
Heuristic	Fully participatory
Life history	Active listener
Ethnographic	Fully participatory
Grounded theory	Fully participatory

By entering into firsthand interaction with people in their everyday lives, ethnographers can reach a better understanding of the beliefs, motivations, and behaviors of their subjects than they can by using any other method.[3]

The investigator as a data-gathering instrument is a logical extension of the primary contention of naturalistic inquiry. This position, shared by many forms of naturalistic inquiry, maintains that the only way to "know" about the "lived" experiences of individuals is to become intimately involved and familiar with the life situations of those who experience them. The extreme of this position is found in heuristic inquiry, in which the investigator investigates his or her personal lived experience. In phenomenological research the investigator develops rapport with study participants but engages in active listening to understand the experiences of others. In ethnography the researcher, as the primary data-gathering instrument, strives for intimate familiarity with the people in the study. By engaging in an active learning process through watching, listening, participating, interviewing, and reviewing materials, the investigator enters the "life world" of others and uncovers what it means to live those experiences.

In endogenous and participatory action research, the level of investigator involvement in data collection varies depending on the way in which the study team chooses to proceed. In these forms of naturalistic inquiry, the investigator tends to serve more as a facilitator of the research process and may or may not be directly involved in the various data collection strategies implemented by the team of participants.

Naturalistic forms of inquiry may employ others in the data-gathering process in addition to the primary investigators. This strategy is particularly useful in studies involving multiple field sites or when the volume of interviews is high and requires assistance from others, who may be researchers, the subjects of the inquiry, or individuals trained in the rigorous procedures that characterize the study. In these cases the investigator and data gatherers form a team and work together to develop a common interview style to ensure similarity and consistency in the use of techniques for building rapport, as well as for probing and eliciting responses. To obtain a comprehensive understanding of the data, the team must also work together to share field impressions, notes, and emerging analytical categories and themes.

Information Collection and Analysis

In naturalistic inquiry the act of gathering information is intimately entwined with analysis; that is, collecting data and conducting analysis reciprocally inform one another. Thus, once established in the field, the investigator evaluates the information obtained through observation, examination of artifacts in taped interviews, and participation in activities. These initial analytical efforts detail the "who, what, when, and where" aspects of the context, which in turn are used to further define and refine subsequent data collection efforts.

The dynamic process of ongoing data gathering, analysis, and more data gathering can be graphically represented by the "spiral" design used in this text. In the spiral, as analysis and data collection are refined, the investigator moves from a broad conception of the field to a more in-depth, richer, and "thick" understanding and interpretation of multiple field "realities."[4]

Time Commitment in the Field

The amount of time spent immersed in a field setting varies greatly across the types of naturalistic inquiry. In some studies, understanding a natural or virtual setting can be time-consuming because of the complexity of the initial query and the context that is being studied. In any type of naturalistic inquiry, however, the investigator must become totally immersed in the setting or involved with the phenomenon of study. "Immersion" means that the investigator must spend sufficient time in the field to ensure that a complete description is produced. In ethnographic research, spending time "hanging out"—interviewing, observing, and participating—has traditionally been called "prolonged engagement" in the field. Prolonged engagement is essential to ensure that the investigator reaches an in-depth understanding of the particular cultural group of focus.[5]

But how much time is necessary? The amount of time spent in the field may vary from a few months to years, depending on the nature of the initial query and its scope, the availability of resources that support the investigator in the endeavor, the amount of time available to the investigator, and the specific design strategy that is followed.

> Assume that you want to examine the initial meanings attributed to the diagnosis of breast cancer among women in their twenties. This approach represents a rather focused query that may require only a few months of interviewing women in this age group who have recently learned of their diagnosis. Even if you plan to observe physicians interacting with these patients, your observations will be confined to this early treatment phase.
>
> On the other hand, assume you want to examine the experiences of women as they move through the stages of biopsy, diagnosis, surgery, chemotherapy, and the uncertainty of the future. Compared with the first approach, this query is broader in scope and will require following a group of women over time. It may require up to 9 months or 1 year of the investigator's time to interview women at each of these different stages, as well as to conduct interviews with their significant others and physicians, to understand the full impact of the sequence of events.

Whether spending a short period or a long time in the field, the investigator must determine the point at which sufficient information has been obtained. At that point the investigator leaves the field and engages in a final interpretive process that involves preparing one or more final reports. This point is sometimes referred to as "saturation." Indications of saturation include the investigator no longer being puzzled or surprised by events or by what people say in the field, the investigator predicting behaviors or outcomes, and information becoming redundant compared with information already collected and learned by the investigator. When the investigator begins to hear the same story or can predict what a respondent is going to say, it is time to leave the field (see later discussion on saturation).

Multiple Information-Gathering Strategies

Some methodologists suggest that by its nature, all naturalistic inquiry is multimethod.[6] We do not see the naturalistic tradition as multimethod in itself, but we do highlight the typical use of numerous data collection methods in a single study. Because different strategies are designed to derive information from numerous sources, the use of multiple approaches to obtaining information enhances the investigator's capacity to obtain a complex and rich understanding of the phenomenon under study. It is therefore common practice to use more than one data collection strategy even if a query is small in scope. Throughout and at the end of the data collection process, all sources of information are analyzed to ensure that they support an interpretive scheme and set of conclusions.

Investigators can use many different data-gathering strategies, some of which are discussed later. In most types of naturalistic inquiry, investigators may not know exactly which strategy they will use before entering the field. Although thought and planning occur in all phases of naturalistic inquiry, the final decision to use a particular approach to collecting information occurs as the research progresses. As noted, an important part of the naturalistic process of data collection occurs during fieldwork, throughout which the investigator must decide which data collection technique to use and at which point it should be introduced.

No standard approach is available to indicate which strategy should be used and when it should be introduced across the different forms of naturalistic inquiry. Data collection decisions are specific to the research query, the preferred way of knowing by the investigator, and the contextual opportunities that emerge while in the field. In a phenomenological study, for example, some investigators prefer to interview respondents first and then review written documents, virtual sources, journals, medical records, and other materials. In this type of study, it is considered critical initially to listen in an interview to the emotions and feelings naturally expressed by individuals asked to reflect on their experiences. Reading the literature or other textual sources before the interviewing process may introduce analytical frames that may prevent attentive listening to the experiences of individuals. In contrast, some ethnographers prefer to initially "hang out" in the field and use the data collection strategy of observation before introducing interviewing or other collection strategies. Still other ethnographers initially conduct open-ended interviews with key informants and then engage in participant observation. Other strategies, such as recordings, standardized questionnaires, or review of documents, may be introduced at subsequent stages of fieldwork.[5]

Overview of Principles

The hallmark of gathering information for the naturalistic researcher is that this action process occurs in and is responsive to the context in which the investigation is taking place. Data-gathering actions are designed to examine the context and all that occurs within it. No standardized data collection procedures structure studies or set criteria for rigor. Rather, the critical components of information-gathering actions tend to be diverse, based on the particular form of inquiry and the investigator's ongoing judgments about what approaches can elicit the most relevant and illuminating data. Usually, the investigator is actively involved in the context over a prolonged time to ensure sufficient immersion in the phenomena under study. However, the level of investigator involvement varies depending on the form of inquiry. In all forms of naturalistic inquiry, best practice involves the use of multiple strategies to obtain information in an ongoing and integrated data collection and analytical process.

These basic components or guiding principles in data gathering yield interpretations and understandings of phenomena that are embedded in specific contexts and complex interrelationships. The complexity of phenomena is preserved in all representations and reports by the nature of the data-gathering process. Let us examine how these principles are implemented and how naturalistic inquiry actually works.

INFORMATION-GATHERING PROCESS

What is the process of conducting fieldwork or gathering information? Although the process has been variably defined, we have borrowed the structure suggested by Shaffir and Stebbins[7] in the early 1990s because of its simplicity and comprehensiveness and continued relevance to the range of designs within the naturalistic tradition. Shaffir and Stebbins view the action process of data collection in naturalistic inquiry as four interrelated parts or considerations: context selection and "getting in the field," "learning the ropes" or obtaining meanings of the setting,

"maintaining relations," and "leaving the field."[7] Although these actions appear to represent distinct phases or research steps, the process is truly integrated; each component overlaps and shapes the other.

Selecting the Context

The first decision about data collection in naturalistic research is where or in what context information should be obtained. The researcher must "bound" the study by depicting a context that is conceptual, virtual, or locational (see Chapters 12 and 14). Because naturalistic research focuses on the natural research context, as well as what happens in it, selection of a context is an important factor in gathering data. The context may be the private lives of famous people, the interrelationships of a surgical team, the world of hospice specialists, the meaning of disability to subscribers of a disability website (listserv), or the meanings of caregiving to Hispanic families.

Context selection may sound simple, but there are several important considerations. First, the specification of a context must be practical or realistic to study. For example, how realistic is it to propose an inquiry to study the private lives of famous people? Will you be able to gain access to such individuals? Will these people choose to participate in this type of study, since agreement will jeopardize their privacy?

Second, in bounding a study to a particular context, the researcher must be careful not to limit the focus and thus the opportunity to obtain a full picture of the phenomenon under investigation. Consider the following examples:

Assume you want to study how children with learning disabilities learn to cope with and adapt to their differences. Identifying the classroom as the main context of the investigation may be too narrow. It may enable you to identify and describe the strategies that children use in that context, but it may not enable you to understand the full range of adaptive mechanisms that are used in learning in other contexts and how these mechanisms are obtained.

You are interested in studying the interrelationships and behaviors of a surgical team. You initially plan to examine the interactions of the surgical team during surgery. However, observations of this context may be too limiting. It may not yield a complete understanding of the interprofessional relationships that inform interactions in the specific context of surgery. Examining professional behaviors in other contexts, such as in the cafeteria, at staff meetings, or in social engagements, may provide important insights.

You are interested in examining the functional capacities of persons with traumatic brain injuries. If the context for the study is functional capacity in a clinical setting, the informant may be maximally functional in this particular setting. The investigator who does not expand the context to include other environments may not discover the functional incapacity that the person with traumatic brain injury often exhibits in less structured settings.

It is important to recognize that identifying the context of a naturalistic study will depend, in part, on the nature of the query, the design strategy, and the characteristics of the persons being studied.

Gaining Access

Once the context for the research endeavor is identified, the investigator must gain access to it. This is not as simple as it may sound. *Gaining access* to the context of the study requires strategizing, negotiating with key individuals who may serve as gatekeepers, and perhaps renegotiating once initial entry has occurred. In some cases the investigator may already be a part of the natural context.

Suppose you are a student and want to understand the process of becoming a health professional. As a student in health care, you are actually an "insider" of this particular context. Although access is not a problem, other aspects to fieldwork will be challenging. As an "insider," you will have to work hard to understand how your knowledge and previous experiences influence the information you gather and interpret.

Consider a situation in which you are a regular reader of a "listserv" devoted to the discussion of disability rights and are examining the texts of postings to determine how rights are conceptualized and experienced. As a regular "lurker," you

are knowledgeable about the lives and experiences of those who post. However, you must be careful to identify this information as different from analysis of the actual posted texts as you analyze the textual data for meanings. Moreover, as an insider, you will also need to analyze how your understandings, biases, values, and experiences influence your interpretation of web-based text.

If the investigator is an "outsider," access must be obtained. Mechanisms for gaining access have been extensively discussed in the literature, particularly by ethnographers.[5,8] How the researcher gains access into a context can influence the entire course of the research process. Gaining access involves obtaining permission to enter and become part of the social or cultural setting. Investigators may use different strategies, depending on the nature of the context and their initial relationship to it. Formal introduction to an informant by another, slowly building rapport through participation, joining a club or virtual context, and gift giving are techniques used by investigators to enter a field.

You want to conduct a study in a medical setting. To gain access, initially it will be important to discuss the nature of your study with the directors of the departments you want to include. This discussion will be followed by a more formal introduction to medical personnel in staff meetings.

Gaining access may be simple but can also take time and hard work. You need to clarify the ways you intend to be involved in the context and the implications of your study for the participants.

An important consideration in obtaining access is the degree to and the way in which the intent of your study is presented to participants (Box 17-1). The

---

BOX 17-1
CONSIDERATIONS IN GAINING ACCESS

1. Presenting study to participants.
2. Ensuring confidentiality.
3. Minimizing impact of investigator on natural context.

researcher must decide on the extent to which the research activity is revealed to those being observed or interviewed. Although disclosure of the purpose and scope of the research is most often made clear to those informants who provide initial access, the specifics of the research activity may remain vague to others who are either observed or interviewed at different times in the course of fieldwork. The extent of overt or covert research activities varies in any type of inquiry depending on the context, varies from study to study, and has important ethical concerns for researchers.

The other aspect of disclosure of research purpose is to ensure your informants that the information they provide will remain confidential. Stearns discusses this issue for physicians in her descriptive study of how health management organizations (HMOs) structure the professional relationship between physician and patient:

> Only a few physicians refused to allow me to tape the interview. However, many expressed concerns that the interview remains confidential. This concern as well as their hesitancy to be interviewed meant that I had to be especially careful not to reveal who I had interviewed or what they had said. Confidentiality of physician (and other) responses was thus of great concern in the research.[9]

As Internet-based research becomes increasingly used, investigators must consider confidentiality in different ways. As mentioned, websites can be easily accessed without the knowledge of those who post messages or interact online. Even if you gain access through registering to become part of a listserv and remain an anonymous participant, you still must take all measures to uphold the same ethic of confidentiality that you would exercise in all other environments.[10]

Another consideration in gaining access is the impact of the investigator on the investigated. Whether the researcher is initially an insider or outsider, his or her presence may change the nature of the field and how people present and live their experiences. The reactive effect of the investigator's presence on the phenomenon being observed is a major methodological dilemma for this type of research.

In his classic study of black men who frequented urban street corners, Liebow describes the effect of his presence:

> All in all, I felt I was making steady progress. There was still plenty of suspicion and mistrust, however. At least two men who hung around Carry Out— one of them the local numbers man—had seen me dozens of times in close quarters but kept their distance and I kept mine.[11]

"Learning the Ropes"

Once initial entry into the context has been made, the investigator must gain access to different informants, personal stories and experiences, texts, and types of observations. Thus, gaining access remains an ongoing process that involves continued negotiation and renegotiation with members of the site or the individual or groups of individuals who are the focus of the study. This ongoing access process is part of the active work of doing fieldwork and has been referred to as "learning the ropes,"[7] "obtaining meanings," or obtaining an "intimate familiarity"[12] with the setting or study phenomena. In classic ethnography this process may appear as if the investigator is simply "hanging out." However, a range of data-gathering strategies, including watching and listening, asking questions, recording, and examining materials, is brought into play to learn meanings within a setting. These strategies are purposely chosen, combined, and integrated and are all part of the unfolding process of learning about the field.

The choice of strategy depends on the ebb and flow of the fieldwork situation and the particular issue on which the investigator is focused. Any data-gathering strategy is designed to move the investigator from being an outsider to an insider capable of understanding and experiencing the meanings of symbols, language, and behavior within the setting. The movement from outside to inside involves a reflexive process in which the investigator is constantly comparing and analyzing pieces of information. Data collection strategies are designed to reveal the unknown and examine phenomena that the investigator does not understand or finds puzzling.

Suppose you are studying families who are experiencing stress as a result of their efforts to provide daily care to a family member with dementia. As you interview a particular family, you are certain that the family will soon choose nursing home placement for the individual with dementia. You become surprised to learn, however, that institutionalization has never been considered by the family.

This example represents what Agar referred to as a "rich point."[2] A *rich point* represents a problem in your understanding and is the point at which you learn that your assumptions are not adequate to explain how things are working. Rich points reflect the active work of the investigator that bridges the distance between his or her world and the world of the people who are the focus of the study. Learning the ropes involves using different data collection strategies that give rise to these rich points.

An investigator has joined an online chat room to learn about the experiences and meanings of marriage to individuals who are gay and lesbian. In anonymous reading of the postings, the investigator is confused by the diversity of opinions about the value of marriage. To move further in the research process, the investigator must make a decision to identify herself, her purpose, and the acceptable actions that should ensue in order to be a more active participant in the listserv.

INFORMATION-GATHERING STRATEGIES

Many different information-gathering strategies are used in naturalistic inquiry. The three main strategies introduced in Chapter 15—watching and listening, asking, and examining materials—have a different purpose and structure when used in naturalistic inquiry than when used in experimental-type designs.

Watching and Listening

The process of watching and listening is often referred to as "observation." In naturalistic research, observation occurs within the natural context or field. In this data collection strategy the investigator can be either a passive observer or a participant. Passive observation involves the investigators situating themselves in the field or particular activity and simply observing what occurs. On the other hand, active involvement or participation in combination with observation has been classically defined

as "the process in which the investigator establishes and sustains a many-sided and relatively long-term relationship with a human association in its natural setting for the purpose of developing a scientific understanding of that association."[12]

More recently, Tedlock (in Denzin and Lincoln[3]) has suggested that the process of *participant observation,* rather than being characterized as the intersection of scientific inquiry with investment in relationships, is a complex human interaction in which meaning and knowledge are generated by the interaction of the investigator, those investigated, and those who hear and read the research report. In participant observation the investigator is not a passive observer but actively engages in the research context to come to know about it. The investigator begins with broad observations to describe what is seen and then narrows the focus to discover the meaning of what has been described. In descriptive observation it is often helpful to think of the investigator as a video camera that records what it sees as it scans the boundaries of the research setting. This technique reminds the researcher that description, not interpretation, is the first step in participant observation.

Participant observation, which Tedlock renames "observation of participation" to remind us of the need to observe ourselves in the process of the investigation, is based on the assumption that an important way of learning about a context and group of people is to participate with them in their daily activities and personally experience and observe what transpires. Participant observation has many behaviors in common with what we do in newly encountered social situations. All of us participate and observe in social situations. As an investigator engaged in participant observation, however, the researcher seeks to become explicitly aware of the way things are. The researcher remains introspective and examines the "self" in the situation and his or her experiences as both the insider participating in the event and the outsider observing the actions.

As described by Rodwell,[13] "It is in the doing of data collection that the understanding of the subject of interest is achieved."

Gubrium summarizes the advantages of this approach as follows:

The goal is to wind up with a depiction of "the way it is," as it were, in a particular setting. [W]e can represent the meanings of a setting in terms more relevant to our subjects than other methods permit. "I've been there," the participant observer likes to put it, "seen what actually happens, and this is the way it is."[14]

In one of his early ethnographies on nursing homes, Gubrium described the multiple roles he assumed over several months as a participant observer:

I took many roles, ranging from doing the rather menial work called "toileting" by people there to serving as gerontologist at staff meetings. I attempted to spend sufficient time in the setting to establish trust, to interact with as many people as possible, and to observe the varied facts of life at Murray Manor in their natural states.[15]

Some types of designs or fieldwork situations warrant less participation in the observation process. Nonparticipatory observation can be used to obtain an understanding of a natural context without the influence of the observer.

> Consider the previous of the investigator examining the meaning of marriage to people of diverse sexual orientation. "Lurking," or reading web postings without identifying oneself, would leave the interactive context of the chat room intact. However, once the investigator actively enters the interaction, the virtual group and all subsequent interaction have been expanded and changed.

During the fieldwork process, watching and listening tend to move from broad, descriptive observations to a narrow focus in which the observer looks for not only more descriptive data but also specific understanding of the meanings of what he or she has observed. The degree of participation in the context and the extent of immersion vary throughout fieldwork and are based on the nature of the inquiry, access to the setting, and practical limitations.

Asking

As a method of data collection, asking in the form of interviewing is another essential strategy used in most types of naturalistic inquiry. Often, asking information

from key informants is the initial and primary data collection strategy in phenomenology, ethnography, and grounded-theory approaches. The investigator may use an asking strategy to obtain an example of a social interchange to clarify or verify the accuracy of observations or to obtain the informant's experience with and view of the phenomenon under study. Asking, unlike observation, involves direct contact with persons who are capable of providing information. Thus, to collect data by asking, the researcher must establish a relationship appropriate to the level of involvement with the informant.

Asking can take many forms in naturalistic research, from an informal, open-ended conversation to a focused or long in-depth interview.[16] The timing of the interview in the research process, the purpose of the asking, and the nature of the relationship with the informant all influence the type of asking the investigator chooses.

The most common form of asking in naturalistic design is unstructured, open-ended interviewing. This type of interviewing is particularly important in the beginning stages of fieldwork when the investigator is trying to become familiar with the language of the group and everyday occurrences.

> In the investigation of the meaning of marriage to chat room members, the investigator might post a broad question such as, "Tell me more about what the term 'marriage' means to each of you."

The open-ended interview may consist of informal conversation recorded by the investigator; face-to-face, telephone, or online "twosomes"; or small groups in which the investigator sets the context for the interview and the informants offer their knowledge.

The ethnographic interview and life history are frequently used face-to-face interviews. In ethnographic interview the investigator seeks to understand culture through talking with insiders in the culture.[17] The investigator not only attends to the content of the interview but also examines the structural and symbolic elements of the social exchange between the investigator and the informant. Contemporary ethnographic interview acknowledges that meanings may be changed and may be made not only within the context of the interview itself, but also at any point from the initial communication through the consumption of the research report.[3]

Life history, or biography,[18] is a form of naturalistic interview that chronicles an individual's life within a social context. In the case of an investigator telling all or part of his or her own life story, the term memoir is used to name the data source. The investigator elicits information not only on the important events or "turnings" in an individual's life, but also on the meaning of those events within the contexts in which they occur. This form of interviewing can also be an independent design structure.

Common forms of group questioning include focus groups and group interviews with social units, such as families with more than one individual or a cohort of individuals who share a diagnostic condition.

> Focus groups are groups that are special in terms of purpose, size, composition, and procedures. Their purpose is to thoughtfully explore through discussion a topic or phenomena of interest to researchers, marketers, or consultants.[19]

In a *focus group* the investigator sets the parameters for the conversation. The participants, usually a group of 6 to 12 individuals, then address the specified topic by responding to guiding probes or questions posed by the investigator. This approach is used when it is believed that the interactions and group discussions will yield more meaningful understanding than single, independent interviews.[20]

Group interviews with small social units are also useful in observing group dynamics and symbolic meanings exchanged among group members. In cultural descriptions, questioning social units can be most valuable in understanding the structural groups of a society. This form of interviewing can also be an independent design structure.

Although the structured questionnaire is primarily used in experimental-type designs, it is occasionally incorporated into certain naturalistic inquiries. Investigators have found that structured or even semi-structured questionnaires can provide important insights into specific questions that emerge in the course of conducting fieldwork. The use of a standardized instrument or structured questionnaire also enables the investigator to determine the distribution of a particular phenomenon. Consider the following example.

> You are conducting a study of the meaning of breast cancer among young women. In open-ended interviewing, you detect that many of the women may be depressed because their recurring statements suggest evidence of depressive symptomatology. To test your "hunch" or emerging hypothesis, you decide to administer a standardized depression scale. The scores that result provide an additional source of data that may or may not support your initial impressions. Also, the use of the scale will enable you to determine the distribution of depression among the study group.

The use of a structured set of questions or standardized scale represents a purposeful and focused approach to asking. This approach is introduced only in naturalistic inquiry when the investigator has been in the field for some time and has developed rapport and "learned the ropes."

Four Components of Asking Strategies

Although we do it every day, asking clear questions that beget the answers we are seeking is not an easy task. We have all been in situations in which the answers to our questions seemed to come from "left field" until we realized that our questions were not understood as we had intended. So now we turn to a more detailed discussion of asking. In naturalistic inquiry, there are four interrelated components of an asking strategy: access, description, focus, and verification.

Access

Asking begins with access. The investigator initially wants to meet and select one or more individuals who can articulate information about the people or phenomenon that is the focus of the study. You may ask who would be willing to speak to a stranger about personal history, events, experiences, and feelings. It is important to know the reasons someone is willing to speak to you so that you have a context to understand what the person relates. Sometimes the first key informant is someone who is formally or informally designated by the cultural group to speak to an outsider. At other times the informant may be a person who is considered a "deviant" within the cultural group or a person who has nothing to lose by "hanging out" with a stranger. In other cases the informant may represent the person with the most knowledge, experience, or seniority in a group.

Regardless of the informant's status, the investigator initially seeks to speak to a number of persons who can orient the researcher to the context or field of inquiry. As the research progresses, the investigator may want to select specific individuals to interview who possess distinct knowledge important to the study. Consider the following examples.

> In her study of homeless, middle-aged women, Butler[21] entered the field with broad criteria for selecting informants. These criteria included those willing to speak with her over a 3-month period and those willing and able to articulate their experiences. Much of her time was spent "hanging out" and establishing rapport with informants. Once a level of rapport and confidence was established, she was able to apply more purposeful and structured interviewing approaches.

> In the classic ethnographic study of urban black men by Liebow,[11] access was initially gained through "hanging out" on the street corner where men were likely to congregate. Liebow describes his first entry into the social scene as occurring serendipitously. On his first day in the field, he noticed a commotion and immediately went to the site where it was occurring. As a result of being there, Liebow was able to introduce himself into the culture of the street corner.

Description

Once access is obtained, the initial goal of asking is to describe. Description begins with asking broad questions that become more focused as trends, recurrent patterns, and themes emerge. Frequently the investigator begins the asking process with a broad probe such as, "Tell me about . . . ."

> In Liebow's study, asking began informally when he invited a man whom he had met on the street corner to have coffee. Liebow clarified his task as a researcher and "sat at the bar for several hours talking over coffee."[11]

Focus

Based on emerging descriptive knowledge, the researcher's asking becomes more focused and probing. Asking questions requires intense listening, a show of respect, and great interest in each aspect of what the informant is saying. The investigator wants to ask questions that yield answers that are detailed and that go into depth about the phenomena of interest. If an informant shows or articulates disinterest or boredom with the interview, the investigator knows the questions are not salient or do not focus on the aspects of the experience or phenomenon important to the interviewee.

In developing an open-ended or semistructured interview in which you want to focus on details and elicit rich description, consider the guidelines listed in Box 17-2.

Verification

As the investigator gains an understanding of the context, asking strategies serve to verify impressions and clarify details of the setting. Verification is the process of checking the accuracy of impressions with informants.

Throughout fieldwork, the interview process may occur in one session, several sessions, or many sessions. It is usually combined with one or more of the other primary data collection strategies of observation and review of existing materials. The decision about length and frequency of asking strategies depends on the nature and scope of the query, the purpose of the

---

BOX 17-2
GUIDELINES FOR OBTAINING RICH DESCRIPTION

1. Do not use questions that yield "yes" or "no" responses.
2. Ask informants for examples to explain their statements.
3. Obtain more details from the examples by asking specific follow-up questions.
4. Use follow-up questions to seek elaborations of statements by probing.
■ "Is this how it always happens?"
■ "How typical is this for you?"
■ "What would have happened if . . .?"
■ "How did you feel when . . .?"

interviews, and the practical limitations that influence the conduct of the study.

Examining Materials

Examining source materials such as texts (records, diaries, journals, e-mails, articles, narratives, letters) is another essential data collection strategy in contemporary naturalistic research. This is particularly the case in health and human service research, where textual records (e.g., charts, progress notes, minutes) are routinely maintained as a natural part of the context.

Similar to watching, listening, and asking, review of materials usually begins with a broad examination of items. Then the investigator moves to a more focused evaluation to explore recurring themes and emerging patterns. Knowledge about what materials are available may occur at any point in the research process. It is not unusual to plan to examine objects and texts at the beginning of a project.

> Assume you are interested in determining the extent to which a behavioral program for persons with mental retardation improves social behavior in sheltered work environments. You may begin by observing workplace behavior. However, there are times throughout the day when you cannot observe. You may examine progress notes written by the sheltered workshop staff to obtain additional information about behavior and better understand behavioral patterns at different times of the day. You will analyze the perceptions of staff in light of your own observations and the other information you obtain.

For the most part, to access text documents, the investigator should obtain appropriate consent, even if he or she is an insider. Exceptions to this principle include unobtrusive data collection in which identity of the individuals studied will not be revealed and cases when consent may not be desirable or possible. The primary aim of unobtrusively collecting information will be to keep the research role covert, with the ethical boundaries of protection of human subjects.

> Consider the researcher asked to evaluate the impact of a community-based intervention designed to decrease drug use in a particular neighborhood. One indicator of drug use in the area is the presence of drug paraphernalia, such as the vials and needles strewn in a small, centrally located park. Examining the contents of the trash and the grounds of the community park may shed light on substance abuse patterns without causing harm to individual substance users. Further, unobtrusive approaches might be the most accurate method (or the only method) of obtaining data to ascertain the outcome of the intervention, especially in light of reluctance or refusal to self-report drug abuse behaviors. Positive changes in the environment may provide an important source of evidence that the intervention is having an impact.

RECORDING INFORMATION

While in the field, an investigator can use several different strategies to record the information that is obtained by watching and listening, asking, or reviewing materials. Recording information is an important aspect of collecting information. The record of information serves as a data set that is analyzed by the investigator in the process of doing fieldwork and then more formally after leaving the field. An investigator must decide how he or she will record information while watching and listening, asking, and reviewing material. Usually, multiple recording strategies are used in fieldwork. The decision about which strategy to use is based on the purpose of the study and the resources of the investigator. Let us examine three primary mechanisms for recording information.

Field Notes

Field notes are a basic way in which investigators record information. This type of recording has been a popular topic in the research literature on naturalistic inquiry and has been described in many ways. Usually, field notes have two basic components: (1) recordings of events, observations, and occurrences and (2) recordings of the investigator's own impressions of events, personal feelings, hunches, and expectations. Some investigators separate these two components. They maintain one set of field notes that carefully document major field activities and events. In a separate notebook or computer file, they keep a running account or personal diary of their own feelings and personal dilemmas encountered in the field.

Numerous formats are suggested in the literature for recording descriptive field notes. According to Spradley,[22] a matrix design can be used to examine the interaction of persons, places, and objects. Other formats are equally useful. Lofland and Lofland[12] suggest recording description and bracketing impressions and interpretation within the context of the description. We have found it useful to use a laptop computer or handheld device on which the screen is divided into two longitudinal columns either through the creation of a table or through using a template. The left side is used to describe, and the right side is used to record the investigator's immediate thoughts, impressions, hunches, and questions as the observation or interview occurs. The ability to separate a description from an interpretation is important in order to clarify and distinguish among observation, impression, one's emotive responses to the context of inquiry and what occurs within it, and thoughts and queries to guide future inquiry.

When to record field notes has also been discussed in the literature. This decision is an important consideration in doing fieldwork and will depend on the nature of the inquiry. Some investigators find it useful to keep a pencil and pad or electronic device available at all times during participant observation activities.

> You are studying homeless adolescents in a shelter setting as the basis for ascertaining their service, health, nutrition, and other support needs. To record your observations as you pass through the building, you carry a personal digital assistant (PDA) to capture the informal interactions of the spontaneous shelter culture, which might give you important insights into the needs of the adolescents.

Other investigators find the act of recording while participating in an event too intrusive and recommend documenting at the conclusion of the day and in privacy. Waiting until the end of the day, however, carries the risk of depending on long-term memory and losing details that may later prove to be important.

Field notes are only one way of recording information and are used in conjunction with other mechanisms.

Voice Recording

Voice recording is a fundamental data-recording strategy in naturalistic inquiry primarily used when conducting on-site or virtual face-to face interviews. To capture and retain communication as precisely as possible, it is especially important to use voice recording when conducting an open-ended interview. In such interviews, informants provide long, detailed accounts that are usually difficult for the investigator to write verbatim. Naturalistic investigators use two primary technologies to record sound: audiotape and digital recording.

Audiotape requires the use of a microphone, tape recorder, and tape. When using an audiotape, remember to test the equipment before an interview to make certain that it will adequately record both your voice and that of the respondent. We have learned from experience that once you lose a taped interview, it cannot be recreated from memory. You should plan to have a backup tape recorder in case there is equipment failure during the interview. You must plan for every contingency to avoid the risk of losing data.

Because recent technological innovations allow transfer of digital sound to text, naturalistic investigators are increasingly turning to digital recording. Various types of recording equipment can be used, including a digital microphone hooked into a computer, a PDA with recording capacity, and even a cellular phone. As with audiotape, ensure that all connections are made and that the equipment is operating both before you start and throughout the interview. Because glitches occur in keeping electronic records, make sure that you back up your digital data. After you record an interview, your next step is to label the tape or data file carefully and make a backup file. If using audiotape or digital recording that cannot be automatically translated to text, you will need to transcribe the recording. If you do have a voice-to-text program, make sure that the format for translation provides you with a useful and well-structured transcript.

Transcription is an important step that involves translating the entire recording to text, usually in a word-processing file. In transcribing, you will need to decide if every utterance should be recorded, such as "uh hum" or laughter. You will need to decide how pauses and silences will be noted in the transcript. Voice-to-text technology is still new, so if you make a determination that all utterances and silences are important, you might want to type a transcript from the voice recording rather than use a computer program to create a text data file.

Typing a transcript takes time but usually is worth the effort, and it is essential when you are searching for nuances of meaning beyond actual words. Every hour of dense interview can take 6 to 8 hours of transcribing. After transcribing a voice recording, you need to compare the written record with the recording to ensure accuracy. Finally, you will want to listen to the voice recording to examine the nuances in vocalization, as well as read the transcript to analyze the narrative.

There are several considerations in using voice recording. First, you must decide whether recording will be intrusive in your field setting and will prevent informants from expressing private thoughts. Second, when using voice recording, informants must be informed that their conversations with you are being recorded. In most cases, obtaining consent from study participants is not a problem. If you are studying issues that are highly sensitive, however, such as sexual practices of teenagers or drug use among businessmen, concerns may be expressed by informants. You will need to explain your plan for maintaining confidentiality and decide who will have access to the voice recordings and where they will be kept. Also, it is important to inform research participants that they can request that recording cease at any point in the interview process.

The third consideration in using voice recordings is their analysis. In the beginning phases of fieldwork, some investigators find that it is important to transcribe voice to text immediately after completing an interview. Reviewing these early recordings often informs the initial development of analytical categories, subsequent data collection efforts, and type of follow-up questions that need to be pursued. As throughout all thinking and action processes in research, your study purpose is foremost in guiding your choice of voice-recording method and transcription. Practical considerations, such as cost, time, and available technological capacity, are other important factors in helping you decide how to proceed.

Video Imaging

Video imaging is another data-recording strategy that is being increasingly used in naturalistic inquiry.[23] Video imaging is particularly useful in studies that focus on interactions between individuals (e.g., mental health professionals and clients) and when observations of both nonverbal and verbal behaviors are the focus of the research study. In participant observation the investigator is involved with both nonverbal and verbal exchanges and may have difficulty monitoring the details of actions. Video imaging enables the investigator to record such details of behaviors that may not be detected at the time of the observation. With imaging, the investigator obtains a permanent record that can be viewed and reviewed multiple times.

As in voice recording, many considerations and decisions must be made when using video imaging. Choice of and familiarity with the equipment and ability to manage it efficiently in the field setting are clearly important. Video imaging devices range from a simple camera on your cell phone or wristwatch to complex digital video camera equipment. Purpose and practical issues will help you decide the best technology and approach.

With video imaging, the issue of "reactivity" needs to be considered. Do individuals monitor their behavior because of the camera? Investigators use various strategies to reduce discomfort and reactivity. Some recommend that the camera be introduced into the field environment before recording the events that are of interest. Having a camera present but not turning it on for several occasions can reduce fear or reluctance of participants to be filmed. Using a small, unobtrusive camera can also be used to create less interference in the natural setting. Another consideration is the angle of the setting and the behaviors that are captured by the camera. The video image may capture only a set of activities that are performed in front of the lens, and thus other movements and exchanges that occur simultaneously but outside its range of vision will be lost.

As in voice recording, the investigator must carefully review each video image many times. Initial review of a video image helps inform the investigator as to how to proceed in the field and which questions to pursue. After leaving the field, formal analysis of the video images may proceed incrementally through the action if the investigator has the appropriate equipment. The use and analysis of images can become quite complex, time-consuming, and expensive.

Video imaging can be used in combination with other techniques, such as participant observation, interviewing, and voice recording.

ACCURACY IN COLLECTING INFORMATION

At this point, you may be asking how an investigator involved with naturalistic inquiry becomes confident that the information he or she has obtained is accurate and reflects empirically shared observations of the field. This concern has been labeled as the issue of "trustworthiness."[24] After all, the investigator wants to obtain information that correctly captures the experiences, meanings, and events of the field. How are we to know if the final interpretation is not simply a fabrication of the investigator or a reflection of his or her personal biases and presuppositions? A number of techniques in naturalistic inquiry are designed to enhance the "truth value" of the investigator's data collection and initial analytical efforts.

Multiple Data Gatherers

One technique used in naturalistic inquiry is the involvement of two or more investigators in the data-gathering and analytical process. The old adage "Two heads are better than one" is also true in naturalistic inquiry. If possible, two or more investigators should observe and record their own field notes independently. This technique checks the accuracy of the observations; more than one pair of eyes and ears are examining and recording the same context. Careful training of both observers is essential to ensure that each observer practice skilled recording and reporting and that all investigators understand the purpose and intent of the study.

Consider an investigator who is studying the culture of a group of hospitalized adolescents. The purpose of such a study may be to determine the norms of the culture as they emerge within the boundaries of the hospital unit. Using the technique of multiple observers, two or more investigators will keep field notes independently of one another and will initially analyze these data separately. The investigators will then meet to compare notes and impressions and reconcile any differences through in-depth discourse about the data set. Not only are multiple observers used, but multiple analyzers ensure accurate data collection as well.

Triangulation (Crystallization)

Another technique that increases the accuracy of information gathering is called *triangulation.*[25] Recently, to reflect the complexity of multiple approaches to obtaining information, some have suggested replacing triangulation with "crystallization."[8] To dispel the two-dimensional and linear image of a triangle, the metaphor of a crystal has become useful in depicting the multifaceted data collection methods and analysis in naturalistic inquiry.

However, because of the frequency of its current use, we refer to multiple methods of data collection with the traditional term "triangulation." By triangulation we mean multiple approaches that bear on the same phenomenon. For example, the use of observation with interviewing, the examination of materials, or the use of all three is characteristic of triangulation in traditional naturalistic research. More recently, quantitative measures and analytical techniques such as "content analysis" have also been introduced to provide the meaning of a phenomenon from a different angle. In triangulating, the investigator collects information from different sources to derive and validate a particular finding. The investigator may observe an event and combine observations with textual, narrative materials to develop a comprehensive and accurate description.

Saturation

Saturation is another way in which the investigator ensures rigor in conducting a naturalistic study. *Saturation* refers to the point at which an investigator has obtained sufficient information from which to obtain an understanding of the phenomenon under study. As previously discussed, when the information gathered by the investigator does not provide new insights or understandings, it is a signal that saturation has been achieved. If you can guess what your respondent is going to do or say in a particular situation, you have probably obtained saturation.[5] In *Tally's Corner* Liebow's prolonged engagement in the field ensured that the investigator obtained a point of saturation.[11]

However, lengthy immersion in the field may not be practical for service provider researchers, who may have limited time and funds to support such an endeavor.

> Suppose that you were constrained by time and money in conducting your study of the service and support needs of homeless adolescents. You would have to use other strategies such as triangulation to heighten the accuracy and rigor of your understandings and interpretations.

You might also use random observation as a strategy to ensure saturation. In this technique an investigator randomly selects times throughout the investigative period to increase the likelihood of obtaining a total picture of the phenomenon of interest.

> You might select random times during the week, including morning, afternoon, and night, to observe in the shelter. In this way you could approximate full immersion in the culture of the shelter. Through random observation, it is theoretically possible to sample the total cycle of the phenomenon of interest.

Member Checking

Member checking is a technique whereby the investigator checks out his or her assumptions with one or more informants. For example, if your analysis identified that the adolescents in the shelter were in need of alternative high school settings, you might verify this with your informants by asking them if your interpretations were accurate. This type of affirmation decreases the potential for the imposition of the investigator's bias where it does not belong. Member checking is used throughout the data collection process to confirm the truth value or accuracy of the investigator's observations and interpretations as they emerge. The informants' ability to correct the vision of their stories is critical to this technique.

> The importance of routinely using member checking is highlighted by our experience in conducting a needs assessment. We took on the task from a rural state health department to develop a grant proposal to obtain funding to restructure "personal care assistant" services. After a number of focus group interviews with diverse stakeholder groups, we analyzed our data and developed a series of principles to guide the preparation of a grant proposal. The primary principle that we identified was the need for adequate training and supervision of personal care assistants. However, when we submitted our preliminary ideas to the stakeholder groups, only the professionals agreed with our priority sequence. For families, consumers, and personal care assistants, the primary need was recruitment, since there were insufficient personnel to meet even basic service needs of the community. If we had not conducted member checks, we might have sought and obtained funding for training that would be unattended.

Reflexivity

Although investigator bias cannot be eliminated, it can be identified and examined in terms of its impact on data collection processes and interpretive accounts. *Reflexivity* refers to the process of self-examination. In reflexive analysis the investigator examines his or her own perspective and determines how this perspective has influenced not only what is learned but also *how* it is learned. Using our needs assessment example, had we conducted reflexive analysis more rigorously when we initially examined the data set, we may have identified the bias toward training that we held as health professional educators and researchers. Through reflection, investigators evaluate how understanding and knowledge are developed within the context of their own thinking processes.

In discussing the importance of reflexive analysis in his research on disabled persons and sexuality, Shakespeare and his colleagues state:

> [P]erhaps we might have misrepresented disabled people's experiences or desires or distorted the evidence to provide an account which is unduly negative or positive. It is unusual to be given the opportunity to reflect on the research process, to justify our work, or to correct any misapprehensions which have arisen.[26]

A personal diary or method of noting personal feelings, moods, attitudes, and reactions to each step of the data collection process is a critical aspect of the process in naturalistic inquiry. These personal notes form the backdrop from which to understand how a particular meaning or analysis may have emerged at the data collection stage. Fetterman[27] suggests that keeping a personal diary is an effective quality control mechanism.

As an example, let us look at the reflexivity issues that Shakespeare addressed when conducting research on "disability sexuality." As an insider in the disability community, Shakespeare worked with his colleagues to find out how he sought to identify the influence of his insider status, his experiences, and his own biases on the research process and outcome. Discussing how he identified and made use of his insider status, Shakespeare says:

> We looked at what little was already available, and we brainstormed from our own experience: we felt that our own lives and experiences were very relevant to the process. Rather than trying to achieve some spurious objectivity or distance, we acted as key informants and research participants.[26]

Now read how Shakespeare and his colleagues used reflexive analysis to identify and respond to sources of disagreement emerging from the diverse roles of each of the three researchers:

> One of us is predominantly a trainer, organizer and activist; another is a psychotherapist and counseling lecturer; a third is an academic. These differences meant that we approached the material in different ways.
>
> I do not believe that academics should be spokespeople for the disability movement. . . . However, academics do have a valuable part to play in the development of our understanding of the world as experienced by disabled people. It is a privileged position.[26]

By explicating and reflecting on his position as an academic, Shakespeare therefore acknowledged the limits and values of his perspective with regard to advancing an understanding of disability sexuality.

Audit Trail

Another way to increase rigor is to maintain an *audit trail* as the researcher proceeds analytically. Some suggest leaving a path of thinking and action processes so that others can clearly follow the logic and manner in which knowledge was developed. In this approach the investigator is responsible not only for reporting results, but also for explaining how the results are obtained. By explaining the thinking and action processes of an inquiry, the investigator allows others to agree or disagree with each analytical decision and to confirm, refute, or modify interpretations. Shakespeare and colleagues[26] clearly identified not only this method, but also how the thinking and action processes unfolded to yield data, impressions, and theory.

Peer Debriefing

One technique to ensure that data analysis represents the phenomena under investigation is the use of more than one investigator as a participant in the analytical process. Throughout a co-investigated study, researchers frequently conduct analytical actions independent of one another to determine the extent of their agreement. Synthesis of analysis and examination of areas of disagreement provide additional understanding on the research query. When only one investigator engages in a project, he or she will often ask an external analyzer to function in the capacity of a co-investigator. In some cases a panel of experts or advisors is used to evaluate the analytical process. This form of *peer debriefing* provides an opportunity for the investigator to reflect on competing interpretations offered in the peer review process, thus strengthening the legitimacy of the final interpretation. Shakespeare and colleagues[26] used peer debriefing at multiple time intervals throughout their study to modify and affirm their interpretations.

SUMMARY

The main purpose of the action process of data collection in naturalistic inquiry is to obtain information that incrementally leads to the investigator's ability to reveal a story, a set of descriptive principles or understandings, hypotheses, or theories. Each piece of information is a building block that the investigator inductively collects, analyzes, and puts together to accomplish one or more of the purposes just stated. The researcher begins with a broad query that gradually narrows, like a funnel, as data collection proceeds and the context becomes clearer to the investigator.

In naturalistic research, the organization and analysis of data collection go hand in hand. Data collection and data management continues to unfold dynamically (see Chapter 18) as analysis reveals further direction for information gathering (see Chapter 20). The investigator is the main vehicle for data collection, although the researcher's involvement may vary among design strategies. To enhance the accuracy of data collection, multiple observers and triangulation of collection methods are two action processes often used by naturalistic investigators.

The naturalistic researcher uses one or more of three basic methods to gather information: watching and listening, asking, and examining materials. Watching and listening occurs in the form of observation and ranges on a continuum from full to no participation in the context that is being observed. Asking also varies in structure, with interviewing as the primary asking process in naturalistic design. Examination of materials occurs in an inductive way and is intended to reveal patterns related to the phenomena under study. Naturalistic data collection occurs along with analysis and moves from broad information gathering to more focused collection of information. The combination of these approaches is critical to obtain breadth and depth of analysis.

As descriptive data are collected to illuminate the answer to "what, where, and when," the next step in the process is to focus data collection efforts based on the ongoing analytical process. The process of information collection continues with "why and how" questions. In ethnography this effort is called "thick" description, or focused observation, in which meanings are sought.

Focused observation hones in on examining the patterns and themes that emerge from descriptive information. The investigator may choose to examine one pattern at a time or may focus on more than one. The investigator narrows the scope of inquiry to themes and the interaction between patterns and themes while remaining open to further discovery. In general, collection strategies provide information that answers the "where, who, how, when, and why" questions. Answers to these five questions yield description, understanding of the context, occurrences within the context, and timing.

EXERCISES

1. Select a public place, such as a shopping mall, outpatient clinic, public transportation station, or Internet chat room. Use unobtrusive methods first and then participatory observation to determine behavioral patterns that characterize the human experience in each setting. Compare your experiences using both forms of observation and what you learned from each.

2. Conduct an open-ended interview with a colleague to obtain an understanding of career choices and his or her career path. What other information-gathering techniques can you use to understand this phenomenon?

3. Select a research article that uses naturalistic inquiry. Identify the information-gathering techniques used and determine the ethical issues involved for each technique.

REFERENCES

1. Hodge R, Kress G: *Social semiotics,* Ithaca, NY, 1988, Cornell University Press.
2. Agar MH: *The professional stranger: an informal introduction to ethnography,* ed 2, San Diego, Calif, 1996, Academic Press.
3. Denzin NK, Lincoln YS: *Handbook of qualitative research,* ed 2, Thousand Oaks, Calif, 2000, Sage.
4. Geertz C: *Interpretation of cultures,* New York, 1973, Basic Books.
5. Pole C: *Fieldwork,* Thousand Oaks, Calif, 2004, Sage.
6. Tashakkori A, Teddlie C : *Handbook of mixed methods social and behavioral research,* Thousand Oaks, Calif, 2003, Sage.
7. Shaffir W, Stebbins R, editors: *Experiencing fieldwork: an inside view of qualitative research,* Newbury Park, Calif, 1991, Sage.
8. Maxwell J: *Qualitative research design,* Thousand Oaks, Calif, 2004, Sage.
9. Stearns CA: Physicians in restraints: HMO gatekeepers and their perceptions of demanding patients, *Qualitative Health Res* 1:326-348, 1991.
10. Mann C, Stewart F: *Internet communication and qualitative research: a handbook for researching on-line,* Thousand Oaks, Calif, 2000, Sage.
11. Liebow E: *Tally's corner,* Boston, 1967, Little, Brown.
12. Lofland J, Lofland L: *Analyzing social settings: a guide to qualitative research,* Belmont, Calif, 1984, Wadsworth.
13. Rodwell MK: *Social work constructivist research,* New York, 1998, Garland.
14. Gubrium J: Recognizing and analyzing local cultures. In Shaffir W, Stebbins R, editors: *Experiencing fieldwork: an inside view of qualitative research,* Newbury Park, Calif, 1991, Sage.
15. Gubrium, J: *Living and dying at Murray Manor,* New York, 1975, St Martin's Press.

16. Rubin H, Rubin IS: *Qualitative interviewing: the art of hearing data*, ed 2, Thousand Oaks, Calif, 2004, Sage.

17. Spradley JP: *The ethnographic interview*, New York, 1979, Holt, Rinehart & Winston.

18. Goodley D, Lawthom R, Clough P, et al: *Researching life stories*, New York, 2004, Routeledge.

19. Williams E: Focus groups, 2004; http://www.hmi.missouri.edu/focus_groups.htm.

20. Bloor M: *Focus groups in social research*, Thousand Oaks, Calif, 2000, Sage.

21. Butler S: *Homeless women*, Seattle, 1991, University of Washington (dissertation).

22. Spradley JP: *Participant observation*, New York, 1980, Holt, Rinehart & Winston.

23. Bottorff, Joan L: Using videotaped recordings in qualitative research. In Morse JM: *Critical issues in qualitative research methods*, Thousand Oaks, Calif, 1994, Sage.

24. Guba EG: Criteria for assessing the trustworthiness of naturalistic inquiries, *Educ Commun Technol J* 29:75-92, 1981.

25. Bluebond-Langner M: *The private worlds of dying children*, Princeton, NJ, 1978, Princeton University Press.

26. Shakespeare T, Barners C, Mercer G: *Doing disability research*, Leeds, UK, 1997, Disability Press.

27. Fetterman DL: *Ethnography step by step*, Newbury Park, Calif, 1989, Sage.

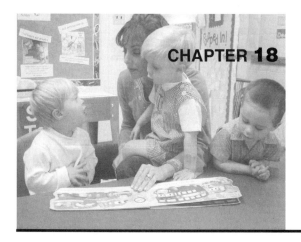

CHAPTER 18

Preparing and Organizing Data

KEY TERMS

Codebook
Data reduction
Database management
Memoing
Narrative
Raw data file
Transcription
Variable label

CHAPTER OUTLINE

Managing Data in Experimental-Type Research
Managing Data in Naturalistic Inquiry
Practical Considerations
Summary

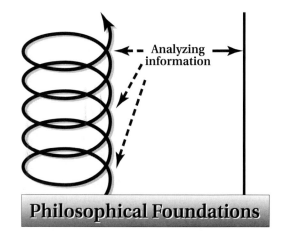

Philosophical Foundations

After learning about the many different strategies that researchers use to collect information, you may be asking what exactly the investigator does with all this collected information.

When you begin to collect information, you will find that you quickly obtain a massive amount of data and that you need to organize and account for every piece of data in a meaningful way. In experimental-type research, even a small survey study may yield more than 100 variables for analysis. Think about all the items you need to ask about even for a pilot study. Information concerning the person's age, gender, relevant personal characteristics, and living status are all

important and common data points. Likewise, in naturalistic inquiry, a 1-hour interview may yield up to 50 or more pages of single-spaced type.

Organizing, or what we refer to as "managing," all this information, whether the data take a numerical or narrative form, is an important action but is not usually discussed or written up by researchers. Most researchers learn to manage data through trial and error or by participating in the research process as mentored students or in postdoctoral training programs. Nevertheless, researchers in both traditions must engage in specific actions to prepare information for analyses that can be described and learned. This chapter discusses this specific action process—the action of preparing and managing information in each of the research traditions.

MANAGING DATA IN EXPERIMENTAL-TYPE RESEARCH

If you are conducting an experimental-type study, what type of data will you be collecting? Because you will be primarily interested in obtaining a quantitative understanding of phenomenon, your data will be numerical. The analysis of numerical data is an action process that is performed after all the data have been collected for the study. That is, at the conclusion of collecting data, you will have many numerical responses to each of your questionnaires, interviews, and observations.

> Consider a somewhat small study involving a survey of 100 students in a college of health professions. Assume the survey is designed to examine student satisfaction with the quality of health profession education. The survey will likely include a number of background questions, such as gender, level of education, financial assistance, marital status, and living arrangement of students. The survey will also include some type of scale that measures satisfaction with education, as well as a series of questions about other aspects of college life. As you will see, this type of study may have 50 to 100 items or variables that will be measured. In a study involving 100 students, this may represent a total of 10,000 data points that will be submitted to statistical analysis. Even in a small study, the amount of information obtained can be enormous and usually requires the assistance of computer technology.

After collecting all this information, what does the researcher do next? For experimental-type researchers, the primary action process is to prepare and organize the data first for entry into a computer program and then for statistical analyses. The researcher follows seven basic steps (Box 18-1).

First, the researcher must examine each interview or data collection form to check for missing information, double-coded responses, or unclear demarcations of responses. This information reflects possible interviewer errors that must be corrected before entering the numerical values into a computer program. The researcher should attempt to address all missing data before data entry. This step may require contacting respondents and seeking answers to missed questions or clarification for double-coded responses.

BOX 18-1

STEPS IN PREPARING DATA FOR STATISTICAL ANALYSIS

1. Check data collection instrument for accuracy and completeness of information.
2. Label each variable on instrument.
3. Assign variable labels to computer locations.
4. Develop codebook and control file.
5. Enter data using double verification or other quality control procedures.
6. Clean raw data files.
7. Develop summative scores.

Second, the researcher must label each variable on the data collection instrument using a convention specified by the statistical package used. For example, Statistical Package for the Social Sciences (SPSS) is a popular, menu-driven, statistical computer program that runs on a personal computer. In SPSS, *variable labels* (names assigned to each variable for ease of identification) must not exceed eight characters, and the first character cannot be a number or a symbol. The labeling of a variable is usually logical and straightforward.

Third, the researcher must decide the order in which the variables will be entered into a data entry computer program. Most researchers use the convention of placing each observation along an 80- to 120-column format (Table 18-1). Usually, each subject or research participant is assigned a unique identification number located in the first 10 columns of a line or row,

---

TABLE 18-1

Example of Raw Data Set

10291	17823123333828288384234343501293124224
10291	2221132000021231
10291	301924302 010212212736572524761
20822	1572122211272931888398479389842654746
20822	2634152346520012354365415142534256342 6234323
20822	368013223 65427234254654 6545212
12311	22342123523642465256415642 65346235
12311	1812235552516617263555527435441325423
12311	381726357 647652763674500000000
21071	18321122112535645625334132432 4342323
21071	2122242442424244231313322525252511111 22344
21071	318723648 723461987234687112333

depending on the length of the case identifier. If there is more than one line of data for a case, the subject identification number is repeated for each row of data. In Table 18-1, each number represents a response to a data collection instrument, in this case a closed-ended questionnaire. These numbers are often referred to as a "raw data set" and form the foundation from which the experimental-type researcher performs statistical manipulations. A data set merely consists of all the numbers obtained through data collection, which are organized in the data entry program according to the format designed by the researcher. Data are usually entered in the order in which the items are sequenced on the data collection form.

> In Table 18-1, the first column on each line refers to the subject's group assignment (i.e., experimental or control group). Columns 02 through 04 refer to the personal identification number. Column 05 indicates the subject's gender (1 = male; 2 = female). Column 06 is blank, and 07 refers to the line number.

In the fourth step the researcher establishes a computer-based control file that consists of a list of the variable labels. Also, a written or electronic record is generated, usually referred to as a *codebook* or "data definition record." This written record is a hard or electronic copy of the variable labels and the range or values that they represent. SPSS provides a separate window in which you can prepare a codebook simply by entering code information about your data set into menu-driven formats.

The fifth step involves entering the numerical values into a computer-based program by a scanner, automatically from web-based data collection protocols (if you have the technology) or by manual entry. Although there are a variety of data-entry programs, they are basically similar. For small data sets (e.g., those under 50 variables), data entry can be conducted using a spreadsheet or *database management* program (e.g., Lotus 1-2-3, Microsoft Excel, FoxPro, Microsoft Access). For large data sets, it is preferable to use a computer-based program that has been specifically developed for the purpose of entering data. Most data entry computer programs enable the investigator to check for out-of-range codes, and

some programs provide double verification. These are important quality control features. Wild codes and out-of-range codes refer to errors in entering data in which characters or numbers entered in the program do not reflect the possible numerical scores assigned to the variable.

> Assume the only responses to a question regarding marital status are 1 for "not married" or 2 for "married." The data entry operator, however, inadvertently types a 3. The data entry program will signal the operator that an error has been made.

Double verification refers to the process of entering the same set of data into the computer program on two separate occasions. The program checks each numerical entry against itself. The program either alerts the key operator when a discrepancy between two entries occurs, or it allows the operator to inspect the two entries visually to determine discrepancies. When this occurs, the keyed responses must be manually checked against the original hard copy of the instrument to determine the correct value.

The sixth step in preparing experimental-type data involves a process of "cleaning" the data that have been entered into the computer. Cleaning data is an action process whereby the investigator checks the inputted data set to ensure that all data have been accurately transcribed from the data collection instrument to the computer entry program. This action step is essential to determine the extent of missing information, to ensure that each response has been correctly coded, and to confirm that no errors were made in entering the numerical scores into the computer.

> If the age of a subject was entered in a data entry program as 27 years rather than the true age of 57, this error would certainly skew an understanding of the mean age and the range of ages represented in the study sample.

In Chapter 15, we discuss the possibility of having either random or systematic errors. Data entry represents a possible source of random error.

Think about a particular study you plan to conduct or you have just read in a journal. What are the possible data errors that might occur, and how can the researcher address them? Researchers use many techniques to clean data and reduce sources of random error. One important way to inspect the data for errors is computing the frequencies of responses for each variable in the data set.

Assume you use a scale to ascertain the level of dependence in basic activities of daily living. The possible responses for each self-care item range from 4 for "completely independent" to 1 for "completely dependent." When you compute the frequencies for each self-care item, you discover that "bathing" has two responses with a value of 5. You will immediately know by inspecting the frequencies that the data are not correct. You will need to identify the subject identification numbers of the two individuals with the out-of-range values, then manually check their interview forms to determine the source of the error. The error may have been inadvertently made by the interviewer or data entry operator.

In addition to checking frequencies, some researchers manually check a random number of lines of data against the original hard copy of the data collection instrument. Others use these methods in combination with printing *raw data files* sorted both by line and subject identification numbers. These printouts allow the researcher to visually inspect for misaligned data, as well as wild and out-of-range codes.

As you can see, there are a number of ways of ensuring quality of the data that are collected and entered and minimizing the possibility of random error at this stage of the research process. At the minimum it is important for the investigator to conduct a careful and systematic examination of the raw data set and the initial frequencies of key variables. Although this examination is often a time-consuming task, it minimizes random error and increases the accuracy of the data set. You should not perform any statistical manipulations until the data have been thoroughly cleaned and are error free. Unfortunately, not every researcher will spend time cleaning data, but we recommend that, as in every other thinking and action process, careful thought be given to this action process as well.

The seventh step and final action to prepare data for analysis involves reducing the vast quantity of information to general categories, summated scores, or single numerical indicators. As you can see from the small excerpt of a larger data set (see Table 18-1), most studies generate an enormous amount of information. One of the first statistical actions taken by experimental-type researchers is to summarize information. Index development and descriptive statistical indicators, such as the mean, mode, median, standard deviation, variance, and other statistically derived values, reduce and summarize individual responses and scores. This summary process is often referred to as *data reduction* and is discussed in greater detail in Chapter 19. These scores are submitted to other types of statistical manipulations to test hypotheses and make inferences and associations.

Before the popular use of desktop computers, only huge data sets were analyzed on mainframe computers. In the past decade, however, superior hardware and software have made computerized data analysis available to most researchers. There are many statistical analytical programs on the market, some more "user-friendly" than others and some more capable of complex computations. Among the most popular and powerful are SPSS (McGraw-Hill, New York) and SYSTAT (SYSTAT, Evanston, Ill.). SPSS is a software program that can run many types of statistical computations on large data sets. Both SPSS and SYSTAT are menu driven and relatively easy to use. In SPSS and SYSTAT the user selects a statistical computation from a menu, then is prompted with a series of branches to perform the next step. Each program has its advantages and disadvantages.

There are many other statistical programs. You can even find statistical software online for free. We advise that you carefully select one that fits your data analysis needs with the assistance of a statistician. Even with the use of computers, it is necessary to have a conceptual understanding of the range of available statistics.

Quantitative approaches to the analysis of data are well developed (see Chapter 19). Each statistical test has been developed and refined as computer technologies and the field of mathematics have advanced. There are clear and explicit rules as to when, how, and under what circumstances specific statistical analyses can be used. Because data must fit specific criteria for any analytical technique, you must be concerned with how you intend to measure concepts. As discussed in Chapter 16, the measurement process will determine the type of data you will obtain and, subsequently, the type of analyses you can perform.

MANAGING DATA IN NATURALISTIC INQUIRY

As you can see, preparing a data set in experimental-type research is an action process that is somewhat independent from analytical actions. Although certain analytical actions require the data to be set up in specific ways, data sets represent a necessary action step before analytical actions, and as such, they are relatively independent of analysis. This is not the case for naturalistic inquiry. In this tradition, organizing data is integral to the analytical process and is in fact an analytical action.[1] Thus the separation of data setup from analysis, as we have done here, is an artifact of book writing rather than a representation of what actually occurs in the conduct of naturalistic inquiry. As such, we discuss aspects of organizing information and return to this action in Chapter 20, which focuses on analysis.

Therefore, as you can surmise, if your research involves naturalistic inquiry, your approach to data management, data cleaning, and data reduction and analysis is different from that used in experimental-type research. In what ways do you think naturalistic data management will differ from quantitative approaches?

First, you will be primarily interested in obtaining a qualitative understanding of phenomena. Your data will be primarily *narrative,* or text based, but can also include other types of data, such as artifacts or video frames of nonverbal behaviors. Second, the process of analysis will be ongoing and linked to the process of collecting information. The integration of the actions of data collection and analysis is a critical aspect of naturalistic designs and is referred to as the "interactive process." Third, you must manage the enormous amounts of information that you obtain as you conduct fieldwork and engage in the process of collecting information. The type of analysis that will be conducted influences how the data are set up and managed.

The analytical strategies employed by researchers who use naturalistic inquiry are varied and explored in Chapter 20. Most analytical strategies are designed to transform the volumes of interview transcripts, audio recordings, video recordings, field notes, and other written electronic and observational information into meaningful categories, taxonomies, or themes that explain the meaning and underlying patterns of the phenomenon of interest. Other analytical strategies are designed to explicate the essence of personal experiences as told to the investigator. As discussed in previous chapters, the information gathered in the different forms of naturalistic inquiry is not numerical but rather verbal and nonverbal manifestations that have been transcribed from a variety of information-gathering techniques and sources.

As shown in Chapters 15 and 17, there are many sources of data in naturalistic inquiry and, likewise, many different analytical strategies. Furthermore, each data source and analytical approach requires a somewhat different approach to managing the information that is gathered. For example, information that is derived from audio recordings is usually transcribed into written text or narrative. On the other hand, data involving video recordings are visually examined and usually marked in terms of frames for repeated reviewing and interpretation. The most frequent approach to analysis, however, involves the written word or narrative; thus the transcription of voice recording from interviews or field notes is an important aspect of most types of designs involving naturalistic inquiry.

Let us examine the process of managing the voluminous amount of narrative information that is obtained in a naturalistic study. It is important to note that in naturalistic inquiry, managing data is also an essential part of the analytical process. As we discuss here, some of the steps in managing qualitative data involve applying analytical techniques. *Transcription* is the first step in analyzing narrative and involves transforming an audiotape into a verbatim written record. The interviewer, the investigator, or a professional transcriber may transcribe an interview. One advantage of having the interviewer or investigator do the transcription is that the act immediately immerses the researcher into the narrative and informs the analytical process. Transcribing can be tedious, however, and a slow typist or someone unfamiliar with the transcription process may find it difficult and not a good use of their time. Although there are voice-to-text software packages now available, we have found that they are not yet accurate enough for rigorous transcription. We expect that soon this software will be perfected so that it can be used in transcription, significantly reducing the time burden of this important action process.

Transcription can be a time-consuming activity. You can expect an average of 6 to 10 hours of typing for each hour of interview recording, depending on the clarity of the tape, the density of the interview, and the typist's familiarity with the task. Explicit directions need to be given to a typist on how to handle the components of the voice recording. For example, you may want to record the number and length of pauses, silences, laughter, or repetitive phrases such as "uh huh." The decision as to what to transcribe will depend on the purpose of the study.

After the completion of a transcription, you must check its accuracy; you will want to ensure that the typed version accurately represents the voice recording verbatim. In checking the transcription, you will also need to resolve misspellings and missing sections attributed to poor sound reproduction.

After cleaning the transcription, the investigator must become immersed in the data; that is, the transcription must be read multiple times to begin the analytical process. In the initial stages of any type of fieldwork, most investigators transcribe all voice recordings. As fieldwork progresses, however, the investigator may transcribe a random selection from each voice recording or a sample for complete transcription.[2] Random selection is particularly useful for large-scale projects, such as in the tradition of classic ethnography, where the investigator increasingly selects which voice-recorded interviews are to be transcribed as the study unfolds.

The short excerpt in Box 18-2 is taken from more than 100 pages of narrative derived from a transcription of a 2-hour voice recording. The voice recordings were generated from a focus group discussion involving six occupational therapists practicing in rehabilitation hospitals in Pennsylvania.[3] In the focus group, therapists were asked to review a case vignette

---

BOX 18-2
EXCERPTS FROM TRANSCRIPT

Ms. K: I personally would probably start off trying to figure out where his left upper extremity was and its recovery and seeing if I could work with that to get it more functional first versus whether I would go ahead right away and start issuing the suction things that would stabilize so that he could use his right hand.

Mr. S: The things that struck me are that, one, he had a stroke. So I started going through a list of equipment that he might use. But then a 67-year-old Italian gentleman from south Philadelphia starts to put other things in my mind. The fact that he lives alone made an impression, and that he had been a butcher. That starts to generate ideas for me.*

Ms. V: You can sort of generally think for the most part that he was within functional limits in other perceptual cognitive areas. I guess from looking at the diagnosis end, that he is a right CVA and he does have a neglect. I would want to really assess his perceptual cognitive deficits a little further, especially in light of a nonfunctional left upper extremity, at that. So looking at the component end, I would want to further examine those areas.

Ms. P: Sensation! Also because it does not mention [in the vignette] anything about any sensation at all. It would be extremely important with neglect.

*See Table 18-3.

---

that involved an older man in rehabilitation after experiencing a cerebrovascular accident (CVA). Therapists were specifically asked to discuss the process by which they would select and provide instruction to this patient in the use of assistive devices.

These excerpts represent precoded, corrected versions of the transcript and illustrate one type of data in naturalistic inquiry. Consider this transcript and the other types of data that could have been collected from in-depth interviews and personal field notes. Think about all these written words; you can quickly obtain an appreciation of the volume of information that is generated in this type of research. These written forms of data can quickly become voluminous, and the researcher must set up multiple files that are cataloged to facilitate cross-referencing and easy access to its "bits and pieces."

Transcription is only one aspect of preparing data for analysis. It is also critical to establish a system to organize information. On the most basic level, you will need to establish a log of each voice recording and the date of its recording. As you begin to identify categories of information, you will need to establish a system for easy retrieval of key passages that reflect these categories. It is also important to keep track of coding and analytical decisions as you read and review materials. Researchers use a variety of organizational schemes, depending on their personal style and preferences and the scope and needs of the research project. Some researchers use note cards and hand-code collected information. Others prefer to use word-processing programs or computer-assisted coding programs (e.g., Nudist, Zyindex, Ethnograph).

In experimental-type research, computer-based statistical programs are a necessity and have facilitated the development of more sophisticated statistical tests. In naturalistic inquiry, computer-based coding programs assist the investigator in organizing, sorting, and manipulating the arrangement of materials to facilitate the analytical process. Obviously, the programs cannot develop an analytical scheme or engage in the interpretive process. Nothing can replace the need for the investigator to be immersed in reading and coding the narrative. Word-processing programs and specially designed qualitative software packages only enable the researcher to catalog, store, and rearrange large sets of information in different sorted files more efficiently. Even when computer assistance is used, many investigators also depend on index cards or loose-leaf notebooks with tabs to separate and identify major topics and emerging themes. Some investigators establish multiple copies of narratives and cut and paste materials to organize and reorganize each written segment into meaningful segments.

In any case, researchers usually maintain a codebook in the form of index cards, word-processing files, or a notebook that summarizes the codes that are used to describe major passages and themes and their location in a transcript. An index or codebook system can be developed in many different ways.

A code, its definition, and its line location in the transcript are recorded in Table 18-2. This excerpt from a codebook reflects three broad analytical categories (medical, individual, and situational) that emerged from the focus group study. Each category has subcodes; the category of "individual" considerations involved up to 14 different subcategories, such as self-care, previous roles, and future roles. The listing of the location of each code in the transcript provides a quick guide to the text. The text can then be sorted by codes, and smaller files can be created that reflect any category of interest (Table 18-3).

As part of the information collection and storage process, the researcher may keep personal notes and diary-like comments and emerging insights that provide a context from which to view and understand field notes at each stage of engagement in the field. This is an example of how data management and data analysis are interrelated in naturalistic research. In most forms of naturalistic inquiry, the investigator is an integral part of the entire research process. It is through the investigator and his or her interaction with informants in the field that knowledge emerges and

TABLE 18-2

Excerpt from Codebook for Focus Group Transcripts (as it relates to Table 18-3)

Code	Definition	Line Location
MED	Medical factors	1282
(DIAG)	1. Diagnosis	
(FUNCT)	2. Function	
(HS)	3. Health status	
(PERC)	4. Perceptual	
INDV	Individual factors	
	1. Background characteristics	
(AGE)	a. Age	1284
(GEND)	b. Gender	
(SES)	c. Socioeconomic status	
(ETHN)	d. Ethnicity	1284
(REL)	e. Religion	
(ROLE)	2. Role	
	a. Past	1287
	b. Present	
	c. Future	
SITUAT	Situational factors	
(LIV)	1. Living situation	1286
(COM)	2. Community	1285
DEC-MAK	Decision-making process	
	1. Reference of order to thoughts	1281-1282
	2. Reflection	1288

TABLE 18-3

Excerpt from Focus Group Transcript with Preliminary Analytical Codes

Line	Codes
	MED: DIAG
	INDV: AGE/GEND/ETHN/ROLE
	SITUAT: LIV/COM DEC-MAK:
1281	The things that struck me are that, one,
1282	he had a stroke. So I started going through
1283	a list of equipment that he might use. But then
1284	a 67-year-old Italian gentleman from
1285	south Philadelphia starts to put other things in
1286	my mind. The fact that he lives alone made an
1287	impression, and that he had been a butcher. That
1288	starts to generate ideas for me.

develops. Thus, these personal comments are critical to the investigator's self-reflections, which occur as part of both the management and the analytical processes. Taking field notes and using them in data collection and analysis are important areas of study.[4]

Reflecting on personal feelings, moods, and attitudes at each juncture of data collection and recording, the investigator can begin to understand the lens through which to interpret the cultural scene or slice of behavior at that point in the fieldwork. The organization of these notes and their emergent interpretations is an important technique. The investigator can develop questions to guide further data collection and to explain observations as they occur. Summarizing or *memoing*[4] as the researcher proceeds is both a management and an analytical technique that produces an "audit trail."[5] An audit trail indicates the key turning points in an inquiry in which the researcher has uncovered and revealed new understandings or meanings of the phenomenon of interest. Others can review the audit trail as a way of determining the credibility of the investigator's interpretations (see Chapter 17).

PRACTICAL CONSIDERATIONS

Another part of the action process of preparing data for analysis, whether for naturalistic or quantitative-type research, involves practical considerations in manging data that potentially can impact the science of your investigation. One consideration is finding a safe place to store data in your office. Data (e.g., questionnaires, voice recordings) should be stored in fireproof or metal cabinets that can be secured by lock and key. Also, you should derive office policies as to who has access to your data, whether the data can be taken out of the office, and by whom. Even within an office, data can be lost. Identify a safe drop-in box, and establish a storage system for completed interviews and interviews that have been entered and cleaned.

Another consideration is to develop a backup disaster plan. You should always have a backup of all data that have been entered or transformed. Keep one backup file in a fireproof metal cabinet and one backup file at home or in a location other than the office. Also, choose a safe place to keep your field notes and other ongoing documentation you may need to use in the field. If theft is a threat, you might want to establish the rule that interviewers should not keep data in their car. Also, interviews can easily be lost, so you may want to establish a rule as to how soon following the completion of an interview it must be brought into the office or storage location.

Besides a backup and disaster recovery plan, you also must make sure that you keep any identifying information and informed consents separate from and not traceable to the data. Your office may in fact be audited by your institutional review board or research committee to make sure that you are compliant with all HIPAA and human subject regulations (see Chapter 12).

Although these are very practical considerations, they are part of the action of research. Consider the consequences for the analytical and reporting stages of your research if your completed audiotapes or interviews are mislabeled, misplaced, or lost.

SUMMARY

Organizing or managing the information collected in a study is an important research task that is not often explicitly discussed in the research literature. Techniques for effectively organizing information for analysis tend to be learned through mentorship opportunities. Nevertheless, data management represents a potential source of random error in both naturalistic inquiry and experimental-type research and therefore warrants careful consideration.

Researchers in experimental-type research proceed with a series of actions to manage and prepare data for statistical analysis. As in all previous research steps, the approach in experimental-type research is linear; it follows data collection and precedes statistical testing. In contrast, analysis is an ongoing and integral part of data collection actions in naturalistic inquiry. Likewise, the management of data and its cleaning and reduction into meaningful interpretive categories occur iteratively, first as part of data collection and then as part of a more formal analysis and report-generating process. In keeping with the different philosophical foundations that make up naturalist inquiry, researchers pursue diverse ways of storing, managing, and preparing information for ongoing analysis and final report writing.

EXERCISES

1. Contact two researchers at a university who work in the experimental-type tradition. Through interviewing, determine their data management arrangements, data entry programs, and types of codebooks.
2. Repeat exercise 1 with two researchers who use naturalistic inquiry.
3. Compare and contrast the different styles of managing information in the experimental-type and naturalistic research traditions.

REFERENCES

1. Glaser B, Strauss A: *The discovery of grounded theory: strategies for qualitative research,* Chicago, 1967, Aldine.
2. Agar MH: *The professional stranger: an informal introduction to ethnography,* ed 2, San Diego, 1996, Academic Press.
3. Gitlin LN, Burgh D, Durham D: *Factors influencing therapists selection of adaptive technology for older adults in rehabilitation: legacies and lifestyles for mature adults,* Philadelphia, 1992, Temple University.
4. Sanjek R, editor: *Fieldnotes: the makings of anthropology,* Ithaca, NY, 1990, Cornell University Press.
5. Guba EG: Criteria for assessing the trustworthiness of naturalistic inquiry, *Educ Commun Technol J* 29:75-92, 1981.

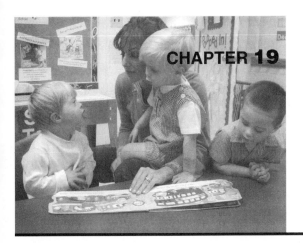

CHAPTER 19

Statistical Analysis for Experimental-Type Research

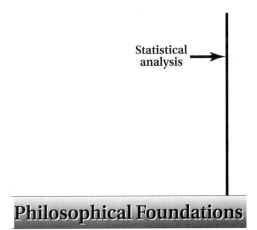

Statistical analysis

Philosophical Foundations

Many newcomers to the research process often equate "statistics" with "research" and are intimidated by this phase of research. You should now understand, however, that conducting statistical analysis is simply one of a number of important action processes in experimental-type research. You do not have to be a mathematician or memorize mathematical formulas to engage effectively in this research step. Statistical analysis is based on a logical set of principles that you can easily learn. In addition, you can always consult a statistical book or website for formulas, calculations, and assistance. Because there are hundreds of different statistical procedures that range from simple to extremely complex, some researchers specialize in *statistics* and thus provide another source of assistance if you should need it. However, except for complex calculations and statistical modeling, you should easily be able to understand, calculate, and interpret basic statistical tests.

The primary objective of this chapter is to familiarize you with three levels of statistical analyses and the logic of choosing a statistical approach. An understanding of this action process is important and will enhance your ability to pose appropriate research questions and design experimental-type strategies. Thus, our purpose here is to provide an orientation to some of the basic principles and decision-making processes in this action phase rather than describe a particular statistical test in detail or discuss advanced statistical procedures. We refer you to user-friendly websites and the references at the end of the chapter for other resources that discuss the range of available statistical analyses. Also, refer to the interactive statistical pages at http://www.statpages.net.

WHAT IS STATISTICAL ANALYSIS?

Statistical analysis is concerned with the organization and interpretation of data according to well-defined, systematic, and mathematical procedures and rules. The term "data" refers to information obtained through data collection to answer such research questions as, "How much?" "How many?" "How long?" and "How fast?" In statistical analysis, data are represented by numbers. The value of numerical representation lies largely in the clarity of numbers. This property cannot always be exhibited in words.

Assume you visit your physician, and he indicates that you need a surgical procedure. If the physician says that most patients survive the operation, you will want to know what is meant by "most." Does it mean 58 out of 100 patients survive the operation, or 80 out of 100?

Numerical data provide a precise language to describe phenomena. As tools, statistical analyses provide a method for systematically analyzing and drawing conclusions to tell a quantitative story. Statistical analyses can be viewed as the stepping-stones used by the experimental-type researcher to cross a stream from one bank (the question) to the other (the answer).

You now can see that there are no surprises in the tradition of experimental-type research. Statistical analysis in this tradition is guided by and dependent on all the previous steps of the research process, including the level of knowledge development, research problem, study design, number of study variables, level of measurement, sampling procedures, and sample size. Each of these steps logically leads to the selection of appropriate statistical actions. We discuss each of these later in the chapter.

First, it is important to understand three categories of analysis in the field of statistics: descriptive, inferential, and associational. Each level of statistical analysis corresponds to the particular level of knowledge about the topic, the specific type of question asked by the researcher, and whether the data are derived from the population as a whole or are a subset or sample. Experimental-type researchers aim to predict the cause of phenomena. Thus the three levels of statistical analysis are hierarchical, with description being the most basic level.

Descriptive statistics make up the first level of statistical analysis and are used to reduce large sets of observations into more compact and interpretable forms.[1] If study subjects make up the entire research population, descriptive statistics can be primarily used; however, descriptive statistics are also used to summarize the data derived from a sample. Description is the first step of any analytical process and typically involves counting occurrences, proportions, or distributions of phenomena. The investigator must descriptively examine the data before proceeding to the next levels of analysis.

The second level of statistics involves making inferences. *Inferential statistics* are used to draw conclusions about population parameters based on findings from a sample.[2] The statistics in this category are concerned with tests of significance to generalize findings to the population from which the sample is drawn. Inferential statistics are also used to examine group differences within a sample. If the study subjects make up a sample, both descriptive and inferential statistics can be used. There is no need to use inferential statistics when analyzing results from an entire population, since the purpose of inferential statistics is to estimate population characteristics and phenomena from the study of a smaller group, a sample. Inferential statistics, by their nature, account for errors that may occur when drawing conclusions about a large group based on a smaller segment of that group. You can therefore see, when studying a population in which every element is represented in the study, why no sampling error will occur and thus why there is no need to draw inferences.

Associational statistics are the third level of statistical analysis.[2] These statistics refer to a set of procedures designed to identify relationships between multiple variables and to determine whether knowledge of one set of data allows the investigator to infer or predict the characteristics of another set. The primary purpose of these multivariate types of statistical analyses is to make causal statements and predictions.

Table 19-1 summarizes the primary statistical procedures associated with each level of analysis. Table 19-2 summarizes the relationship among the level of knowledge, type of question, and level of statistical analysis. Let us examine the purpose and logic of each level of statistical analysis in greater detail.

LEVEL 1: DESCRIPTIVE STATISTICS

Consider all the numbers that are generated in a research study such as a survey. Each number provides information about an individual phenomenon but does not provide an understanding of a group of individuals as a whole. Recall our discussion in Chapter 16 of the four levels of measurement (nominal, ordinal, interval, and ratio). Large masses of unorganized numbers, regardless of the level of measurement, are not comprehensible and cannot in themselves answer a research question.

TABLE 19-1

Primary Tools Used at Each Level of Statistical Analysis

Level	Purpose	Selected Primary Statistical Tools

Descriptive statistics	Data reduction	Measures of central tendency
		  Mode
		  Median
		  Mean
		Measures of variability
		  Range
		  Interquartile range
		  Sum of squares
		  Variance
		  Standard deviation
		Bivariate descriptive statistics
		  Contingency tables
		  Correlational analysis

Inferential statistics	Inference to known population	Parametric statistics Nonparametric statistics

Associational statistics	Causality	Multivariate analysis
		Multiple regression
		  Discriminant analysis
		  Path analysis

TABLE 19-2

Relationship of Level of Knowledge to Type of Question and Level of Statistical Analysis

Level of Knowledge	Type of Question	Level of Statistical Analysis
Little to nothing is known	Descriptive Exploratory	Descriptive
Descriptive information is known, but little to nothing is known about relationships	Explanatory	Descriptive Inferential
Relationships are known, and well-defined theory needs to be tested	Predictive Hypothesis testing	Descriptive Inferential Associational

Descriptive statistical analyses provide techniques to reduce large sets of data into smaller sets without sacrificing critical information. The data are more comprehensible if summarized into a more compact and interpretable form. This action process is referred to as data reduction and involves the summary of data and their reduction to singular numerical scores. These smaller numerical sets are used to describe the original observations. A descriptive analysis is the first action a researcher takes to understand the data that have been collected. The techniques or descriptive statistics for reducing data include frequency distribution, measures of central tendency (mode, median, and mean), variances, contingency tables, and correlational analyses. These descriptive statistics involve direct measures of characteristics of the actual group studied.

Frequency Distribution

The first and most basic descriptive statistic is the *frequency distribution.* This term refers to both the distribution of values for a given variable and the number of times each value occurs. The distribution reflects a simple tally or count of how frequently each value of the variable occurs in the set of measured objects. As discussed in Chapter 18, frequencies are used to clean raw data files and to ensure accuracy in data entry. Frequencies are also used to describe the sample or population, depending on which has participated in the actual study.

Frequency distributions are usually arranged in table format, with the values of a variable arranged from lowest to highest or highest to lowest. Frequencies provide information about two basic aspects of the data collected. They allow the researcher to identify the most frequently occurring class of scores and any pattern in the distribution of scores. In addition to a count, frequencies can produce "relative frequencies," which are the observed frequencies converted into percentages based on the total number of observations. For example, relative frequencies tell us immediately what percentage of subjects has a score on any given value.

Assume you want to develop a drug prevention program in a high school. To plan adequately, you need to know the ages of the students who will participate. You obtain a list of ages of 20 participants (Table 19-3); the ages are measured at the interval level and are listed in the order in which the students register. However, the list is difficult to derive meaning from or to interpret. For example, the average age of the group, the age distribution among the categories, and the youngest

TABLE 19-3

Ages of High School Students

18	15	14	16	17
17	17	15	17	18
16	15	14	15	16
15	17	16	14	18

TABLE 19-4

Frequency Distribution of Ages of Students (N = 20)

Age	Frequency	Percent
14	3	15
15	5	25
16	4	20
17	5	25
18	3	15

and oldest ages of those who signed up for the program are not immediately apparent on the list. To understand the data, you can develop a simple frequency table (Table 19-4). This table organizes the ages of the sample in ascending order and indicates the number and percentage of students at each age. There is only one variable presented, and its level of measure is interval. This simple rearrangement of the data provides important information that you can immediately understand. From this table, it is readily apparent that ages range from 14 to 18 years and the most frequently occurring ages are 15 and 17 years.

You can reduce the data further by grouping the ages to reflect an ordinal or nominal level of measurement.

You may want to know how many students fall within the age range of 14 to 16 and 17 to 18 years (ordinal; Table 19-5) or young and old (categorical or nominal).

It is often more efficient to group data on a theoretical basis for variables with a large number of response categories. Frequencies are typically used with categorical data rather than with continuous data, in which the possible number of scores is high,

TABLE 19-5		
Frequency Distribution by Age Interval (in years)		
Age interval	Frequency	Percent
14 to 16	12	60
17 to 18	8	40

such as test grades or income. It is difficult to derive any immediate understanding from a table with a large distribution of numbers.

In addition to a table format, frequencies can be visually represented by graphs, such as a pie chart, histogram or bar graph, and polygon (dots connected by lines). Let us use another hypothetical data set to illustrate the value of representing frequencies using some of these formats. Assume you conducted a study with 1000 persons 65 years of age or older in which you obtained scores on a measure of "life satisfaction." If you examine the raw scores, you will be at a loss to understand patterns or how the group behaves on this measure. One way to begin will be to examine the frequency of scores for each response category of the life satisfaction scale using a histogram. There are five response categories: 5 = very satisfied, 4 = satisfied, 3 = neutral, 2 = unsatisfied, and 1 = very unsatisfied. Figure 19-1 depicts the dis-

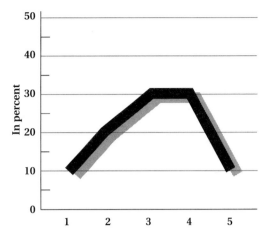

Figure 19-2   Polygon depicts distribution of scores by percentage of responses in each category.

tribution of the scores by percentage of responses in each category (relative frequency).

You can also visually represent the same data using a polygon. A dot is plotted for the percentage value, and lines are drawn among the dots to yield a picture of the shape of the distribution, as well as the frequency of responses in each category (Figure 19-2).

Frequencies can be described by the nature of their distribution. There are several different shapes of distributions. Distributions can be symmetrical (Figure 19-3, *A* and *B*), in which both halves of the distribution are identical. This distribution is referred to as a normal distribution. Distributions can also be nonsymmetrical (Figure 19-3, *C* and *D*) and are characterized as positively or negatively skewed. A distribution that has a positive skew has a curve that is high on the left and a tail to the right (Figure 19-3, *E*). A distribution that has a negative skew has a curve that is high on the right and a tail to the left (Figure 19-3, *F*). A distribution can be characterized by its shape, or what is called kurtosis, and is either characterized by its flatness (platykurtic; Figure 19-3, *G*) or peakedness (leptokurtic; Figure 19-3, *H*). Not shown is a bimodal distribution, which is characterized by two high points. If you plot the age of the 20 students who registered for the drug prevention course (data shown in Table 19-4), you will have a bimodal distribution.

It is good practice to examine the shape of a distribution before proceeding with other statistical approaches. The shape of the distribution will have

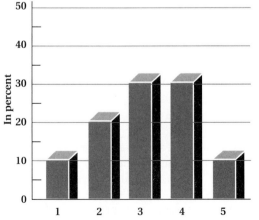

Figure 19-1   Histogram depicts distribution of scores by percentage of responses in each category.

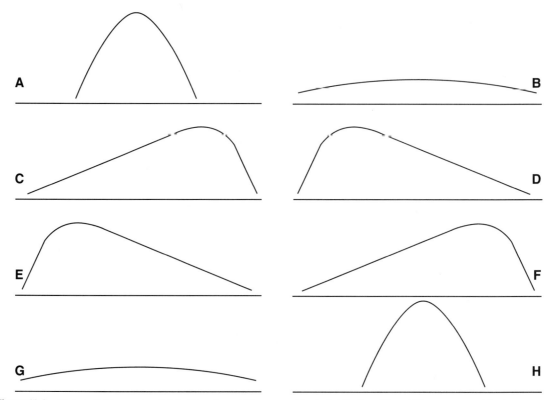

Figure 19-3 Types of frequency distribution: **A** and **B,** symmetrical distribution; **C** and **D,** nonsymmetrical distribution; **E,** positively skewed distribution; **F,** negatively skewed distribution; **G,** platykurtosis (flatness); **H,** leptokurtosis (peakedness).

important implications for determining central tendency and the other types of analysis that can be performed.

Measures of Central Tendency

A frequency distribution reduces a large collection of data into a relatively compact form. Although we can use terms to describe a frequency distribution (e.g., bell shaped, kurtosis, or skewed to the right), we can also summarize the frequency distribution by using specific numerical values. These values are called *measures of central tendency* and provide important information regarding the most typical or representative scores in a group. The three basic measures of central tendency are the mode, median, and mean.

Mode

In most data distributions, observations tend to cluster heavily around certain values. One logical measure of central tendency is the value that occurs most frequently. This value is referred to as the "modal value" or the *mode*. For example, consider the data collection of nine observations, such as the following values:

9	12	15	15	15	16	16	20	26

In the above distribution of scores, the modal value is 15 because it occurs more than any other score. The mode therefore represents the actual value of the variable that occurs most often. It does not refer to the frequency associated with that value.

Some distributions can be characterized as "bimodal" in that two values occur with the same frequency. Let us use the age distribution of the 20 students who plan to attend the drug abuse prevention class (see Table 19-4). In this distribution, two categories have the same high frequency. This is a bimodal distribution; 14 is the value of one mode, and 17 is the value of the second mode.

In a distribution based on data that have been grouped into intervals, the mode is often considered to be the numerical midpoint of the interval that contains the highest frequency of observations. For example, let us reexamine the frequency distribution of the students' ages (see Table 19-5). The first category of ages, 14 to 16 years, represents the highest frequency. However, because the exact ages of the individuals in that category are not known, we select 15 as our mode because it is the midway point of the numerical values contained within this category.

The advantage of the mode is that it can be easily obtained as a single indicator of a large distribution. Also, the mode can be used for statistical procedures with categorical (nominal) variables (numbers assigned to a category; e.g., 15 male and 25 female).

Median

The second measure of central tendency is the *median*. The median is the point on a scale above or below which 50% of the cases fall. It lies at the midpoint of the distribution. To determine the median, arrange a set of observations from lowest to highest in value. The middle value is singled out so that 50% of the observations fall above and below that value. Consider the following values:

22	24	24	25	27	30	31	35	40

The median is 27, because half the scores fall below the number 27 and half are above. In an odd number of values, as in the above case of nine, the median is one of the values in the distribution. When an even number of values occurs in a distribution, the median may or may not be one of the actual values, since there is no middle number; in other words, an even number of values exist on both sides of the median. Consider the following values:

22	24	24	25	27	30	31	35	40	47

The median lies between the fifth and sixth values. The median is therefore calculated as an average of the scores surrounding it. In this case the median is 28.5 because it lies halfway between the values of

27 and 30. If the sixth value had been 27, the median would have been 27. Look at Table 19-4 again. Can you determine the median value? Write out the complete array of ages based on the frequency of their occurrence. For example, the age of 14 occurs three times, so you list 14 three times; the age of 15 occurs five times, so you list 15 five times; and so forth. Count until the 10th and 11th value. What age did you obtain? If you identified 16, you are correct. The age of 16 years occurs in the 10th and 11th value and is therefore the median value of this group of students.

In the case of a frequency distribution based on grouped data, the median can be reported as the interval in which the cumulative frequency equals 50% (or midpoint of that interval).

The major advantage of the median is that it is insensitive to extreme scores in a distribution; that is, if the highest score in the set of numbers shown had been 85 instead of 47, the median would not be affected. Income is an example of how the median is a good indicator of central tendency because it is not affected by extreme values.

Mean

The *mean,* as a measure of central tendency, is the most fundamental concept in statistical analysis used with continuous data. Remember that different from the mode and median, which do not require mathematical calculations (with the exceptions discussed), the mean is derived from manipulating numbers mathematically. Thus the data must have the properties that will allow them to be subjected to addition, subtraction, multiplication, and division.

Suppose that you were doing a study in which you were interested in comparing how young adult males and females responded to a smoking prevention program. You assign the number "1" to code male gender and "2" to code female gender. It would not make sense to calculate a mean score for gender because 1 and 2 are nominal and used to identify categories rather than magnitude. Similarly, if you coded ages as 1= ages 18 to 21, 2 = ages 22 to 25, and 3 = ages 26+, you would not be able to subject your ordinal data (1, 2, 3) to the calculation of the mean because these numbers denote order, not mathematical magnitude.

The mean serves two purposes. First, it serves as a data reduction technique in that it provides a summary value for an entire distribution. Second and most important, the mean serves as a building block for many other statistical techniques. As such, the mean is the most important measure of central tendency. There are many common symbols for the mean (Box 19-1).

BOX 19-1
COMMON SYMBOLS FOR THE MEAN

Mx = mean of variable *x*
My = mean of variable *y*
X̄ = x bar or mean value of a variable
M = mu, mean of a sample

The formula for calculating the mean is simple:

$$M = \frac{\Sigma X_i}{N}$$

where ΣX_i = sum of all values, M = mean, and N = total number of observations. You may recognize this formula as the one that you learned to calculate averages.

The major advantage of the mean over the mode and median is that in calculating the mean, the numerical value of every observation in the data distribution is considered and used. When the mean is calculated, all values are summed and then divided by the number of values. However, this strength can be a drawback with highly skewed data in which there are outliers or extreme scores, as stated in our discussion of the median. Consider the following example.

Suppose you have just completed teaching a continuing education course in cardiopulmonary resuscitation (CPR). You test your students to determine their competence in CPR knowledge and skill. Of a possible 100, the following scores were obtained:

100	100	100	95	95

To calculate the mean, you will add each value and divide the sum by the total number of values (100 + 100 + 100 + 95 + 95 = 490/5 = 98). The mean score of your group is 98. You

---

are satisfied with the scores and with the high level of knowledge and skill. Now let us see what happens in the following distribution of test scores:

100	100	100	90	35

The mean is calculated as 100 + 100 + 100 + 90 + 35 = 425/5 = 85. The mean (85) presents quite a different picture, even though only one member of the group scored poorly. If only the mean were reported, you would have no way of knowing that the majority of your class did well and that one individual or outlier score was responsible for the lower mean.

Which Measure(s) to Calculate?

Although investigators often calculate all three measures of central tendency for continuous data, all may not be useful. Their usefulness depends on the purpose of the analysis and the nature of the distribution of scores. In a normal curve, the mean, median, and mode are in the same location (Figure 19-4). In this case it is most efficient to use the mean, because it is the most widely used measure of central tendency and forms the foundation for subsequent statistical calculations.

However, in a skewed distribution the three measures of central tendency fall in different places (Figure 19-5). In this case you will need to examine all three measures and select the one that most reasonably answers your question without providing a misleading picture of the findings.

Measures of Variability

We have learned that a single numerical index, such as the mean, median, or mode, can be used to describe a large frequency of scores. However, each has certain limitations, especially in the case of a distribution

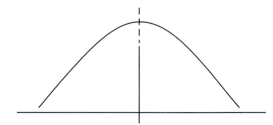

Figure 19-4 Normal curve, where mean, median, and mode are in same location.

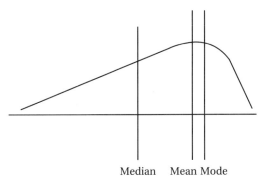

Figure 19-5 Skewed distribution, where the three measures of central tendency fall in different places.

TABLE 19-6	
Life Satisfaction Scores for Two Groups*	
Group 1	Group 2
102	128
99	78
103	93
96	101

*See Figure 19-6.

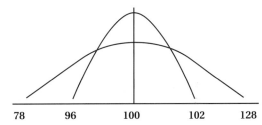

Figure 19-6 Dispersion of homogeneous and heterogeneous life satisfaction scores in two groups (see Table 19-6).

with extreme scores. Most groups of scores on a scale or index differ from one another, or have what is termed "variability" (also called spread or dispersion.) Variability is another way of summarizing and characterizing large data sets. By variability we simply mean the degree of *dispersion* or the differences among scores. If scores are similar, there is little dispersion, spread, or variability across response categories. On the other hand, if scores are dissimilar, there is a high degree of dispersion.

Even though a measure of central tendency provides a numerical index of the average score in a group, it is also important to know how the scores vary or how they are dispersed around the measure of central tendency. Measures of variability provide additional information about the scoring patterns of the entire group.

> Consider two groups of life satisfaction scores measured as continuous data, as shown in Table 19-6. In both groups the mean satisfaction score is equal to 100. However, the variability, or dispersion, of scores around the mean is quite different. The scores in group 1 are more homogeneous. In the second group the scores are more variable, dispersed, or heterogeneous. The dispersion of scores for the two groups is shown in Figure 19-6. Therefore, knowing the mean will not help ascertain differences in the two groups, even though they exist. Let us assume you had to develop a support group educational program for both groups. You would approach the focus of each group differently, based on your knowledge of the variability in scores.

To describe a data distribution more fully, a summary measure of the variation or dispersion of the observed values is important. We discuss five basic measures of variability: range, interquartile range, sum of squares, variance, and standard deviation.

Range

The *range* represents the simplest measure of variation. It refers to the difference between the highest and lowest observed value in a collection of data. The range is a crude measure because it does not take into account all values of a distribution, only the lowest and highest. It does not indicate anything about the values that lie between these two extremes. In the group 1 data listed in Table 19-6, the range is 96 to 103, or a range of 7 points. In group 2 data the range is 78 to 128, or a range of 50 points.

Interquartile Range

A more meaningful measure of variability is called the *interquartile range* (IQR). The IQR refers to the range of the middle 50% of subjects. This range describes the middle of the sample or the range of a majority of subjects. By using the range of 50% of subjects, the investigator ignores the extreme scores or outliers. Assume your study sample ranges in age from 20 to 90 years, as follows:

20	20	21	34	35	35	35	38	39	45	85	90

If you only use the range, you will report a range of 20 to 90 with a 70-point spread. However, most individuals are approximately 35 years of age. By using the IQR, you will separate the lowest 25% (ages 20, 20, and 21 years) and the highest 25% (45, 85, and 90 years) from the middle 50% (34, 35, 35, 35, 38, and 39 years). You will report the range of scores that fall within 50th percentile. In this way you ignore the outliers of 85 and 90. Usually, when reporting the median score for a distribution, the IQR is also used. To calculate the median, you will count to the middle of the distribution. Similarly, with IQR, you will count off the top and bottom quarters.

Sum of Squares

Another way of interpreting variability is by squaring the difference between each score and the mean. These squared scores are then summed and referred to statistically as the *sum of squares* (SS). The larger the value of SS, the greater the variance. The SS is used in many other statistical manipulations. The equation for SS is as follows:

$$SS + \Sigma(X_M - X)^2$$

Variance

The *variance* (V) is another measure of variability and is calculated using the following equation:

$$V = \frac{\Sigma(X_M - X)^2}{N}$$

As the equation shows, variance is simply the mean or average of the sum of squares. The larger the variance, the larger is the spread of scores.

Standard Deviation

The *standard deviation* (SD) is the most widely used measure of dispersion. It is an indicator of the average deviation of scores around the mean or, simply, the square root of the variance. In reporting the SD, researchers often use lowercase sigma (σ) or *S*. Similar to the mean, SD is calculated by taking

into consideration every score in a distribution. The SD is based on distances of sample scores away from the mean score and equals the square root of the mean of the squared deviations. SD is derived by computing the variation of each value from the mean, squaring the variation, and taking the square root of that calculation. The SD represents the sample estimate of the population standard deviation and is calculated by the following formula:

$$S = \sqrt{\frac{\Sigma(y - y)^2}{n-1}}$$

Examine the following calculation of the SD for these observations and a mean of 15.5 (or 16):

14	21	15	12

$$S = \sqrt{\frac{(16-14)^2 + (21-16)^2 + (16-15)^2 + (16-12)^2}{4-1}}$$

$$S = \sqrt{\frac{4 + 25 + 1 + 16}{4-1}}$$

$$S = \sqrt{\frac{46}{3}}$$

$$S = 3.9$$

The first step is to compute deviation scores for each subject. Deviation scores refer to the difference between an individual score and the mean. Second, each deviation score is squared. If the deviation scores were added without being squared, the sum would equal zero, because the deviations above the mean always exactly balance the deviations below the mean. The standard deviation overcomes this problem by squaring each deviation score before adding. Third, the squared deviations are added; the result is divided by one less than the number of cases, and then the square root is obtained. The square root takes the index back to the original units; in other words, the standard deviation is expressed in the units that are being measured.

The standard deviation is an index of variability of scores in a data set. It tells the investigator how scores deviate on the average from the mean. For example, if two distributions have a mean of 25 but one sample has an SD of 70 and the other sample an SD of 30, we know the second sample is more

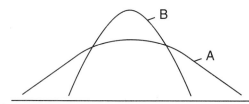

Figure 19-7   Comparison between small and large standard deviation. *A*, Large standard deviation. *B*, Small standard deviation.

homogeneous because we know that the scores more closely cluster around the mean or that there is less dispersion (Figure 19-7).

Based on a normal curve, approximately 68% of the means from samples in a population will fall within one standard deviation from the mean of means, 95% will fall within two standard deviations, and 99% will fall within three standard deviations.

The mean and standard deviation are often reported together in a data table.

It is important to know the measure of central tendency for a particular variable, as well as its measure of dispersion, to understand fully the distribution that is presented.

Bivariate Descriptive Statistics

Thus far we have discussed descriptive data reduction approaches for one variable (univariate); the procedures described are conducted for a univariate distribution. Another aspect of describing data involves looking for relationships among two or more variables. We describe two methods: contingency tables and correlational analysis.

Contingency Tables

One method for describing a relationship between two variables (bivariate relationship) is a "contingency table," also referred to as a "cross-tabulation." A contingency table is a two-dimensional frequency distribution that is primarily used with categorical (nominal) data. In a contingency table, the attributes of one variable are related to the attributes of another.

Returning to an earlier example, you want to know the number of male and female students for each age category of the 20 high school students registered for a drug abuse

TABLE 19-7

Contingency Table of Age by Gender (N = 20)

Age	Gender Male	Female	Total
14	2	1	3
15	3	2	5
16	2	2	4
17	4	1	5
18	1	2	3
Total	**12**	**8**	**20**

prevention program. You can easily develop a contingency table that displays the number of male and female students for each age category (Table 19-7).

Table 19-7 shows an unequal distribution, with more male than female students registered for the course. You can add a column on the table that indicates the percentage of male and female students for each age. Also, you can use a number of statistical procedures to determine the nature of the relationships displayed in a contingency table. You can determine whether the number of male students is significantly greater than the number of female students and not a chance occurrence. These procedures are called "nonparametric statistics" and are discussed later.

Correlational Analysis

A second method of determining relationships among variables is correlational analysis. This approach examines the extent to which two variables are related to each other across a group of subjects. There are numerous correlational statistics. Selection depends primarily on the level of measurement and sample size. In a correlational statistic, an index is calculated that describes the direction and magnitude of a relationship.

Three types of directional relationships can exist among variables: positive correlation, negative correlation, and zero correlation (no correlation). A positive correlation indicates that as the numerical values of one variable increase or decrease, the values for the other variable also change in the same direction. Conversely, a negative correlation indicates that numerical values for each variable are related in an opposing direction; as the values for one variable increase, the values for the other variable decrease.

> 🔍 The relationship between age and height in children younger than 12 years demonstrates a positive correlation, whereas the relationship between illiteracy and years of education represents a negative correlation.

To indicate the magnitude or strength of a relationship, the value that is calculated in correlational statistics ranges from −1 to +1. The value of −1 indicates a perfect negative correlation, and +1 signifies a perfect positive correlation. By "perfect," we mean that the calculated values for each variable change at the same rate as another.

> 🔍 Assume you find a perfect positive correlation (+1) between years of education and reading level. This statistic will tell you that for each year (measured as a single unit) of education, reading level will improve 1 unit.

A zero correlation is demonstrated in Table 19-6, which displays the relationship between life satisfaction and age. The closer a correlational statistical value falls to |1| (absolute value of 1), the stronger the relationship (Figure 19-8). As the value approaches zero, the relationship weakens.

Two correlation statistics are frequently used in social science literature: the Pearson product–moment correlation, known as the Pearson r, and the Spearman rho. Both statistics yield a value between −1 and +1. The Pearson r is calculated on interval level data, whereas the Spearman rho is used with ordinal data.

> 🔍 To illustrate the use of the Pearson r, suppose you were interested in investigating research productivity in health and social work faculty. You examine numerous variables measured with interval level data to determine which were related to productivity in a sample of 200 faculty members. To ascertain the extent of the relationships among selected demographic variables and publication productivity, you would conduct a series of Pearson r calculations. Assume you find that the strongest correlation (r = − 0.38) existed between the

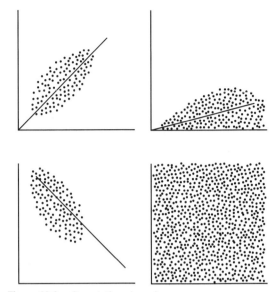

Figure 19-8   Correlational analyses.

> hours spent in the classroom and the productivity. Note the negative association. That is to say, more hours in the classroom are related to lower productivity. The weakest correlation (r = .014) existed between desire to publish and actual publication productivity. Note that the second correlation is positive.
>
> If you had used ordinal data in your measurements, you would have used the Spearman rho to examine these relationships.

Are these findings valuable? Could the relationships be a function of chance? Are these important in light of such seemingly low correlations? To answer these questions, the investigator must first submit the data to a test of significance, which determines the extent to which a finding occurs by chance. The investigator selects a *level of significance,* which is a statement of the expected degree of accuracy of the findings based on the sample size and on the convention in the relevant literature. The investigator locates the correlation coefficient in a table in the back of a statistics book or examines a computer printout. If the correlation value exceeds the number listed in the table, or if the computer presents an acceptable level of significance, the investigator can assume with a degree of certainty that the relationship was not caused by chance.

Consider how this is done. Let us suppose that you select 0.05 as your confidence level. This number means the results will be caused by chance 5 times out of 100. You locate a table of critical values and find that the absolute value of your number of 0.38 exceeds the value you need to determine that the finding is significant or not caused by chance. Therefore you conclude that –0.38 is significant at the 0.05 level and report it to the reader as such. It is more likely that you will conduct your analysis on a computer using statistical software. If so, you would search a computer file to determine the corresponding level of significance, calculated for the value of $r = -0.38$. If it was 0.05 or smaller, you would conclude that this finding was significant.

Other statistical tests of association are used with different levels of measurement. For example, investigators often calculate the point biserial statistic to examine a relationship between a nominal variable and an interval level measure. When two nominal variables are calculated, the phi correlation statistic is often selected by researchers as an appropriate technique.[3] You can read about these tests and others in a text on statistical analysis.

LEVEL 2: DRAWING INFERENCES

Descriptive statistics are useful for summarizing univariate and bivariate sets of data obtained from either a population or a sample. In many experimental-type studies, however, researchers also want to determine the extent to which observations of the sample are representative of the population from which the sample was selected. Inferential statistics provide the action processes for drawing conclusions about a population, based on the data that are obtained from a sample. Remember, the purpose of testing or measuring a sample is to gather data that allow statements to be made about the characteristics of the population from which the sample has been obtained (Figure 19-9).

Statistical inference, which is based on probability theory, is the process of generalizing from samples to populations from which the samples are derived. The tools of statistics help identify valid generalizations and those that are likely to stand up under further study. Thus, the second major role of statistical analysis is to make inferences. Inferential statistics include

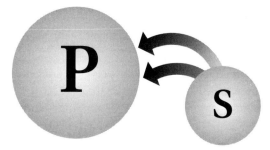

Figure 19-9   Relationship between sample *(S)* and population *(P)*.

statistical techniques for evaluating many properties of populations, such as ascertaining differences among sets of data and predicting scores on one variable by knowing about others.

Two major concepts are fundamental to understanding inferential statistics: confidence levels and confidence intervals.

Because we are now interested in making estimates and predictions about a larger group from observations drawn from a subset of that group, we cannot be certain that what we observe in our smaller group is accurate for all members of the larger group. This statement is the basis of using probability theory to guide inferential statistical analysis. By specifying a confidence level and a confidence interval, we make a prediction of the range of observations we can expect to find and how accurate we expect these to be. This set of predictions also specifies the degree of error that we are willing to accept, and it guides the researcher and consumer in the interpretation of statistical findings.

A *confidence interval* is defined as the range of values that we observe in our sample and for which we expect to find the value that accurately reflects the population. Consider the following example.

> You are interested in predicting the percentage of inpatients on your rehabilitation unit who will use adaptive equipment after discharge. You randomly select a sample from your population of inpatients, and after surveying them for 3 months postdischarge, you find that 20% are still using their equipment. Should you expect that 20% of your population would follow the same pattern? This percentage would be your best guess, but it is derived from a subset of population members. Therefore you need to expand your estimate to

specify an interval of scores that you are confident will include the "true value" of the larger population, in this case an interval of 15% to 30%.

However, deriving a confidence interval is only the first step. Because we are now in the world of probability, specifying a confidence interval must contain a statement about the level of uncertainty as well. This is where confidence level comes into play. A *confidence level* is simply the degree of certainty (or expected uncertainty) that your confidence interval is accurate for your population. So you might be 50% confident or 99% confident that your findings will be accurate. In the previous example, if you specified a confidence level of 99%, you would be 99% certain that 15% to 30% of your population would use adaptive equipment 3 months after discharge from the rehabilitation unit. The degree of assuredness, or level of confidence, that your sample values are accurate for the population is what constitutes the confidence level.

Before we discuss some of the most frequently used statistical tests and the sequence of action processes necessary to use them, consider another example.

You are a mental health provider and are interested in testing the effect of a new rehabilitation technique on the functional level of persons with schizophrenia who are hospitalized in long-term care institutions. In this study, you will evaluate the rehabilitation technique for its effectiveness on one unique group. You will also evaluate its value for the population of persons with schizophrenia residing in institutional settings, which the sample represents. First, you will need to define your population carefully in terms of specific inclusion and exclusion criteria. You will randomly select a sample from your defined or targeted population using an appropriate random sampling technique. Next, you will randomly assign the obtained sample to either an experimental group or a control group condition. You will pretest all subjects, expose the experimental group to the intervention, and posttest all subjects. Hypothetically, the scores on your measure of functional status range from 1 to 10, with 1 the least functional and 10 the most functional. Now you have a series of scores: pretest scores from both groups and posttest scores from both groups.

Let us assign hypothetical means to each group to illustrate the point. The experimental group has a pretest mean of 2 and a posttest mean of 6, whereas the control group has a pretest mean of 3 and a posttest mean of 5. In a real study, you would calculate measures of dispersion as well, but for instructive purposes, we will omit this measure from our discussion. To answer your research question, you must examine these scores at several levels. First, you will want to know if the groups are equivalent before the intervention. You hypothesize that there will be no difference between the two groups before participation in the intervention. Also, you will hypothesize that the groups adequately represent the population. Visual inspection of your pretest mean scores shows different scores. Is this difference occurring by chance, or as a result of actual group differences? To determine whether the difference in mean scores is caused by chance, you will select a statistical analysis (e.g., independent t-test) to compare the two sets of pretest data (e.g., experimental and control group mean scores). At this point, you will hope to find that the scores are equivalent, and that therefore both sample groups represent the population.

Second, you will want to know whether the change in scores at the posttest is a function of chance or what is anticipated to occur in the population. You will therefore choose a statistical analysis to evaluate these changes. The analysis of covariance (ANCOVA) is the statistic of choice for the true-experimental design. In actuality, you will hope that the experimental group demonstrates change on the dependent or outcome variable at posttest time. You will hypothesize that the change will be greater than that which may occur in the control group and greater than the scores observed at pretest time.

Thus, as a consequence of participating in the experimental group condition, you will want to show that the sample is significantly different than the control group and thus the population from which the sample was drawn. In actuality, you will be testing two phenomena: inference, or the extent to which the samples reflect the population at both pretest and posttest time, and significance, or the extent to which group differences are a function of chance.

As you may recall, the "population" refers to all possible members of a group as defined by the researcher (see Chapter 13). A "sample" refers to a subset of a population to which the researcher wants to generalize. The accuracy of inferences from samples to populations depends on how representative the sample is of the population. The best way to ensure "representativeness" is to use probability sampling techniques. To use an inferential statistic, you will follow the five action processes introduced in Chapter 13 and summarized in Box 19-2.

Action 1: State the Hypothesis

Stating a hypothesis is both simple and complex. In experimental-type designs that test the differences between population and sample, most researchers state a "hunch" of what they expect to occur. This statement is called a working hypothesis. For statistical analysis, however, a working hypothesis is transformed into the null hypothesis. The null hypothesis is a statement of no difference between or among groups. In some studies, the investigator hopes to accept the null hypothesis, whereas in other studies, the researcher is hoping to fail to accept the null hypothesis.

Initially, as in the example of the experimental design given earlier, we hope to accept the null hypothesis between the pretest mean scores of the experimental and control groups to ensure that our experimental and control groups are equivalent. We do not want our sample scores to differ from the population scores or the experimental and control groups to differ from one another at baseline before the introduction of the treatment intervention. We pose and test the null hypothesis and hope, that in testing it, the probability at which our statistical value is significant will be unacceptable (we describe significance in detail in the next section). For our posttest and change scores, however, we hope to reject (fail to accept) the null hypothesis. We want to find differences between the posttest scores of each

group and a change between pretest and posttest scores only in the experimental group. These findings will tell us that the experimental group, after being exposed to the experimental condition (the intervention), is no longer representative of the population who did not receive the intervention. In other words, the intervention appears to have produced a difference in the scores of the individuals who participated in that group.

Why is the null hypothesis used? Theoretically, it is impossible to prove a relationship among two or more variables.[3] It is only possible to negate the null hypothesis of "no difference."[4,5] Nonsupport for the null hypothesis is similar to stating a double negative. If it is not "not raining," it logically follows that it is raining. Applied to research, if there is no "no difference among groups," differences among groups can be assumed, although not proven.

Action 2: Select a Significance Level

A level of significance defines how rare or unlikely the sample data must be before the researcher can reject the null hypothesis. The level of significance is a cutoff point that indicates whether the samples being tested are from the same population or from a different population. It indicates how confident the researcher is that the findings regarding the sample are not attributed to chance. For example, if you select a significance level of 0.05, you are 95% confident that your statistical findings did not occur by chance. If you repeatedly draw different samples from the same population, theoretically you will find similar scores 95 out of 100 times. Similarly, a confidence level of 0.1 indicates that the findings may be caused by chance 1 of every 10 times.

As you can see, the smaller the number, the more confidence the researcher has in the findings and the more credible the results. Because of the nature of probability theory, the researcher can never be certain that the findings are 100% accurate. Significance levels are selected by the researcher on the basis of sample size, level of measurement, and conventional norms in the literature. As a general rule, the larger the sample size, the smaller is the numerical value in the level of significance. If you have a small sample size, you risk obtaining a study group that is not highly representative of the population, and thus your confidence level drops. A large sample size includes more elements from the population, and thus the chances of representation and confidence of findings increase. You therefore can use a stringent level of significance (0.01 or smaller).

One-Tailed and Two-Tailed Levels of Significance

Consider the normal curve in distribution of scores (see Figure 19-4). Extreme scores can occur either to the left or to the right of the bell shape. The extremes of the curve are called "tails." If a hypothesis is nondirectional, it usually assumes that extreme scores can occur at either end of the curve or in either tail. If this is the case, the researcher will use a two-tailed test of significance. The investigator uses a test to determine whether the 5% of statistical values that are considered statistically significant are distributed between the two tails of the curve. If, on the other hand, the hypothesis is directional, the researcher will use a one-tailed test of significance. The portion of the curve in which statistical values are considered significant is in one side of the curve, either the right or the left tail. It is easier to obtain statistical significance with a one-tailed statistical test, but the researcher will run the risk of a Type I error. A two-tailed test is a more stringent statistical approach.

Type I and II Errors

Because researchers deal with probabilities in statistical inference, two types of statistical inaccuracy or error can contribute to the inability to claim full confidence in findings.

Type I Errors. In a *Type I error,* also called an "alpha error,"[2] the researcher errs by failing to accept the null hypothesis when it is true. In other words, the researcher claims a difference between groups when, if the entire population were measured, there would be no difference. This error can occur when the most extreme members of a population are selected by chance in a sample. Assume, for example, that you set the level of significance at 0.05, indicating that 5 times out of 100 the null hypothesis can be rejected when it is accurate. Because the probability of making a Type I error is equal to the level of significance chosen by the investigator, reducing the level of significance will reduce the chances of making this type of error. Unfortunately, as the probability of making a

Type I error is reduced, the potential to make another type of error increases.

Type II Errors. A *Type II error,* also called a "beta error,"[2] occurs if the null hypothesis is mistakenly accepted when it should be rejected. In other words, the researcher fails to ascertain group differences when they actually have occurred. If you make a Type II error, you will conclude, for example, that the intervention did not have a positive outcome on the dependent variable when it really did. The probability of making a Type II error is not as apparent as making a Type I error.[6] The likelihood of making a Type II error is based in large part on the power of the statistic to detect group differences.[2]

Determination and Consequences of Errors. Type I and II errors are mutually exclusive. However, as you decrease the risk of a Type I error, you increase the chances of a Type II error. Furthermore, it is difficult to determine whether either error has been made because actual population parameters are not known by the researcher. It is often considered more serious to make a Type I error because the researcher is claiming a significant relationship or outcome when there is none. Because other researchers or practitioners may act on that finding, the researcher wants to ensure against Type I errors. On the other hand, failure to recognize a positive effect from an intervention, a Type II error, can also have serious consequences for professional practice.

Action 3: Compute a Calculated Value

To test a hypothesis, the researcher must choose and calculate a statistical formula. The selection of a statistic is based on the research question, level of measurement, number of groups that the researcher is comparing, and sample size. An investigator chooses a statistic from two classifications of inferential statistics: parametric and nonparametric procedures. Both are similar in that they (1) test hypotheses, (2) involve a level of significance, (3) require a calculated value, (4) compare the calculated value against a critical value, and (5) conclude with decisions about the hypotheses.

Parametric Statistics

Parametric statistics are mathematical formulas that test hypotheses based on three assumptions

---

> **BOX 19-3**
> **THREE ASSUMPTIONS IN PARAMETRIC STATISTICS**
>
> ■ Sample is derived from a population with a normal distribution
> ■ Variance is homogeneous
> ■ Data are measured at interval level

(Box 19-3). First, your data must be derived from a population in which the characteristic to be studied is distributed normally. Second, the variances within the groups to be studied must be homogeneous. Homogeneity is displayed by the scores in one group having approximately the same degree of variability as the scores in another group. Third, the data must be measured at the interval level.

Parametric statistics can test the extent to which numerous sample structures are reflected in the population. For example, some statistics test differences between only two groups, whereas others test differences among many groups. Some statistics test main effects (i.e., the direct effect of one variable on another), whereas other statistics have the capacity to test both main and interactive effects (i.e., the combined effects that several variables have on another variable). Furthermore, some statistical action processes test group differences only one time, whereas others test differences over time. Most researchers attempt to use parametric tests when possible because they are the most robust of the inferential statistics. By "robust," we mean statistics that most likely detect a significant effect or increase power and decrease Type II errors.

Although we cannot present the full spectrum of parametric statistics, we examine three frequently used statistical tests to illustrate the power of parametric testing: t-test, one-way analysis of variance, and multiple comparisons. These techniques are used to compare two or more groups to determine whether the differences in the means of the groups are large enough to assume that the corresponding population means are different.

t-Test. The t-test is the most basic statistical procedure in this grouping. It is used to compare two sample means on one variable. Consider the following example.

> You want to compare the life satisfaction level of physical therapy (PT) students with occupational therapy (OT) students. You administer a general life satisfaction scale, scored such that ascending values indicate higher levels of satisfaction, to a randomly selected sample of students and obtain a mean score for each group. Assume the OT students have an average score of 125.6 and PT students an average of 120.3. At first glance it appears the OT group has the larger mean. However, it is not much larger than the mean derived from the PT group. The statistical question follows: Are the two sample means sufficiently different to allow the researcher to conclude, with a high degree of confidence, that the population means are different from one another (even though we will never see the actual population means)?

The t-test provides an answer to this question. If the researcher finds a significant difference between the two sample means, the null hypothesis will be rejected. As a test of the null hypothesis, the *t* value indicates the probability that the null hypothesis is correct.

Three principles influence the t-test. First, the larger the sample size, the less likely a difference between two means is a consequence of an error in sampling. Second, the larger the observed difference between two means, the less likely the difference is a consequence of a sampling error. Third, the smaller the variance, the less likely the difference between the means is also a consequence of a sampling error.

The t-test can be used only when the means of two groups are compared. For studies with more than two groups, the investigator must select other statistical procedures. Similar to all parametric statistics, t-tests must be calculated with interval level data and should be selected only if the researcher believes that the assumptions for the use of parametric statistics have not been violated. The t-test yields a *t* value that is reported as "t = x, p = 0.05"; *x* is the calculated *t* value, and *p* is the level of significance set by the researcher.

There are two types of t-tests. One type is for independent or uncorrelated data, and the other type is for dependent or correlated data. To understand the difference between these two types of t-tests, return to the example of the two-group randomized design to test an experimental intervention for patients with schizophrenia.

We stated that one of the first statistical tests performed determines whether the experimental and control group subjects differ at the first testing occasion, or pretest. The pretest data of experimental and control group subjects reflect two independent samples. A t-test for independent samples will be used to compare the difference between these two groups. However, let us assume we want to compare the pretest scores to posttest scores for only the experimental subjects. In this case we will compare scores from the same subjects at two points in time. The scores will be more similar because they are drawn from the same sample, and pretest scores serve as a good predictor of posttest scores. In this case the scores are drawn from the same group and are highly correlated. Therefore the t-test for dependent data will be used, which considers the correlated nature of the data. To learn the computational procedures for the test, we refer you to statistics texts.

One-Way Analysis of Variance. The "one-way" analysis of variance (ANOVA), or "single-factor" ANOVA, serves the same purpose as the t-test. It is designed to compare sample group means to determine whether a significant difference can be inferred in the population. However, one-way ANOVA, also referred to as the "F-test," can manage two or more groups. It is an extension of the t-test for a two-or-more-groups situation. The null hypothesis for an ANOVA, as in the t-test, states that there is no difference between the means of two or more populations.

The procedure is also similar to the t-test. The original raw data are put into a formula to obtain a calculated value. The resulting calculated value is compared against the critical value, and the null hypothesis is rejected if the calculated value is larger than the tabled critical value or accepted if the calculated value is less than the critical value. Computing the one-way ANOVA yields an F value that may be reported as "F(a,b) = x, p = 0.05"; x is computed F value, a is group degrees of freedom, b is sample degrees of freedom, and p is level of significance. "Degrees of freedom" refers to the "number of values, which are free to vary"[3] in a data set.

There are many variations of ANOVA. Some test relationships when variables have multiple levels, and some examine complex relationships among multiple levels of variables.

> You are interested in determining the effects of rehabilitation intervention, family support, and functional level on the recovery time for persons with closed head injuries. Measuring the relationship between each independent variable and the outcome will be valuable. However, it will seem prudent to consider the interactive effects of the variables on the outcome. Several variations of the ANOVA (e.g., ANCOVA) should be considered.

Multiple Comparisons. When a one-way ANOVA is used to compare three or more groups, a significant F value means that the sample data indicate that the researcher should reject the null hypothesis. However, the F value, in itself, does not tell the investigator which of the group means is significantly different; it only indicates that one or more are different.

Several procedures, referred to as multiple comparisons (*post hoc* comparisons) are used to determine which group difference is greater than the others. These procedures are computed after the occurrence of a significant F value and are capable of identifying which group or groups differ among those being compared.

Nonparametric Statistics

Nonparametric statistics are statistical formulas used to test hypotheses when the data violate one or more of the assumptions for parametric procedures (see Box 19-3). If variance in the population is skewed or asymmetrical, if the data generated from measures are ordinal or nominal, or if the size of the sample is small, the researcher should select a nonparametric statistic.

Each of the parametric tests mentioned has a nonparametric analog. For example, the nonparametric analog of the t-test for categorical data is the chi-square. The chi-square test (X^2) is used when the data are nominal and when computation of a mean is not possible. The chi-square test is a statistical procedure that uses proportions and percentages to evaluate group differences. The test examines differences between observed frequencies and the frequencies that can be expected to occur if the categories were independent of one another. If differences are found, however, the analysis does not indicate where the significant differences are. Consider the following example.

> You want to know whether 100 men and 100 women differ with regard to their political party affiliation (Republican or Democrat). Your first step will be to develop a contingency or "cross-tab" table (a 2 × 2 table) and carry out a chi-square analysis. If there are no differences, you will expect each cell to have the same number of observations. The same number of men and women will have indicated the same party preference (e.g., 50 men indicate Republican, 50 men indicate Democrat, and likewise, 50 women indicate Republican, and 50 women indicate Democrat). However, the actual data look somewhat different, with unequal cells. The chi-square evaluates whether differences in cells are statistically significant, that is, whether the differences are not attributable to chance, but it will not tell you where the significance lies in the table.

The Mann-Whitney U test is another powerful nonparametric test. It is similar to the t-test in that it is designed to test differences between groups, but it is used with data that are ordinal. Many other nonparametric tests are useful as well, and you should consult other texts to learn about these techniques (see References).

For some of the nonparametric tests, the critical value may have to be larger than the computed statistical value for findings to be significant. Nonparametric statistics, as well as parametric statistics, can be used to test hypotheses from a wide variety of designs. Because nonparametric statistics are less robust than parametric tests, researchers tend not to use nonparametric tests unless they believe that the assumptions necessary for the use of parametric statistics have been violated.

Choosing a Statistical Test

The choice of statistical test is based on several considerations (Box 19-4). The answers to these questions guide the researcher to the selection of specific statistical procedures.

The discussion that follows of the tests frequently used by researchers should be used only as a guide. We refer you to other resources to help you select appropriate statistical techniques.[7]

BOX 19-4

QUESTIONS TO CONSIDER IN CHOOSING A STATISTICAL TEST

1. What is the research question?
   - Is it about differences?
   - Is it about degrees of a relationship between variables?
   - Is it an attempt to predict group membership?
2. How many variables are being tested, and what types of variables are they?
   - How many variables do you have?
   - How many independent and dependent variables are you testing?
   - Are variables continuous or discrete?
3. What is the level of measurement? (Interval level can be used with parametric procedures.)
4. What is the nature of the relationship between two or more variables being investigated?
5. How many groups are being compared?
6. What are the underlying assumptions about the distribution of a measurement in the population from which the sample was selected?
7. What is the sample size?

Action 4: Obtain a Critical Value

Before the widespread use of computers, researchers located critical values in an appropriate table in the back of a statistics book. The "critical value" is a criterion related to the level of significance and tells the researcher what number must be derived from the statistical formula to have a significant finding. However, statistical software reports your findings differently. Rather than identifying your probability level and then examining the critical value that you need to use as your criterion for determining significance, the computer printout will tell you at what probability your calculated value is a critical value. So rather than looking at the calculated value of your statistic, you identify significant findings by searching for levels of probability that are smaller in value than the value that you have chosen.

> You are interested in testing the degree to which an obesity prevention program resulted in knowledge acquisition about nutrition and exercise. Table 19-8 presents a hypothetical computer-generated analysis for your inquiry.

Using a pretest-posttest quasi-experimental design, you test your sample of 50 participants before the intervention on a knowledge test scored from 0 to 100, with ascending scores indicating greater knowledge. You then deliver the intervention and administer the posttest to determine the degree to which knowledge increased. To test your working hypothesis that knowledge will increase significantly, you formulate the null hypothesis of no difference between the mean pretest and posttest scores, then test it using a one-tailed t-test for dependent samples. (Remember that one-tailed tests are used if you hypothesize the direction of change, and dependent t-tests are used when the same sample generates the two data sets to be compared).

Action 5: Reject or Fail to Reject the Null Hypothesis

The final action process is the decision about whether to reject or fail to reject the null hypothesis. So far we have indicated that a statistical formula is selected along with a level of significance. The formula is calculated, yielding a numerical value. How do researchers know whether to reject or fail to reject the null hypothesis based on the obtained value?

Before the use of computers, the researcher would set a significance level and calculate degrees of freedom for the sample or number of sample groups (or both). Degrees of freedom are closely related to sample size and number of groups. Calculating degrees of freedom depends on the statistical formula used. By examining the degrees of freedom in a study, the researcher can closely ascertain sample size and number of comparison groups without reading anything else. In the t-test, for example, degrees of freedom are calculated only on the sample size. Group degrees of freedom are not calculated because only two groups are analyzed, and therefore only one group mean is free to vary. When degrees of freedom for sample size are calculated, the number 1 is subtracted from the total sample (DF = n − 1), indicating that all measurement values with the exception of 1 are free to vary. For the F ratio, degrees of freedom are also calculated on group means because more than two groups may be compared.

Once the researcher has calculated the degrees of freedom and the statistical value, he or she locates the table that illustrates the distribution for the statistical values that were conducted. The critical values are located by observing the value that is listed at the intersection of the calculated degrees of freedom and the level of significance. If the critical value is larger than the calculated statistic, in most cases the researcher accepts the null hypothesis (i.e., no significant differences between groups). If the calculated value is larger than the critical value, the researcher rejects the null hypothesis and within the confidence level selected accepts that the groups differ.

With the increasing use of computers, researchers rarely make use of tables. The computer is capable of calculating all values and further identifying the p value at which the calculated statistical value will be significant. In the hypothetical data in Table 19-8, the means and standard deviations are presented for both pretest and posttest scores. The calculated value of t is 10.56, and the probability value at which the calculated value would be a critical value is .004. You would therefore fail to accept the null hypothesis because the probability is smaller than your selected level of .05. Therefore, using a computer to calculate statistics presents the information so that you can immediately identify if your findings are significant by simply examining the probability values.

LEVEL 3: ASSOCIATIONS AND RELATIONSHIPS

The third major role of statistics is the identification of relationships between variables and whether knowledge about one set of data allows the researcher to infer or predict characteristics about another set of data. These statistical tests include factor analyses, discriminant function analysis, multiple regression, and modeling techniques. The commonality among these tests is that they all seek to predict one or more outcomes from multiple variables. Some of the techniques can further identify time factors, interactive

TABLE 19-8

Hypothetical Data from Analysis of Knowledge Acquisition

Pretest Mean/SD	Posttest Mean/SD	t Value	P
67/9.75	89.6/2.63	10.56	.004

SD, Standard deviation; *P*, probability.

effects, and complex relationships among multiple independent and dependent variables.

To illustrate this level of statistical analysis, let us consider a hypothetical study in which you are interested in investigating predictors of outcome of marital counseling.

Given the complexity of the topic marital counseling, you have identified 22 variables from the literature that have the potential of predicting outcomes on two variables: length of counseling and degree of reported improvement in the marital relationship. Included among the independent or predictor variables are the extent of investment in the counseling process on the part of the couple, degree of communication difficulty, current living arrangements of the couple, perceived equality of shared responsibility, and future expectations for success expressed by the couple. To analyze your complex data set, you choose an analysis technique called "automatic interaction detector," a statistical procedure that can reveal predictive relationships and the strength of those relationships to examine the effect of the 22 variables on both outcomes. As you can see, predictive statistics are extremely valuable in that they suggest what might happen in one arena (outcome in counseling), based on knowledge of certain indicators (22 predictive variables).

Multiple regression is used to predict the effect of multiple independent (predictor) variables on one dependent (outcome or criterion) variable. Multiple regression can be used only when all variables are measured at the interval level. Discriminant function analysis is a similar test used with categorical or nominal dependent variables.

In the previous example of an examination of research productivity in health and social work faculty, suppose, as the basis for making decisions about tenure and promotion, you were interested in determining the predictive capacity of hours spent in the classroom, desire to publish, university support for publication, and degree of job satisfaction on publication productivity, the four variables as illustrated. Multiple regression is an equation based on correlational statistics in which each predictor variable is entered into an equation to determine how strongly it is related to the outcome variable and how much variation in the outcome variable can be predicted by each independent variable. In some cases a stepwise multiple regression is performed, in which the predictors are listed from "least related" to "most related" and the cumulative effect of variables is reported. In your study, it was found that all four predictor variables were important influences on the variance of the outcome variable.

Other techniques, such as modeling strategies, are frequently used to understand complex system relationships. Assume you are interested in determining why some persons with chronic disability live independently and others do not. With so many variables, you may choose a modeling technique that will help identify mathematical properties of relationships, allowing you to determine which factor or combination of factors will best predict success in independent living. (See the list of references for further information about these more advanced statistical techniques.)

SUMMARY

Statistical analysis is an important action process in experimental-type research that occurs at the conclusion of data collection and data preparation efforts. Hundreds of statistical tests can be categorized as representing one of three levels of analysis: descriptive, inferential, or associational. The level of statistical analysis used depends on many factors, especially the research question, level of measurement of study variables, sample size, and distribution of scores. Each level of analysis builds on the other. Descriptive analyses are always conducted first, followed by inferential and associational, if the question and data warrant each subsequent form of analysis.

The decisions made in each previous step of the research process determine the specific statistical actions that will be undertaken. Thus, embedded in the investigator's research question, in the operational definitions of key concepts, and in the sampling procedures are the statistical manipulations that the investigator will be able to use.

The statistical stage of the research process represents for many researchers the most exciting action process. It is at this juncture that data become meaningful and lead to knowledge building that is descriptive, inferential, or associational. The researcher does not have to be a mathematician to appreciate and understand the logic of statistical manipulations. If the investigator does not have a strong background in mathematics, he or she should consult an expert or a statistician at the start of the study to ensure that the question and data collection methods are compatible with the statistical approaches that best answer the research question.

The purpose of this chapter is to "jump start" your understanding of this action research process. Many different guides and statistical books and resources describe in detail the hundreds of tests from which to choose.

REFERENCES

1. Royeen C, editor: *Clinical research handbook,* Thorofare, NJ, 1989, Slack.
2. Healey JF: *Statistics: a tool for social research,* ed 7, Belmont, Calif, 2005, Wadsworth.
3. Pilcher D: *Data analysis for the helping professions: a practical guide,* Newbury Park, Calif, 1990, Sage.
4. Mohr L: *Understanding significance testing,* Newbury Park, Calif, 1990, Sage.
5. Henkel RE: *Tests of significance,* Newbury Park, Calif, 1976, Sage.
6. Huck SW, Cormier WH, Bounds WG: *Reading statistics and research,* New York, 1974, Harper & Row.
7. Andrews FM et al: *A guide for selecting statistical techniques for analyzing social science data,* ed 2, Ann Arbor, 1981, University of Michigan.

EXERCISES

1. Select a research article that uses statistical procedures; (a) Determine the level of statistical techniques used; (b) Ascertain the rationale behind the selection of the specific statistics used; (c) Critically analyze the statistical tests and determine whether they were appropriate to answer the question the investigator initially posed and appropriate to the level of measurement and sample size.

2. Given the following scores, develop a frequency table and find the mode, median, mean, range, and standard deviation:

    12 35 34 26 26 13 21 22 22 22 24 35 36 37 39 51 23 42
    41 21 21 22 25 26 27 44 42 13 35 43 12

3. Identify a research article that reported in a table format the mean and standard deviation scores to describe the basic characteristics of the study sample. Examine the table; in your own words, write a description of the study based on the numbers presented. Compare your description with that of the study authors.

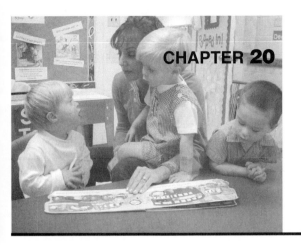

CHAPTER 20

Analysis in Naturalistic Inquiry

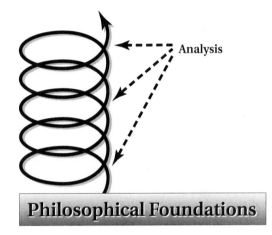

Philosophical Foundations

We now turn our attention to the way in which researchers approach the analysis of data in naturalistic inquiry. As you probably surmise at this point, the action process of conducting analyses in naturalistic inquiry is quite different from the actions taken during statistical decision making in experimental-type research. Analysis in naturalistic research is a dynamic and iterative process. Also, as noted in Chapter 18, keep in mind that organizing information in naturalistic inquiry is an analytical action, and it is difficult to separate organization and management actions from analytical actions.

Although all analytical strategies reflect a logical approach, there is no step-by-step, recipe-like set of rules that can be followed by an investigator in naturalistic inquiry. Many different organizational and analytical strategies can be used at different points in the process. The analytical process also depends on the type of data that are collected, and it will vary depending on whether the data are narrative, observational, visual, musical, diaries, or other data formats.

After you read this chapter, you may want to refer to other literature sources for specific analytical approaches in naturalistic inquiry.[1-4] The following discussion provides an overview of the basic principles that underlie the general thinking and action processes of researchers involved in different forms of analysis across the traditions of naturalistic inquiry.

STRATEGIES AND STAGES IN NATURALISTIC ANALYSIS

Many different purposes inform the analytical process in naturalistic inquiry. The selection of a particular approach to analysis depends on the primary purpose of the research study, the scope of the query, and the particular design. Table 20-1 summarizes the basic purpose and analytical approach used by seven different designs in naturalistic inquiry.

Some analytical strategies in naturalistic inquiry are extremely unstructured and interpretive, such as in phenomenology, heuristic approaches, and some ethnographic studies. Other analytical strategies are highly structured, as in grounded theory. Still other types of naturalistic inquiry may incorporate numerical descriptions and may vary in the type of analysis used, as in certain forms of ethnography, endogenous approaches, and participatory action research. Further, some forms of naturalistic inquiry are highly interpretive but use a specific analytical strategy, such as in life history. In this type of study, the investigator searches for "epiphanies," or key turning points, in the life of the individual(s) under study, using a chronological or biographical account as the basis from which interpretations are derived. Each analytical approach provides a different understanding of the phenomenon under study and reveals a distinct aspect of field experience. Furthermore, in any given study a researcher may use a combination of analytical strategies at different points in the course of fieldwork.

Assume you are conducting a microethnographic study of the meaning of daily life in an assisted-living facility for elder residents. You decide to use several different data collection strategies, such as interviewing residents and family members, observing daily activities, and video-recording staff interactions with residents. The initial purpose of your analysis is to describe daily routines and behaviors of the residents. One analytical strategy may involve counting the number of activities in which residents are engaged, then grouping activities by the categories they represent (e.g., self-care, leisure, social). Another purpose of the analysis is to identify themes that explain the meanings attributed by residents to their daily life in the facility. Analysis will involve an interpretive process to identify statements that reflect core meanings of the experience of assisted living. Based on these two analytical steps, suppose you discover that staff relationships are a

TABLE 20-1

Purpose and Analytical Strategy of Naturalistic Study Designs

Study Design	Main Purpose	Basic Analytical Strategy
Endogenous	Varies	Varies
Participatory action research	Varies	Varies
Phenomenology	Identifies essence of personal experiences	Groups statements based on meaning; develops textual description
Heuristic	Discovers personal experiences	Describes meaning of experience for researcher and others
Life history	Provides biographical account	Describes chronological events; identifies turning points
Ethnography	Describes and explains cultural patterns	Identifies themes and develops interpretive schema
Grounded theory	Constructs or modifies theory	Provides constant comparative method to name and frame theoretical constructs and relationships

salient factor in the experiences of residents. To better understand this particular finding, you may add another analytical strategy, such as frame-by-frame video analysis of staff-resident verbal interactions.

Therefore, you would need to use three different analytical approaches in this study. Each approach would reflect a specific purpose and yield a particular understanding of the phenomenon of interest. The findings from each approach would then be integrated to contribute to a comprehensive and integrative understanding of the initial research query (e.g., "What is the experience and meaning of living in assisted living?").

Although each type of naturalistic design uses a different analytical strategy, the basic process across any type of naturalistic design can essentially be conceptualized as occurring in two overlapping and interrelated stages. The first stage of analysis occurs at the exact moment the investigator enters the field. It involves the attempt to make immediate sense of what is being observed and heard, or what is referred to as "learning the ropes."[2] At this stage the purpose of analysis is primarily descriptive and yields "hunches" or initial interpretations that guide data collection decisions made in the field. The second stage follows the conclusion of fieldwork and involves a more formal review and analysis of all the information that has been collected. The investigator refines or evolves an interpretation that is recorded in a written report for dissemination to the scientific community.

In each stage the researcher may use a different analytical approach. The actions in each stage are best conceptualized as a "spiral" in which each loop of the spiral involves a set of analytical tasks that lead to the next loop in successive fashion until a complete understanding of the field or phenomenon under study is derived.

STAGE ONE: ANALYSIS IN THE FIELD

As shown in previous chapters, the process of naturalistic inquiry is iterative. Let us examine what this means in the initial analytical stage. First, data analysis occurs immediately as the researcher enters the field, and analysis continues throughout the investigator's engagement in the field. Analysis is the basis from which all subsequent field decisions are made: who to interview, what to observe, and which piece of information to explore further. Data collection efforts are inextricably connected to the initial impressions and hunches that are formulated by the investigator; that is, an observation, or datum, gives rise to an initial understanding of the phenomenon under study. This initial understanding informs or shapes the next data collection decision. Each collection–analytical action builds successively on the previous action.

Thus, during fieldwork, the researcher begins the process of systematically examining data—field notes, recorded observations, and transcriptions of interviews—to obtain initial descriptions, impressions, and hunches. It is important to note that transcriptions are usually completed immediately or shortly after the completion of an interview or observation to enable the investigator to evaluate the data and make subsequent field decisions to further the data collection efforts. The investigator also keeps careful records of his or her perceptions, biases, or opinions and begins to group information into meaningful categories that describe the phenomenon of interest. This descriptive analysis is especially critical in the early stages of fieldwork. It is essential to the process of reframing the initial query and setting limits or boundaries as to who and what should be investigated.

This initial set of analytical steps involves four interrelated thinking and action processes (Box 20-1). Keep in mind that these interrelated thinking and action processes are dynamic. That is, the four processes are not neat, separate steps or entities that occur in sequence at a particular time in fieldwork. Rather, they are ongoing, overlapping processes that lead to refinement of interpretations throughout the data-gathering effort.

BOX 20-1
ANALYTICAL THINKING AND ACTION PROCESSES

- Engaging in inductive and abductive thinking
- Developing categories
- Grouping categories into higher levels of abstraction
- Discovering meanings and underlying themes

Investigators, particularly those new to this type of inquiry, may feel overwhelmed and initially lost in this process. The sheer quantity of information generated in a short time also can make the investigator feel inundated. However, these feelings are a natural part of the experience of conducting naturalistic inquiry. The researcher must be able to feel comfortable with being in "limbo" at first, or not knowing the whole story and just letting it unfold.

Engaging in Thinking Process

Naturalistic inquiry is based on either an inductive or an abductive thinking process (see Chapter 1). This thinking process is key to all the analytical approaches of naturalistic inquiry. One of the first analytical efforts of the researcher is to engage in a thoughtful process. This may seem basic to any research endeavor, but the active engagement of the investigator in thinking about each datum in naturalistic inquiry assumes a different quality and level of importance than in other research endeavors. David Fetterman describes this basic analytical effort in ethnographic research as follows:

> The best guide through the thickets of analysis is at once the most obvious and most complex of strategies: clear thinking. First and foremost, analysis is a test of the ethnographer's ability to process information in a meaningful and useful manner.[5]

More specifically, an inductive and abductive thinking process is characterized by the development of an initial organizational system and the review of each datum. The organizational system must emerge from the data. The investigator must avoid imposing constructs or theoretical propositions before becoming involved with the data. For example, in the case of data collected through an interview, the researcher will read and reread the transcriptions. From these initial readings, ideas and hunches will be formulated. In a phenomenological, heuristic, or life history approach, the investigator will continue working inductively until all meanings of an experience are explicated.

In an abductive approach the thinking process begins inductively with an idea. The investigator explores information or behavioral actions and formulates a working hypothesis, which is examined in the context of the field to see whether it fits. The investigator works somewhat deductively to draw implications from the working hypothesis as a way of verifying its accuracy. This process characterizes the actions of the investigator throughout the field experience, especially for grounded theory[6] and ethnography.[7]

In ethnography, Fetterman labels this process as "contextualization," or the placement of data into a larger perspective.[5] While in the field, the investigator continually strives to place each piece of data into a context to understand the "bigger picture" or how the parts fit together to make the whole. One way the investigator strives to understand how a datum fits into the larger context is by grouping information into categories.

Developing Categories

A voluminous amount of information is gathered within a short period in the course of fieldwork. The researcher will feel the need to manage the immense amount of data collected so quickly. Consider when you have had to review a large body of literature for a course in college. Perhaps you first went to the library to obtain information from the literature. You probably realized that your notes from the readings soon became overwhelming and that you needed to develop some organization to make sense of the information you gathered. The same principle applies in the initial stages of analysis in naturalistic inquiry. The researcher must find a way to organize analytically and make sense of the information as it is being collected.

One of the first meaningful ways in which the investigator begins to organize information is to develop categories, or "affinities." We prefer the term *categories* for clarity and word recognition. Northcutt and McCoy[8] note the similarities between categories and variables, indicating that categories are single phenomena that can be named and in which multiple elements must occur. This action process represents a major step in naturalistic analysis. How do categories emerge? As Wax describes:

> The student begins "outside" the interaction, confronting behaviors he finds bewildering and inexplicable: the actors are oriented to a world of meanings that the observer does not grasp...and

then gradually he comes to be able to categorize peoples (or relationships) and events.[9]

The researcher enters the field to see and understand phenomena without imposing concepts, labels, categories, or meanings *a priori*. Thus, categories emerge from researcher-field interactions and the initial information that is obtained and synthesized. Preliminary categories are developed and become the tools used to sort and classify subsequent information as it is received.

Spradley and McCurdy[10] describe the process of generating categories as the process of classifying objects according to their similarities and differences from other objects. Categories such as "student," "provider," and "client" make it easier to anticipate the behavior of individuals in these groups and to identify the cultural rules that govern their behavior. Categories are basic cultural elements that enable people to organize experiences. Categories are social inventions, since objects are not grouped in any natural way. These groupings change from culture to culture, time to time, and context to context.

Consider the way in which colors are classified in different cultures. Although most people living in the United States have only one basic category for the color "white," Eskimo Indians refer to numerous categories. This difference is not surprising, considering the prevalence of "white" in the natural environment in Alaska.

Categories are therefore embedded within a cultural context and reveal at the most basic level the way in which a culture classifies objects and establishes its system of meanings.

How do you find or identify categories? In identifying categories, researchers must stay as close to the data as possible and not impose their own cultural categorization and labeling system. One strategy is to search for commonalities among different objects, experiences, or events. Agar[7] suggests that recurrent topics are prime candidates for categories.[7] Consider the following example:

Gitlin et al.[11] examined the meanings attributed to mobility aids and other assistive devices by patients in rehabilitation who had experienced strokes and were first-time users of the equipment. The initial analytical strategy involved using a pile-sorting technique in which two members of the research team independently read each statement about the devices, as generated by patients during brief interviews. These comments were independently sorted by each researcher into basic categories based on perceived similarities and differences. The categories reflected the underlying topics expressed in patient statements. (A statement about a "reacher" device, such as, "It's good for picking up things," was categorized as representing a comment that explicitly focused on instrumental utility and the patient's stance, which in this case was positive toward the device.) Next, the two researchers compared their summary lists of the categories they had generated. Differences were discussed, and the categories identified were refined. A final comprehensive list was prepared and reviewed by all investigators. This process yielded 11 basic topics or categories of meaning.

As the data collection activity proceeds, the naturalistic investigator uses the original categories as the basis for analyzing new data. New data are either classified into existing categories or may serve to modify or create new categories to depict the phenomenon of interest accurately. Lofland and Lofland[12] suggest that the researcher "file" data by placing them into categories based on characteristics that the data share. The researcher decides on the filing scheme and considers both descriptive and analytical cataloging. Data placed in the descriptive categories answer "who, what, where, and when" queries and do not involve interpretation. Analytical or more interpretive categories answer "how and why" queries. Any one datum can be categorized in several ways. Thus, cross-coding or referencing the same excerpt or piece of information in multiple ways is important and adds another level of complexity to the coding process.

The development of categories is based on repeated review and examination of narrative, video, or other types of information that have been collected. The investigator assigns codes to each category. A number of methods can be used, depending on the investigator's personal style and preferences of working. For example, some researchers generate multiple copies of a data set (e.g., transcription from an interview) and literally cut sections from the transcript that reflect the identified categories. Each cut section is pasted in a notebook or on an index card and filed by the category it represents. (As discussed in Chapter 18, some researchers prefer to use word processors to organize data.)

Computer software programs (e.g., Nudist, Zyindex, Ethnograph) facilitate the coding process for large data sets and can help the researcher develop separate files of information that reflect multiple categories. These programs automatically assign codes to similar passages or keywords identified by the investigator. For example, the researcher may program the computer to assign the code "self-care" to every datum that has the term "bathing" in it. Keywords can be selected based on categories that arise from the data set, and the computer can be programmed to assign codes automatically based on a keyword list.

Developing Taxonomies

A *taxonomy* is a system of categories and relationships. Taxonomies have also been called "typologies" and "mindmaps."[8] Developing a taxonomy represents the next level of organizing information. Taxonomic analysis involves two processes: (1) organizing or grouping similar or related categories into larger categories and (2) identifying differences between sets of subcategories and larger or overarching categories.

Related subcategories are grouped together in the taxonomic process. For example, basic categories such as "whales" and "dogs" belong to the larger category of "animals"; basic categories such as "blocks" and "dolls" belong to the larger category of "toys." In taxonomy, sets of categories are grouped on the basis of similarities. The investigator must uncover the threads or inclusionary criteria that link categories. Taxonomic analysis is therefore an analytical procedure that results in an organization of categories and that describes their relationships. In a taxonomic analysis the focus is on identifying the relationship between wholes and parts.

In the Gitlin et al. study[11] of people who recently experienced strokes, the 11 initial categories identified were further grouped into six broader dimensions to reflect the experience of device use among first-time users. For example, one dimension was labeled "issues posed by device use." This dimension included four subcategories that reflected concerns ranging from the physical interface between the equipment and the user to the social consequences of being a device user.

Discovering Underlying Themes

One of the main purposes of naturalistic research is to understand how each observation or part fits into the whole to make sense of the layers of meaning and the multiple perspectives that compose the field experience. The major inductive method to accomplish this task is to search for relationships among categories and to reveal the underlying *theme* or meaning in categories and their components beyond what is immediately visible. Agar suggests that it is from the "simple" process of first establishing topics, categories, and codes that "you begin building a map of the territory that will help you give accounts, and subsequently begin to discuss what 'those people' are like."[7]

According to Glaser and Strauss,[6] the researcher engages in the thinking process of "integrating," in which he or she finds relationships among categories and further searches for overlap, exclusivity, or hidden meanings among categories. Investigators in grounded theory use the term "theoretical sensitivity" to refer to the researcher's sensitivity and ability to detect and give meanings to data, to go beyond the obvious, and to recognize what is important in the field.[13,14]

The ethnographer looks for patterns of behavior by examining repeated actions.[10] Have[15] reminds us that we are not seeking to interpret intrapsychic phenomena; rather, in "ethnomethodology" we focus on activity as the basis for analysis and meaning. Categories and taxonomies are compared, contrasted, and sorted until a discernable thought or behavioral pattern becomes identifiable and the meaning of the pattern is revealed. As exceptions to rules emerge, variations on themes are detectable. As themes are developed based on abstractions (categories and taxonomies), they are examined in light of ongoing observations. At this point, the investigator may use a literature review or other theoretical concepts to derive an understanding and explanation of the categories based on what has already been investigated or theoretically posited.

These rigorous methods are part of an inductive approach to analysis, and they move the researcher up each loop of the spiral toward understanding and interpretation. Each analytical step from category and taxonomy to thematic identification allows the researcher to uncover the multiple meanings and perspectives of individuals and to develop complex understandings of their experiences and interactions.

Savishinsky, in his study of the culture of a nursing home, notes the multiple levels of insights that occur in naturalistic inquiry and the way in which new data can influence previously held notions:

> The lives of the residents were absorbing because beneath the deceptively simple style in which they told their stories, there was often depth of passion, or the moral twists of fable, or one small detail which transformed the meaning of all the other details.[16]

STAGE TWO: FORMAL REPORT PREPARATION

Analysis is a critical and active component of the data collection process. As noted, it begins early in the action process of data collection and continues once the investigator formally leaves the field and has completed collecting information. This final stage of the process is a more formal and analytical step in which the investigator enters into an intensive report preparation effort that furthers the interpretive process. The main objective is to consolidate the investigator's understandings and impressions by writing one or more manuscripts, a final report, or even a book. This reporting effort involves a self-reflective and highly interpretive process, the ease of which often depends on how well the investigator initially organizes and cross-references the voluminous records and field notes. In this more formal analytical stage, the investigator reexamines materials and refines categories, taxonomies, and themes, and derives an *interpretation*. The investigator must also purposely and carefully select quotes and examples to illustrate and highlight each aspect of the refined interpretation. Selections are carefully made (1) to ensure adequate representation of the interpretation or themes the investigator wants to convey, (2) to remain true to the voices and experiences being referenced, and (3) to depict accurately the context in which the narrative occurred.

In the final interpretation, the investigator moves beyond each datum or piece of information to suggest a deeper understanding of the whole through theory development or an explication of the themes and general principles that emerge from the study of the phenomenon of interest.

EXAMPLES OF ANALYTICAL PROCESSES

Researchers use the basic analytical processes somewhat differently and often label these activities distinctly. In this section we examine these similarities and differences in diverse naturalistic approaches. We highlight aspects of the analytical process of grounded theory to demonstrate its highly structured approach in naturalistic inquiry.

Grounded Theory

One of the most formal and systematic analytical approaches is found in grounded theory. The purpose of this approach is to develop theory. Glaser and Strauss[6] suggest specific procedures to examine data. Their approach to grounded theory systematizes the inductive incremental analytical process and the continuous interplay between previously collected and analyzed data and new information. The authors label their analytical approach as the *constant comparative method*. As information is obtained, it is compared and contrasted with previous information to fit all the pieces inductively together into a larger puzzle. Patterns emerge from the data set and are then coded (placed in a category). Data filing occurs by categorizing and coding. In the constant comparative method, researchers not only search for themes to emerge but also code each piece of raw data according to the categories in which it belongs.

Initially, codes are open, which refers to a "process of breaking down, examining, comparing, conceptualizing and categorizing data." Axial coding then occurs, which refers to "a set of procedures whereby data are put back together in new ways after open coding by making connections between categories." Selective coding occurs next, which is the "process of selecting the core category, systematically relating it to other categories."[14] Codes reflect the similarities and differences among themes and continue to test the category system through analysis of each datum and categorical assignment as data are collected. In this way the analysis is grounded in and emerges from each datum. Theory emerges from the data, is intimately linked to the field reality, and reflects a synthesis of the information gathered.

Grounded theory may be the most systematic and procedure-oriented process in naturalistic inquiry. In various books, Strauss and Glaser—together, individually, and with other authors—systematically walk the researcher through each analytical step of coding and categorizing and use a prescribed language to identify each procedure and task (see References).

Ethnography

Most ethnographic field studies use a range of analytical approaches, based on the specific purpose and nature of the study. The researcher may borrow techniques from grounded theory or use a more general thematic analysis, depending on the particular philosophical stance and analytical orientation of the researcher. To illustrate one way in which a field study analysis may be conducted from beginning to end, we examine DePoy and Archer's study,[17] which was designed to discover the meaning of the quality of life and independence to nursing home residents.[17]

Because of the limited theory that explained the quality of life and meaning of independence from the perspective of the elderly residents, DePoy and Archer initially chose a qualitative approach to address their research query.[17] As the primary data collector, Archer began by examining the "social situation" of a nursing home in rural New England, or what Spradley and McCurdy[10] refer to as the place where the research takes place. Archer recorded her data by separating her observational log into two categories: the physical environment and the human environment. This organizational framework is based on an "environmental competence model" that envisions a person's competence as influencing and, in turn, being influenced by aspects of the physical and social surroundings where behaviors occur.

Archer answered three basic queries with this organizing scheme: (1) What bounds the environment in which the residents live? (2) What physical characteristics does the environment display? and (3) What types of interaction occur within the physical environment? Data were collected and preliminary analyses

evolved, determining the similarities between objects to derive descriptive categories. Once Archer was able to collect descriptive data about the environment and who was in it, she and DePoy sampled segments of the data set to examine relationships and types of interaction patterns that occurred within the environment. After reading and rereading observational notes, they identified a pattern of the daily schedule followed by both residents and formal providers in the institution. This schedule was conceived as a category of its own, and Archer returned to the field to observe specific times of the day to elaborate or broaden the meaning of this category. For example, she observed morning care, mealtimes, and visiting hours. This set of observations provided greater insight as to the reasons people acted in the way that they did during these times and the meaning of the activity for these individuals. Thus the initial query became reformulated as, "Why do they do what they do, and what is the meaning of the activity?"

In addition to developing descriptive categories, DePoy and Archer[17] used constant comparison[14] and taxonomic analysis.[4,10] When the constant comparison approach was used, two categories of resident activity emerged from the first set of field notes: self-care and rehabilitation. For example, Archer documented in her field notes an observation of a woman dressing herself with the assistance of an occupational therapist. This datum was initially coded as reflecting two categories of self-care and rehabilitation. The coding occurred as a result of constant comparison in which the observation was compared with previous data in each category and was determined to be sufficiently similar to be included in both.

However, as a consequence of comparing new and previous data, discrepancies emerged. This dissonance required reflection and action involving the revision of the category scheme initially developed to depict the nature of the datum. Further along in fieldwork, DePoy and Archer's constant comparisons revealed that the category of "self-care" was characterized by residents conducting their morning routine with assistance in dressing by the occupational therapist. However, other observations revealed that numerous residents were sitting in their beds during the morning self-care time schedule, calling for nursing staff. Did these observations fit into the category of self-care? Because the residents were exercising their right to obtain help from staff, the data could have been coded as self-care. However, because residents appeared to need and be dependent on requested assistance, the data did not seem to fit the concept of independence inherent in the category of self-care. Self-care was thus reconceptualized to reflect a new meaning and was eliminated as a category by itself. The example of the woman dressing with the assistance of the occupational therapist was now coded as "functional relationships," whereas observations of those remaining in their beds were revised as subcategories of "in waiting" and "confinement" (Figure 20-1).

As categories emerged from the data set and became clarified by constant comparison, DePoy and Archer examined relationships among them. Figure 20-1 depicts the simple taxonomy of nursing home experience that inductively emerged from the full data set. As you can see, the lines demonstrate bidirectional connections among categories of findings. For example, the category of "confinement" was divided into three subcategories, biophysical, social, and environmental confinement. Biophysical confinement was both caused by and resulted in mobility choices that were intimately related to the category of "functional relationships" (relationships between residents and staff based on resident need).

ACCURACY AND RIGOR IN ANALYSIS

In naturalistic research a major concern is obtaining an in-depth, rich description and explanation of phenomena. The investigator may not be concerned with the generalizability or external validity of study findings. Rather, the primary focus is obtaining a comprehensive and truthful representation of a particular context. At this point, however, you may be wondering how you, as a consumer of naturalistic research, can trust an investigator's final interpretations as representing scientific "truth." How can you determine the accuracy or the *truth value* of an investigator's interpretation of field data? How can you be assured

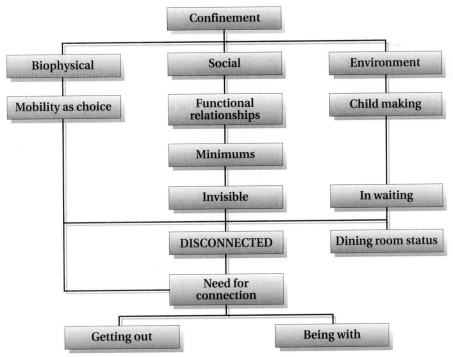

Figure 20-1 Taxonomy for a study of independence and quality of life in nursing home residents. (From DePoy E, Archer L: *Top Geriatr Rehabil* 7:64-74, 1992.)

that the experiences of research participants are "accurately" represented in a final report? The question is whether the findings reveal meanings that will be shared by other researchers if they had conducted the same set of interviews, observations, and analytical orientation. The issue of validity and truth is clearly important.

In naturalistic research the debate continues over how best to construct standards for conducting and evaluating data-gathering and analytical efforts. Lincoln and Guba have labeled this as a concern with the trustworthiness or *credibility* of an account.[18,19] Using a rather structured approach, these authors and others have identified a number of strategies by which an investigator can enhance the confidence in the truth of the findings from naturalistic inquiry.[8] The concern with credibility of an account or interpretive scheme is similar to the issue of internal validity in experimental-type research. In reading a report involving naturalistic inquiry, the critical reader needs to ask two primary questions: (1) To what extent are the biases and personal perspectives of the investigator identified and considered in the data analysis and interpretation? and (2) What actions has the investigator taken to enhance the credibility of the investigation?

To enhance the accuracy of representation of data and the credibility of interpretation, researchers often use six basic actions (Box 20-2). When reading a published study using naturalistic inquiry, check whether the investigator has used any of these strategies. Let us review each approach to see how it applies to the analytical process. (Also see the discussion of these techniques in Chapter 17.)

BOX 20-2

TECHNIQUES TO ENHANCE CREDIBILITY OF ANALYSIS

■ Triangulation (crystallization)
■ Saturation
■ Member checking
■ Reflexivity (self-examination)
■ Audit trail
■ Peer debriefing

Triangulation (Crystallization)

Triangulation, which more recently has been referred to as *crystallization,* is a basic aspect of data gathering that also shapes the action process of data analysis. In triangulation, one source of information is checked against one or more other types of sources to determine the accuracy of hypothetical understandings and to develop complexity of understanding. For example, one approach to triangulation may involve the comparison of a narrative from an interview with published materials such as a journal. Triangulation enables the investigator to validate a particular finding by examining whether different sources provide convergent information. The term "crystallization" has been applied to reflect the comprehensive analytical understanding that occurs as a result of the comparison of different and diverse sources to explain a phenomenon.

Saturation

Saturation refers to the point at which an investigator has obtained sufficient information from fieldwork. As you may recall, there are several indicators that data collection can be terminated (see Chapter 17). For example, the investigator obtains saturation when the information gathered does not provide additional insights or new understandings. Another indication that saturation has been achieved is when the investigator can guess what a respondent is going to say or do in a particular situation. If saturation is not achieved, the investigator reports only partial information that is preliminary, and a credible and comprehensive account or interpretive schema cannot be developed.

Member Checking

Member checking is a technique in which the investigator checks an assumption or a particular understanding with one or more informants. Affirmation of a particular revelation from a research participant strengthens the credibility of the interpretation and decreases the potential of introducing investigator bias. This technique is often used throughout the data collection process. It is also introduced in the formal stage of analysis to confirm the truth value of specific accounts and investigator impressions.

Reflexivity

In the final report or manuscript, it is important for the researcher to discuss his or her personal biases and assumptions in conducting the study and how these affect the research process. Personal biases are revealed in the course of collecting data and during the active process of reflexivity (self-examination). The investigator purposely engages in a reflexive process to examine his or her perspectives and personal biases to determine how these may have influenced not only what is learned but also how it is learned.

Audit Trail

Another way an investigator can increase truth value is by using an audit trail. Lincoln and Guba[18] suggest that an investigator should leave a path of his or her thinking and coding decisions so that others can review the course of logic and decision making that was followed. The principle here is that the investigator needs to be able to clearly articulate the analytical pathways so that others can agree or disagree or question the decisions that have been made. Remember that research is a critical thinking process in both experimental-type and naturalistic traditions.

Peer Debriefing

Peer debriefing is another strategy that can be used to affirm emerging interpretations. In this approach the investigator purposely involves peers in the analytical process. An investigator may convene a group of peers to review his or her audit trail and emerging findings, or the researcher may ask a peer to independently code a randomly selected set of data. The investigator compares the outcomes with his or her coding scheme. Areas of agreement and disagreement are identified and discussed. Either approach provides an opportunity for the investigator to reflect on other possible competing interpretations of the data. Peer debriefing may occur at different junctures in the analytical process.

SUMMARY

Analysis in naturalistic inquiry has many different purposes and strategies. Some researchers seek to generate theory, whereas others aim to reveal and interpret human experiences. Each purpose will yield a different analytical strategy. Regardless of study purpose, however, the essential characteristic of the analytical process is that it involves an ongoing inductive and abductive thinking process that is interspersed with the activity of gathering information. Although the analytical process has well-described essential components, each form of naturalistic inquiry approaches this action process differently.

One of the most difficult aspects of naturalistic inquiry is being prepared for the voluminous amount of data that is obtained. Even in a small-scale study, such as a life history of a single individual, the amount of information obtained and its analysis can initially be overwhelming. The analytical process begins with the simple act of reading and reviewing on multiple occasions the interviews, observational notes, and video images collected. This step begins the thinking process that is essential to the research. Through inductive and abductive reasoning, the boundaries of the study become reformulated and defined, and initial descriptive queries are answered. Further data collection efforts are determined by the need to explore the depth and breadth of categories more fully and to answer "why" and "how" type of queries. As data are obtained, they are coded and organized into meaningful categories. The boundaries and meanings of categories are further refined through the process of establishing relationships among categories. Queries that ask "Why?" and "How?" lead to the development of taxonomies. This in turn leads to emergent patterns, meanings, and interpretations of how observations fit into a larger context. Existing theoretical frameworks or constructs in the literature may be brought into the analytical process to refine emerging interpretations or to serve as points of contrast. A refined and final interpretation is usually derived after the investigator exits the field and begins the writing process. Gubrium eloquently summarizes the analytical process as follows:

> Analysis proceeds incrementally with the aim of making visible the native practice of clarification, from one domain of experience to another, structure upon structure.[3]

Throughout the analytical process, the investigator must remain flexible and open to constantly challenging his or her emerging interpretive framework.

EXERCISES

1. Return to exercise 1 in Chapter 17, which asks you to observe a public place to determine characteristic behavior patterns. Now examine your raw data and search for categories. Based on the categories, code each datum and develop a descriptive taxonomy of behavior.
2. Develop an audit trail for your data collection and analysis activities in the previous inquiry.
3. Give your raw data set from exercise 1 to a colleague for analysis and to establish an audit trail. When your colleague has completed the task, compare your conclusions. Reconcile any differences by reexamining your data and your audit trails.

REFERENCES

1. Wolcott HF: *Transforming qualitative data: description, analysis, and interpretation,* Thousand Oaks, Calif, 1994, Sage.
2. Gubrium JF, Holstein JA: *The new language of qualitative method,* New York, 1997, Oxford University Press.
3. Gubrium J: *Analyzing field reality,* Newbury Park, Calif, 1988, Sage.
4. Miles MB, Huberman AM: *Qualitative data analysis: an expanded sourcebook,* Thousand Oaks, Calif, 1994, Sage.
5. Fetterman DL: *Ethnography step by step,* ed 2, Newbury Park, Calif, 1998, Sage.
6. Glaser B, Strauss A: *The discovery of grounded theory,* Chicago, 1967, Aldine.
7. Agar MH: *The professional stranger: an informal introduction to ethnography,* ed 2, San Diego, 1996, Academic Press.
8. Northcutt, McCoy: *Interactive qualitative analysis,* Thousand Oaks, Calif, 2004, Sage.
9. Wax M: On misunderstanding verstechen: a reply to Abel, *Sociol Soc Res* 51:323-333, 1967.
10. Spradley JP, McCurdy DW: *The cultural experience: ethnography in a complex society,* Prospect Heights, Ill, 1988, Waveland Press.
11. Gitlin LN, Luborsky M, Schemm R: Emerging concerns of older stroke patients about assistive devices in rehabilitation, *Gerontologist* 38(2):169-180, 1998.
12. Lofland J, Lofland L: *Analyzing social settings: a guide to qualitative observation and analysis,* ed 3, Belmont, Calif, 1994, Wadsworth.
13. Glaser BG: *Theoretical sensitivity: advanced in the methodology of grounded theory,* Mill Valley, Calif, 1978, Sociology Press.
14. Strauss AL, Corbin JM: *Basics of qualitative research: grounded theory procedures and techniques,* Newbury Park, Calif, 1990, Sage.
15. Have PT: *Understanding qualitative research and ethnomethodology,* Thousand Oaks, Calif, 2004, Sage.
16. Savishinsky JS: *The ends of time: life and work in a nursing home,* New York, 1991, Bergen & Garvey.
17. DePoy E, Archer L: Quality of life in a nursing home, *Top Geriatr Rehabil* 7:64-74, 1992.
18. Lincoln YS, Guba EG: *Naturalistic inquiry,* Newbury Park, Calif, 1985, Sage.
19. Guba EG: Criteria for assessing the trustworthiness of naturalistic inquiries, *Educ Commun Technol J* 29:75-92, 1981.

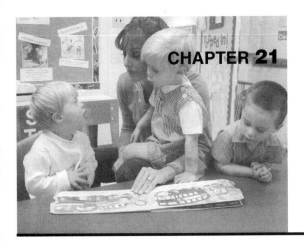

Sharing Research Knowledge Before the Study

The document details the main thinking and action processes you intend to implement. The document describes the significance of your idea and provides justification for the need of your research using supportive literature, a statement as to your specific research question or query, specific hypotheses if applicable, your procedures, analytical plan, and ethical considerations and the informed consent process. This chapter discusses the importance of sharing your research thinking and action processes before entering the field or conducting the inquiry and describes basic approaches.

REASONS FOR SHARING BEFORE FIELD ENGAGEMENT

Writing a document or proposal before engaging in research actions is an important aspect of the research process for several reasons. First, as we discussed in Chapter 12, for any type of research study, you will need to submit a written proposal to a human subject board or research committee of your institution. That is, before starting any type of study, institutional review board (IRB) approval for the conduct of the study must be obtained; otherwise, you are not legally and ethically permitted to implement your research plan. Large health systems, academic institutions, and health and human service settings that have significant research volume usually have their own human subject review committee and establish their own formats for submitting a

$\mathbf{B}$efore actually entering the field or initiating an experimental-type, naturalistic, or mixed-method inquiry, you most likely will have to commit your specific research ideas to paper in the form of a written document. This written document, referred to as a *proposal,* is simply a text or record that describes how you "propose" to carry out your research idea.

proposal. Therefore it is important to contact the research office at your institution to secure their specific instructions for writing and submitting a proposal to their office for their review.

Another important reason for writing a proposal before starting an inquiry is to obtain financial support for the research activity. Most research, regardless of the research tradition and even if it is a pilot study, requires resources to implement. Think of the amount of time and effort that may be required of you and an interviewer, statistical consultant, or others to conduct your study. Consider the costs of materials you may need (e.g., audio or video machine, paper, disks, special computer software programs) or the costs associated with mailings and telephoning. Additionally, you may want to provide a small "honorarium" to study participants as a way of thanking them for their time and effort, a common practice in research. Thus, writing a proposal to request a small or large amount of funds to support the conduct of a study may be critical. Even a small amount of funds (e.g., $150 to $500) can help offset the costs associated with conducting a range of studies and data collection actions, such as conducting a systematic and comprehensive literature review, doing naturalistic or experimental-type meta-analysis, forming a focus group, extracting information from charts, and testing the acceptability of a battery of standardized tests. There are numerous places to seek funding for large or small amounts, including sources internal to your department (e.g., student research funds), referred to as intramural funding programs, and external sources (e.g., federal agency, health foundation), referred to as extramural funding.

Yet another important reason for writing a proposal is to have a written record of the specific thinking and action processes you plan to implement that you can then share with colleagues to obtain their feedback. Obtaining feedback about your research plan before implementation is an important aspect of the research process. It helps to sharpen your thinking and actions and to place your efforts within the larger context of the scientific and consumer communities. Also, a written plan can serve as your own reference or guide as you proceed with a study.

At some point in your student or professional life and involvement in the world of research, you will need to write a research proposal. Writing a proposal is not really as intimidating as it may sound. The document can be as brief as 2 to 5 pages for an IRB submission or as lengthy as 40 or more pages when submitting a detailed research plan for consideration of funding from an external agency. Proposal writing is a technical skill. As such, proposals follow particular formats and structures that can be easily learned and then applied.

Because committing your ideas to paper in the form of a proposal is part of the thinking processes in research, this chapter describes the basic elements of writing a proposal to document a study and to seek funding. Many different types of proposals are written to obtain funding from external sources, such as those written to conduct a conference, purchase equipment, train students or health and human service professionals, and evaluate demonstration projects or service programs. Each type of proposal follows a different format. In this chapter, however, we discuss writing a proposal for research, whether for an experimental-type, naturalistic, or mixed-method study.

A research proposal to secure funding from a particular source is referred to as a "grant." The process of identifying a suitable funding source and writing the proposal is referred to as *grantsmanship*. A research grant will usually provide monies for salary support for the investigator and his or her team, the specific materials needed to carry out the research (e.g., supplies, telephone calls, mailings), data analysis, and travel to professional meetings. Since obtaining money is part of the reality of being involved in research, we start by describing key aspects of grantsmanship.

WHERE TO SEEK SUPPORT FOR A RESEARCH IDEA

Writing a grant to obtain funds to support your research activity is one of the main reasons for writing a research proposal, particularly for large-scale studies or studies requiring specialized or costly equipment or procedures. Finding a funding source for your research idea can be challenging. The funding environment for research is constantly changing, and the priorities and interests of various sources of funding are always being modified in response to advances in health care, new developments in knowledge, societal trends, and congressional activity. Therefore, finding the right *funder* for your particular research idea may take time and require knowledge of multiple sources that provide information about a wide range of funding opportunities. In this section we outline some of the major sources of funding for health and human services research.

Where can you find a potential funding source? Your own department, professional organization, student association, reference librarian, and the Internet are all worthwhile places to begin your search for support of your research idea. For example, your own department may have a research fund to support pilot research efforts of faculty, students, or professionals; this should be the first place in which you inquire. Many professional associations also provide small grants, which may range from $2000 to $50,000 or more, and predoctoral and postdoctoral research stipends. There are also special "listservs" and Internet-based grant-seeking programs that you can join that will help identify sources of funding based on keywords that reflect your research interests.

Funders usually post on their web pages and in newsletters what is known as a *call for proposals,* which is a notice of an opportunity to submit a proposal on a specific topic of interest to an agency or funder. Agencies publish announcements describing a problem area and inviting interested parties to propose ways to investigate all or part of the problem. These announcements vary considerably in the detail used in describing the research they would like to see submitted. The federal government tends to provide explicit descriptions of what needs to be included in grant proposals. Foundations and private companies tend to be much more general as to the format for a research proposal.

The U.S. government remains the largest source of research money available on health-related issues. It is a huge enterprise comprising an array of departments, agencies, institutes, bureaus, and centers. Although there are pockets of money for health and human service professionals throughout the federal government, two departments have a focused interest in health and human services: the Public Health Service within the Department of Health and Human Services (DHHS), which supports the National Institutes of Health (NIH), and the U.S. Department of Education. Within the Department of Education, the Office of Special Education and Rehabilitation Services (OSERS) has a variety of programs of potential interest to the health professions, as does the National Institute on Disability and Rehabilitation Research (NIDRR).

Private foundations are another source of funding for health and human service research. More than 70,000 foundations in the United States offer grants to individuals, institutions, and other not-for-profit groups. The four types are independent foundations, company-sponsored foundations, operating foundations, and community foundations. Generally, only the first two types provide research support to independent investigators, although all four types of foundation offer potential funding opportunities.

Finally, drug companies, equipment manufacturers, and other companies related to health care often have money available for small research projects. Many large corporations have funds for research projects that advance their interests. The main interest of companies in the private sector is the testing or evaluation of their own products. For example, an equipment manufacturer may want a new assistive device evaluated for its utility and acceptability, or a company may pay for the development and evaluation of a patient-education video that promotes their product.

We recommend that you examine the websites of potential funding sources to gain an understanding of the types of research questions and queries they seek to fund and to identify the particular format they require for a proposal submission. As you search for appropriate funding sources, you may discover that your research idea is not of interest to agencies. This does not mean that your idea is without merit, but it does indicate that you will need to rethink or rework your idea to match socially and congressionally sanctioned public health concerns that become embraced by funding agencies. You may find that your research idea is too advanced or "futuristic" to be of interest to funders, or that although it is of great interest to your own profession, it is not considered significant from a broad public health perspective. Thus, it is necessary to cast a wide net and look for funding from a range of sources.

WHO READS A PROPOSAL?

When you write a research proposal, it will be read and evaluated by a particular audience, referred to as the *reviewer*. The reviewer(s) of your proposal may be your research professor; your peers; the head of your clinical or academic department; a diverse committee of consumers, physicians, and researchers who review for an institution's human subject review board; or a group of scientists from various disciplines. As such, you can be assured that the persons who review your proposal will come from diverse backgrounds and have different levels of exposure and knowledge of the phenomenon you seek to investigate, as well as their own professional standards as to what constitutes scientific inquiry.

When you submit a proposal to your professor, department, or institution or to an external source such as a funding agency, reviewers will evaluate it using various criteria. Usually, the evaluative criteria will be specified in your syllabus or in a call for proposals. For the most part, reviewers are asked to evaluate whether your research plan contributes to knowledge building, is feasible, and is scientifically valid. Some reviews are qualitative and you will receive written comments, whereas others are quantitative and you will receive a score. Writing a proposal is a purposeful process and as such must be carefully crafted to match the evaluative criteria and the background and knowledge base of the audience or reviewer. Thus, before writing down your ideas, it is important to know who evaluates your proposal and the evaluative criteria that will be applied.

> Suppose you need to submit a proposal to obtain funding from an agency. By going on the Internet, you identify several potential funding sources that may be appropriate or relevant to your research interest. In reading the directions for proposal development and submission on their web pages, you learn that one agency emphasizes "innovation," whereas another agency is concerned with "dissemination" of research findings. Although your basic research idea may not change, in writing the proposal, you would emphasize different aspects of your research plan based on the evaluative criteria and specific interest of the target audience.

In writing a proposal, you also need to define your key concepts carefully and articulate your ideas clearly so that they can be adequately understood by reviewers from diverse disciplines and life experiences. A concept that is core to your discipline may not be relevant to another or may be defined very differently.

> In most health and human service professions for the term "self-care" refers to the basic activities that people engage in that are essential to daily life, such as bathing, grooming, and dressing. In sociology, however, self-care refers to the study of the actions that persons engage in to take care of themselves, such as what medications they take, who is informed about their symptoms, and when a physician should be contacted and for what reasons.

Thus, in writing a proposal, you need to adapt to the lens of your reviewers and define and reference all key terms. In this respect, writing a proposal is similar to sharing information in the form of a report, which we discuss in Chapter 22. That is, as in report writing, constructing a proposal is purposeful and targets a particular reader or audience, in this case the reviewer.

WRITING A RESEARCH PROPOSAL

The principles and processes involved in writing a proposal are similar to those for sharing information and reporting your study at its completion (see Chapter 22).

Basic Principles

There are four basic principles for writing a research proposal: clarity, precision, parsimony, and attention to structure. Each of these should guide how you write, regardless of the specific purpose of the proposal.

By "clarity," we mean that the proposal needs to be easily understood regardless of the reviewer. If a report is vague, verbose, or overly complex in writing style, your research ideas will not be successfully conveyed. By "precision," we mean explicating each thinking and action plan.

Parsimony is another important principle that should guide your proposal writing. If the proposal is too lengthy or too wordy, it will be difficult for reviewers to understand your key points. So it is important to be "pithy" and keep your proposal to the point. A proposal is written using simple, direct statements. It is not a place to experiment with a creative writing style or prose.

The fourth principle involves the need for "attention to structure," such as ensuring that all references are correctly cited, that proposal instructions are carefully followed, and that the proposal is easy to read, with no typos, incorrect spellings, or glaring grammatical errors.

Common Elements of a Research Proposal

As in sharing information and writing a report, writing a proposal to initiate the research process involves answering a series of questions (Box 21-1).

Although each agency or potential funding source, IRB, or department has its own format for writing a research proposal, there are common elements to such a document. Table 21-1 outlines the basic sections required for most proposals, regardless of the type of research or the research tradition. Each section of a proposal is designed to answer the core questions posed in Box 21-1, which relate to the "who, what, when, where, and how" of your research idea. The basic elements of a proposal ask you to address how your research idea fits into the larger body of knowledge, as well as how you intend to use the findings or knowledge that you generate.

We now examine each of these proposal elements in more detail.

Title

The title of your research study captures the main idea or theme of your proposal in a short phrase. It should not be so brief that it says nothing or so long

TABLE 21-1	
Common Elements of a Proposal	
Necessary Element	**Information Included**
Why	Title
	Abstract
	Introduction/Statement of research problem
What	Specific aims/Study objectives
	Literature review/Significance
How	Action plan/Methodology
	Reporting/Dissemination plan
When	Management of project
	Time line
Who	Investigator credentials
Where	Institutional qualifications
	Resources
Supporting material	Previous experience, publications
	Letters of support
	Formal agreements with consultants, other institutions if applicable

that a person reading your proposal has to work to determine the point of your study.

Assume you want to conduct a study on the health conditions of elder men who are homeless and living in the shelter system. A title such as "Homeless Men" would be too brief and would not capture the main idea of your proposed research. A better title might be "Health Conditions of Older Homeless Men."

Some agencies have specific requirements as to the length of the title. For example, a title of a research proposal submitted to NIH must not exceed 56 typewritten spaces, including punctuation and spaces between words.

Abstract

The abstract is a brief description of each element that is contained in your proposal. It represents an executive summary of the study you propose. Generally, the abstract contains a statement of the purpose of your study or project, your research design, and key actions. If you are submitting your proposal to an external agency, there may be word

BOX 21-1
QUESTIONS TO GUIDE PROPOSAL WRITING

- What is your project about?
- Why is it important?
- What will you do?
- How will you do it?
- What will it cost?
- Why will it cost what it does?
- Why are you the best one to do it?

limitations. In either case, the abstract must be clear and succinct but comprehensive. In addition to the title, the abstract is the first section of the proposal that a reviewer reads and thus provides the framework for reviewing your proposal. An abstract that is not clearly written, that is not comprehensive, or that has typographical errors can be misleading and can give the reviewer a poor impression, potentially influencing how the entire proposal is evaluated.

Because the abstract represents an executive summary of the entire project, it should be the last section you actually write. For NIH grant applications, the title and abstract will be used to assign your proposal to a specific panel of reviewers. Thus, it is essential that both title and abstract reflect the core content of the proposal so that it is given to the appropriate panel.

Introduction

One way to begin your proposal is with an introductory paragraph that provides the reader with a general overview of the project's main idea and its importance. In this section you address the questions regarding what your project is about and why it is important. You state the overall purpose of your study in the introduction.

> Consider your study on the health conditions of homeless men. An opening introductory paragraph would briefly discuss the increasing number of persons who are homeless in the United States, the type of health conditions that have been documented by previous research, and the gap in knowledge that your study will address. You might conclude with your purpose statement.

Although this introductory section is brief, it is necessary to cite data from sources such as national studies or reports.

Specific Aims

"Aims" stem from a research purpose statement and concisely describe what will be tested or evaluated in your research project. In addition to specifying the aims of the study, you might state hypotheses specific to each aim that you intend to test formally, if appropriate. Box 21-2 provides an example of a specific aim and an accompanying hypothesis.

> **BOX 21-2**
> **EXAMPLE OF A SPECIFIC AIM AND HYPOTHESIS**
>
> *Specific aim:* Test the immediate effects (up to 4 months) and long-term effects (at 6 and 12 months) of a life skills training program for men who are homeless.
> *Hypothesis:* Homeless men who participate in the life skills program will report less depressed affect and will achieve goal attainment in specific skill areas in comparison to homeless men in a control group who receive no intervention or treatment.

If you propose to conduct a study using a qualitative methodology in which formal hypothesis testing is inappropriate, you will need to explain this point carefully to reviewers (as we discuss later). Although there is increasing awareness among review panels of the scientific value of naturalistic inquiry, the formats for most proposals favor a quantitative or linear structure to describing the research plan.

"Aim statements" are critical building blocks of a proposal. They provide a mental template or a road map of what you plan to accomplish in the project.

Rationale: Significance and Importance

Next in your proposal, you need to provide a rationale for your study and discuss why it is significant and how it will address a gap in existing knowledge. Providing a brief review of the key literature that informs your research is important (see Chapter 5). Although having an idea that is exciting to you is a necessary starting point in conducting a research study, the idea must also have some merit and must be perceived as significant by the larger scientific community and your audience, whether a human subject board, funding agency, or your professor.

You will address the "so what" question in the rationale. The "so what" question is a response that a reviewer might make after reading this section if you have not convinced the person that your idea is important and relevant to public health. The "so what" response represents a fatal flaw in a research endeavor. If a reviewer cannot answer the "so what" question by reading your rationale, it has a poor chance of being evaluated positively regardless of its methodological rigor or design validity.

The significance of your research idea must be justified with a concise review of other research studies that highlight the level of knowledge of the field, the need for further research, and how your research addresses the gap in knowledge. Your review of previous research should demonstrate that your question or query is important but has not been satisfactorily answered. It should include only the most pertinent and current works and not a long discourse about topics only peripherally related to your project. A theoretical framework should also be clearly and explicitly linked to the variables you propose to examine.

There are at least two ways to organize the writing of the literature review. One approach is to present articles chronologically, with the oldest articles first, to provide a historical perspective. Another approach is to group articles according to common themes that are relevant to your topic.

In your study on the health conditions of men who are homeless, one strategy for reviewing and categorizing the related literature is to identify articles or studies that do the following:

1. Identify national and local statistics about the number of individuals who are homeless.
2. Contain demographic data about the homeless population.
3. Describe the health care needs of homeless persons.
4. Describe the problems faced by this group in accessing the health care system.
5. Discuss the gaps in knowledge about health conditions of men who are homeless and the methodological challenges in sample identification and data collection.

In reviewing the literature, it is important to consider resources outside your own field or profession and to obtain sources where the original work in an area is conducted.

If the topic area of interest to you has not been studied or written about extensively, your review may be relatively brief. You then need to demonstrate that your topic is significant and cite the lack of research as one reason for conducting your study. A critical point to remember in writing a review of relevant literature is that the information you use and report must be from primary sources. A *primary source* is the original article from which this information is reported. It is usually not appropriate to discuss a research article that is described or presented in an article by an author who did not conduct or report on the original study.

At the conclusion of reviewing relevant literature, provide a summary that reflects a synthesis and analysis of the articles. In this concluding section, you should discuss the way in which the literature you cited supports your background, significance, research question, hypotheses, and design. Also, identify the gaps in knowledge and the way in which your study or educational program systematically contributes to knowledge building to address these gaps.

Research Plan

In this section of the research proposal, each action process is described in detail, including plans for bounding your study, identifying and recruiting a sample, collecting information, and analyzing the data you obtain. Also, you will need to provide a justification for each action process. Box 21-3 outlines key aspects of research methodology to present in a proposal.

Common mistakes made in writing this section of a proposal are an inadequate justification for why a particular action process is chosen, poor integration of ideas, lack of design validity, and lack of sufficient detail about the bounding and selecting of research study participants.

BOX 21-3
SECTIONS OF RESEARCH METHODOLOGY TO PRESENT IN A PROPOSAL

1. Overview of research design
2. Sample description and bounding procedures
   a. Inclusion and exclusion criteria
   b. Recruitment plan
3. Action processes
   a. Procedures
   b. Materials
   c. Data collection
   d. Analytical plan
4. Human subjects
   a. Assurance of confidentiality
   b. Informed consent process
5. Study validity and reliability
6. Assumptions and study limitations
7. Timetable of key research activities

Keep in mind that there is no specific order for presenting the subsections of the research methodology discussed next. Rather, your research plan should be presented in a logical order and should reflect an integration of your ideas.

Research Design. As discussed in Part III, the research design is the "blueprint" or plan in experimental-type design or the expression of the tradition that will be followed in a naturalistic inquiry. Each component of the research design must be presented and justified clearly and concisely.

One strategy is to begin this section of the proposal with a brief statement that summarizes or labels the design you intend to implement (e.g., two-group randomized experimental design, retrospective chart review, $2 \times 2 \times 2$ factorial design, ethnography) and explain in what way the design is appropriate to address your specific research question or query.

Then, briefly highlight the major elements of the design. In an experimental-type inquiry, state the independent and dependent variables, the sampling frame, sample size and selection procedures, and the number of testing occasions planned. It is important to be specific in your description. For example, when specifying the independent and dependent variables, include how each is related in the study (e.g., causal, explanatory, mediator, predictor). Box 21-4 provides an example of a design statement for an experimental-type study.

BOX 21-4
DESIGN STATEMENT FOR EXPERIMENTAL-TYPE STUDY

This study will describe the health conditions that present to men living in the shelter system who are 55 years of age or older. A descriptive survey design using a stratified random sample is proposed by which 100 men from 30 homeless shelters in the region will be randomly selected to complete a face-to-face interview designed to assess four areas of health: oral hygiene, mental health, physical aches and pains, and drug and alcohol use. The survey will contain demographic information, multiple-choice questions that tap knowledge of signs and symptoms of each problem, and open-ended questions that ask respondents to describe their approach to dealing with each problem.

BOX 21-5
DESIGN STATEMENT FOR NATURALISTIC QUERY

This study will explore the meaning of health and wellness of men living in the shelter system who are 55 years of age or older. An ethnographic study of a large homeless shelter that houses more than 1000 men per month will be conducted. In-depth interviewing of shelter staff and residents and direct observation of daily life and shelter activities will be carried out over an 18-month period. Areas that will be explored in the interviews will be how residents participate in basic hygiene, when they seek medical care, and what it means to be in good health or feeling good. All interviews will be recorded and transcribed and a thematic analysis conducted.

In a naturalistic inquiry the same level of specificity must be provided as in experimental-type research. (The issues related to this are discussed later.) Specify the basic tradition in which the query is based; the context, field, or geographical location where the inquiry will proceed; the key projected data collection strategies (e.g., key informant, participant observation); and the analytical plan. Box 21-5 provides an example of a design statement for a query in a naturalistic tradition.

Boundary Setting

This section of a proposal describes how you intend to "bound" your study. Consider outlining the following five basic points:

1. Describe the criteria that will be used to select study participants. This involves listing the specific criteria for inclusion and exclusion of study participants and the reason or justification for each of these criteria.
2. Describe the anticipated characteristics of the study participants and the extent to which these are representative of the population to which you plan to generalize the study findings. In discussing the sample characteristics, include a description of age, gender, race, ethnicity, and health status.
3. Describe the procedures you will use for recruiting the sample.
4. Discuss the sample size and the justification for its adequacy using power analysis, if appropriate.
5. Provide evidence of the feasibility of obtaining the required sample.

Collecting Information. This subsection should include a discussion of the procedures you will follow in collecting data and the instruments you will use, if applicable.

Human Subjects. This subsection provides a discussion of the protection of human subjects. The discussion should include (1) your plans to ensure confidentiality of the information or data that you obtain from human subjects, (2) how consent from study participants will be obtained, (3) the potential benefits and risks for a subject associated with participation, and (4) the risk/benefit ratio (see discussion on IRB in Chapter 12).

Validity and Reliability

You also address the validity and reliability of your design. Validity refers to whether a design and its procedures are appropriate and will yield information to answer the research question. You should explain the specific procedures you will use to ensure that your approach is the appropriate way to answer your research question. For example, if your purpose is to demonstrate causality, you might use an experimental design and discuss why the particular design you chose is most appropriate.

You also should explain the reliability of your approach to data collection and analysis. Clearly describe the specific design features you have established that will ensure consistency of procedures in such a way that another investigator could replicate your study.

You plan to make direct observations of a person's physical functioning using a standardized performance-based measure. In your research proposal, you need to discuss how you will ensure reliability and inter-rater agreement among the interviewers making the observations.

Assumptions and Limitations

In this section of the proposal, you discuss the specific limitations of your design. Almost every study has some limitations, either based on features inherent in the design or based in its application to your particular situation. Think about these limitations and how they may introduce possible sources of bias.

Suppose you are conducting a Delphi study. A limitation of this technique is that some respondents may discuss their opinions with others participating in the study. This is a limitation that may have consequences for your findings. Thus, you should identify this limitation and discuss the way you plan to address it.

Timetable

It is important to outline in narrative or table format the basic actions that will be implemented and the time required. This is important because it provides your audience with an understanding of each necessary action and whether it is feasible to accomplish these actions within the planned time frame of the study. Also, the timetable provides a road map and schedule of the actions you will take, which will be a helpful reference as you manage the research study.

Analytical Plan

This section involves a discussion of your analytical strategy and the statistical tests or qualitatively based techniques you plan to use. In your discussion it is helpful to restate the specific aims and hypotheses of your study, if applicable, and then identify the analytical approaches that will be used to address each aim or hypothesis. Also, provide a brief rationale for your choice of analytical approaches, and if it is an experimental-type study, include the significance level that will be used to determine statistical significance.

Dissemination Plan

Sharing your research findings is an essential element of the research process (see Chapter 2). Also, most funding sources want to be sure that their funds are used wisely and that the results of a successful project have a wide impact. From their perspective, it makes little sense to fund a project if only a few people will benefit from a successful outcome. Therefore, many agencies require that you present a systematic plan to show how you will disseminate the results of your project. Two accepted ways to do this are through presentations at national, scientific, and professional meetings and through publications in professional journals. Also, consider other creative and innovative ways to ensure a wide distribution of your findings that target multiple audiences. These methods may include the development and distribution of instructional manuals, plans to develop workshops or continuing education programs, or special ways to reach consumers as well as other professional groups. We discuss this in more detail in Chapter 22.

Plan of Management

In this section you begin to answer the question as to why you are the most appropriate person to conduct the study you are proposing. Although you may have a wonderful idea, you must also assure your readership that you can accomplish the program goals efficiently. This section is particularly important when applying to a funding agency. You can answer this question by showing that you have a clear, logical, and efficient plan of management that will be executed by a project team of well-qualified people at an institution that can provide the necessary support and resources. A clear description of the organizational and management structure will answer the first part of this question. In your management plan, you will need to discuss in detail the roles and responsibilities of key personnel, the amount of time each person will work on the project, and the time frame in which each project task will be implemented. Agencies frequently request that you organize this information in the form of a time line or a detailed Gantt chart of major activities.

An approach to writing this section is to visualize that you have already been funded. Think about exactly what you would have to do implement your action plan if you were to start tomorrow. Who would you need to hire? What contacts would be important? What resources would you need? Logically and rationally think through your plan before you write the section. This process may raise critical points of weakness in your research design, or it may highlight limitations in institutional resources.

Investigative Team Credentials

This section also helps answer the question about your qualifications to carry out the project. Review your plan to determine the special skills necessary to implement each step of the project, then carefully select team members with this expertise. For example, if you are proposing a study that requires a repeated-measures design or statistical modeling techniques, make sure you have a statistician on your team with expertise in these specific analytical strategies. If your study uses naturalistic inquiry, you must ensure that a member of your team is an expert in qualitative methodologies and software programs. In writing an educational grant, make sure you are working with someone who has curriculum development skills. Select individuals with complementary experience and credentials. For example, in an educational grant, you might need two people, one with curriculum development skills and one with experience in curriculum evaluation.

In writing about the credentials of the team, you should include a brief descriptive paragraph highlighting the qualifications of each member. Emphasize their past experience, publications, or presentations that show expertise in the topic of the project. You should also cite funding for other projects, either from sources external to your institution or from sources inside your institution, that you or other members have received. Offices held in professional organizations, teaching, or consulting experiences can provide additional credibility and demonstrate that you have the necessary background to implement the research successfully.

Institutional Qualifications

Just as your team needs to be qualified, your institution needs to have the resources to assist and support you in carrying out your project. You need to include a concise description of your institution's resources and qualifications. For example, has your institution acquired a significant amount of external funding? Does it have a comprehensive library, a learning resource center, or an active research office? What are the computer facilities available for your use?

Budget

This section addresses questions regarding the cost of your project and the reasons for the costs. You need to prepare a budget that is not inflated or wasteful and still sufficient to accomplish all your activities. Do not try to "pad" your budget by inflating costs or adding unnecessary expenses. Also, do not underestimate what it will cost you to carry out the study or educational program. The best rule of thumb is to develop a budget that accurately reflects the cost of the activities you are proposing. Most institutions have budget offices or offices of research administration that can help you as you prepare this budget.

You also are required to justify each expense. This should be included in a budget justification section following the actual budget. In this section, describe what each item will be used for and why it is necessary for your study.

References

As in all scientific work, a reference of your sources of information is required. If the agency does not specify a reference style, we recommend using the style specified by the American Psychological Association (APA). In any case, be sure to be consistent in the presentation of references.

Appendix Material

The appendices usually include information that supplements the narrative portion of the document. Appendix materials may include the complete "curriculum vitae" of key members of the research team, sample questionnaires or examples of open-ended probes, pertinent articles you have authored that relate to the study, and most important, letters of support from consultants or from leaders in your profession.

SPECIAL CONSIDERATIONS

Special considerations in preparing proposals are based on the type of research you plan to conduct.

Preparing an Experimental-Type Proposal

Within the experimental-type tradition, language and structure for presentation are standard across the basic elements of the proposal. The language used is logical and in the active tense. It involves a temporal and logical sequence detailing each step. Usually, ideas are presented in the third person and detached from personal opinion. The experimental-type report usually has six sections in the body of the report, an abstract, and a list of references used to support the inquiry.

The abstract precedes the narrative report and serves as a summary of each section of the proposal. The reference list contains full citations of all literature identified in the proposal. Many citation formats exist. We suggest that you consider the use of a computerized program (e.g., *Procite* or *Endnote*) to keep track of your literature and to format your references automatically in your style of choice. The degree of detail and precision in each section will depend on the purpose and audience for the proposal.

Preparing a Naturalistic Proposal

Because of the many epistemologically and structurally different types of naturalistic designs, we cannot assert a single proposal structure. The proposal, however, usually conforms to the basic elements previously outlined. Unfortunately, this structure favors the linear approach of experimental-type research. The proposal format, particularly the demand for details before entering the field, can present as a challenge to the naturalistic researcher. In addition, most audiences or reviewers of proposals are schooled in the tradition of experimental-type research, and they do not understand the naturalistic tradition or the vast differences in approaches to research design.

In writing a proposal, the naturalistic researcher must be sure not only to lay out the details of the action plans, but also to explain clearly why a particular action will be implemented according to its appropriateness for the tradition in which the research is based. For example, the researcher might want to offer a set of "working" hypotheses and explain why in naturalistic research it is not appropriate to offer testable statements. Or, the researcher may need to specify approaches to data collection (e.g., watching, in-depth interviewing, review of documents) but must explain that the approaches used will unfold at different points in time, to be decided once the investigator is in the field. Again, it is important to provide a detailed justification for each action statement and why it is appropriate in a naturalistic approach. Thus, in writing the proposal, you not only have to provide an explanation of your study, but also help educate the reviewer as to how to evaluate your design within the specific tradition you are following.

Preparing a Mixed-Method Proposal

In developing a proposal for a study that uses mixed methods, care must be taken to provide sufficient justification and details for each methodological component. Because a mixed-method study may involve different research traditions, there is an added level of complexity to the proposal writing process. As in any proposal, the writer must strive for clarity and precision in presentation as well as completeness. Each component of the designs and how and why methods are being mixed must be carefully detailed.

SUMMARY

You now should have a basic understanding of how and why researchers share their thinking and actions before engaging in the field. One important reason for sharing before the conduct of a study is to secure financial support for the activity. Grantsmanship is a critical component of the thinking processes in which researchers engage, and we refer you to other books that provide more comprehensive and focused discussions of grantsmanship that you may find useful.[1,2] Key to writing a research proposal is careful consideration of format, audience, and detail. Use of technical language and direct, clear simple statements is optimal. Each statement in a proposal will be scrutinized by readers, usually a group of the investigator's peers, that is, persons knowledgeable in the content of the research question or query. Most critical in justifying the research question or query and proposed action plan is to provide supporting evidence that is compelling and credible. By knowing the audience (e.g., who will be reading your proposal), you can also select the evidence that is most credible for that group. If you are writing for a medical audience, you might emphasize the significance of your research for quality of care; if you are writing for a health policy audience, emphasizing costeffectiveness may be more important. No matter what research tradition you are working in or which proposal format you use, four principles should guide its development: clarity, precision, parsimony, and attention to structure.

EXERCISES

1. Obtain a grant proposal from a funded investigator or from your school's office of research and outline its basic structure; provide a critique of each section. Did the investigator explain the terms adequately? Did the investigator justify key aspects of the action plan? Did the investigator convince you that the proposed research question or query will significantly contribute to knowledge building?
2. Write a "mini" proposal (up to 5 pages) that contains the essential structure as outlined in Table 21-1. What aspects of the proposal were challenging? Show your proposal to a colleague and ask for critical feedback.

REFERENCES

1. Gitlin LN, Lyons KJ: *Successful grant writing: strategies for health and human service professionals,* ed 2, New York, 2004, Springer.
2. DePoy E, Gilmer D: Adolescents with disabilities and chronic illness in transition: a community action needs assessment, *Disabilities Studies Quarterly,* Spring, 2000.

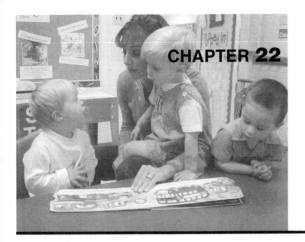

CHAPTER 22

Sharing Research Knowledge During and After the Study

KEY TERMS
Accessible
Dissemination
Linguistic sensitivity
Reporting

CHAPTER OUTLINE

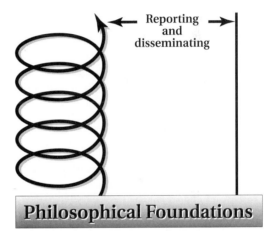

Reporting and disseminating

Philosophical Foundations

Although you may have completed the collection and analysis of information for a study, your efforts as a researcher are not quite complete. The tenth essential of research, "sharing research knowledge," involves two important action processes: purposeful reporting and dissemination of knowledge gained from a study. Unless you report and disseminate, you have not completed the research process. Sharing knowledge is critical to knowledge building. Also, communicating knowledge gained from an inquiry with those who can benefit is an important ethical action.

By *reporting* research knowledge, we mean the preparation of a communication of all or part of an inquiry to one or more audiences. *Dissemination* follows reporting and is defined as the action process of purposely sharing the report. These action processes usually occur at the conclusion of a research project. Often, however, there are opportunities to communicate the progress of a study or report some

265

of the methodological challenges before completing the actions of data collection and analysis.

Think about our definition of research in Chapter 1. Do you remember the four criteria to which a study must conform? These four criteria, which apply to any type of research inquiry, are the following: logical, understandable, confirmable, and useful. Reporting and disseminating are two research action processes that also reflect these criteria. However, "usefulness" is the one research criterion that cannot be accomplished without communicating to others the findings of a completed study and their meaning.

Reports are designed to fit a particular avenue or context that is chosen for the dissemination of research findings. The methods chosen for reporting research are purposeful. They are driven by several factors, the most important of which are the question or query and the particular audience or community on whom the researcher wants to have an impact. We believe that three basic principles should inform the action process of reporting: writing guidelines, accessibility, and linguistic sensitivity.

WRITING GUIDELINES

We begin our discussion with writing because it is the most typical way that reporting is accomplished. Any research study may generate one or more reports.

As you probably have surmised by now, each type of inquiry has a distinct language or set of languages and structures that organize the reporting action process. However, all written reporting, regardless of the research tradition that the report will reflect, is based in a common set of guidelines.[1] These include issues related to clarity, purpose, knowledge of target audience, and citation style.

Clarity

Writing a report serves little purpose if it is not understood.[2] Therefore an investigator should be certain that his or her report is clear and well written. There are many books on writing and many ways of approaching this task, which is often difficult, particularly for the new investigator. As in any professional activity, the more you do it, the more proficient you will be and easier the task will become. It is important to recognize that writing is an important aspect of the research process; it takes time, thought, and creative energy.

Purpose

As we have stated throughout this book, multiple purposes drive the selection of research action processes. These purposes also structure the nature of the reporting action process.[3] Consider, for example, two different purposes for writing a report: a publication in a professional journal and a written evaluation for a community organization. Researchers who write for the purpose of publishing their research in scholarly journals must conform to the style and expectations of the journal to which the manuscript is submitted. The researcher may also consider writing an article for practitioners and thus will present results and interpretations somewhat differently. The researcher who has just completed an evaluation of a community program may need to write a report to the board of directors or the funding agency to ensure continuation of financial support. In this case the researcher may emphasize positive programmatic outcomes and write the research report consistent with the expectations of the funding agency. Each purpose for conducting and reporting research must be carefully considered.

Multiple Audiences

As stated earlier, being aware of the many audiences who can benefit from an inquiry is critical to meet the "useful" criterion in our definition of research. Audiences are diverse in their languages, the meanings they attribute to language, and their values regarding credibility. Thus, along with purpose, the audiences for whom the report is written will determine, in large part, how the written report will be structured and the degree of specificity that will be included. The audience may vary in areas of expertise and knowledge of research methodology. The important point is to identify your reason for writing a report to a particular audience and to assess how that purpose can be communicated to that audience. You need to write in a style that is consistent with the level of understanding and knowledge of the targeted reader. To this end, the concepts of accessibility and linguistic sensitivity are important, as discussed later.

Citations

You need to be aware of several other important points as you develop written reports. The first is the issue of plagiarism. We realize that most researchers who plagiarize do not intend to do so. To avoid this potential and devastating mistake, you need to be aware of the norms for citation and credit. All work written by another person, even if not directly quoted in your work, must be cited. Many different citation formats are used in health and human service research. We refer you to your publication source for the correct format and urge you to become familiar with it. If necessary, have someone else check your work to ensure that you have properly credited other authors.

Another important point to remember in report writing is that it is not an acceptable practice to quote from other research studies in the literature review of an article for a journal. Many students of research like to review a body of literature by stringing together a series of quotes from different articles. However, the review of the literature section in a report must reflect a summation and critical analysis of the most salient aspects of existing studies.

Another common error among newcomers to formal writing is the use of citations that you have not directly read. Consider the following example:

You read an article by an author, Dr. Smith, and in her review of the literature, she cited a number of other authors and their studies. You are interested in these other studies and include them in your study based on your reading of Dr. Smith's article, and you cite them in your reference list. However, you have never obtained and read the original articles. In this case you are actually using Dr. Smith's interpretations of these studies. Remember, Dr. Smith selected the most salient points from these studies that supported her particular approach. Therefore, her interpretation may be different from the intent of the original work. If you had read the articles yourself, you may have derived a different understanding. In writing a research report, only primary citations are acceptable.

Therefore you have two choices. You can report Dr. Smith's interpretation of the studies she reviewed and cite her article in your reference list. For example, you may say, "According to Dr. Smith, the literature on the adequacy of home care for elders is underdeveloped." A second strategy is to retrieve the articles cited in Dr. Smith's report, read them, and report your interpretation of this body of literature. In this case you will then cite each study you read and include it in your reference list.

With these commonsense principles, let us now consider the specific writing considerations for each tradition.

WRITING AN EXPERIMENTAL-TYPE REPORT

Reports of experimental-type research use a common language and follow a standard format and structure for presenting a study and its findings. The language used by the experimental-type researcher is "scientific" in nature. It is logical and detached from personal opinion. Interpretations are supported by numerical data. There are usually seven major sections of an experimental-type report (Box 22-1). Although investigators sometimes deviate from this order of presentation, these sections are usually considered the critical components of a scientific report. Let us examine each section.

The abstract appears before the full report and briefly summarizes or highlights the major points in each subsequent section of the report. It includes a statement of the research purpose, brief overview of method, and summary of the major findings and

---

BOX 22-1
MAJOR SECTIONS OF AN
EXPERIMENTAL-TYPE REPORT

1. Abstract
2. Introduction
3. Background and significance
4. Method
   - Design
   - Research question(s)
   - Population and sample
   - Measures
   - Data analysis strategies
   - Procedures
5. Results
6. Discussion
7. Conclusion

implications of the study. Usually the abstract does not exceed one or two paragraphs. Professional journals usually specify the length of the abstract; some journals require brief abstracts that are no longer than 100 words.

The introduction presents the problem statement, the purpose statement, and an overview of the questions that the study addresses. In this section the researcher embeds the study in a particular body of literature and highlights the study's specific intended contribution to professional knowledge and practice.

The background and significance section reviews the literature that provides the conceptual foundation for your research study. In this section, key concepts, constructs, principles, and theory of the study are critically summarized. (Refer to your literature chart or concept matrix to help organize the background and significance section.) The degree of detail in presenting the literature will depend on the researcher's purpose and intended audience. For example, in a journal article the researcher usually limits the literature review to the seminal works that precede the study, whereas in a doctoral dissertation all previous work that directly or indirectly informs the research question is included. Some researchers combine the introduction and literature review into one section. Grinnell[3] has named the combined introduction and literature review "the problem statement."

The method section consists of several subsections, including a clear description of the design, an explication of the research question or questions, the population and sample, the measures or instrumentation, the specific data analysis strategies, and the procedures used to conduct the research. The degree of detail and specificity is once again determined by the purpose and audience. However, sufficient information must be provided in each subsection of methods so that the reader has a clear understanding of how data were collected and the specific procedures that were implemented.

The analyzed data are presented in the results section. Usually, researchers begin by presenting descriptive statistics of their sample, then proceed to a presentation of inferential and associational types of statistical analysis. A rationale for statistical analysis is presented, and the findings are usually explained. However, interpretation of the data is not usually presented in this section. Data may be presented in narrative, chart, graph, or table form. You should be aware that there are prescribed formats for presenting statistical analyses. Ary et al.[4] provide excellent information to guide both the preparation and the evaluation of written reports.

The discussion section may be the most creative part of the experimental-type research report. In this section the researcher discusses the implications and meanings of the findings, poses alternative explanations, relates the findings to published work, and suggests the potential application or use of the research results. Most researchers include a statement of the limitations of the study in this section as well, although this can also be found in the sections that discuss methods or findings.

The conclusion section is a short summary that provides interpretations and application of the study findings to future research directions or health care practices.

As you can see, writing an experimental-type report follows a logical, well-accepted sequence that includes seven essential sections. The degree of detail and precision in each section depends on the purpose and audience for the report.

Also, it is important to note that there is a specific reporting structure for the true experimental design, the randomized controlled trial. Because this design strategy requires highly specified elements, such as randomization, a control group, a treatment group, and analysis and interpretation of treatment effects, the reporting follows a rather uniform presentation. To enhance the scientific utility and transparency of each action process in this design strategy, efforts have been made to standardize the reporting of trials. In the 1990s an international body of researchers engaged in clinical trials put forth the Consolidated Standards of Reporting Trials (CONSORT) in an effort to provide standard language and structure and enhance the ability of readers to evaluate the validity of trials. The CONSORT includes a checklist of the items that should be included in a report of a trial and a flow diagram indicating enrollment and participation status of study subjects. It has been adopted by many medical journals, including *The Lancet* and the *Journal of the American Medical Association,* which now require written manuscript submissions that are reporting trials to use the checklist and flow diagram.[5] For example, the checklist for the method section indicates the need to report the following design elements: participants, interventions, study and intervention objectives, outcome measures, sample size, randomization procedures, blinding techniques, and statistical methods.

WRITING A NATURALISTIC REPORT

Because of the many epistemologically and structurally different types of research designs that reflect naturalistic inquiry, there is no single, accepted format for writing a final report. However, some basic commonalties among the varied designs can guide report writing in this tradition. Unlike experimental-type reporting, naturalistic reporting does not follow a prescribed format with clear expectations for language and structure. Written reports tend to be rich in detail and description and draw on data in the form of narratives to illustrate major themes and interpretations. The structure of the presentation is not standardized, and there is great variation in the format, sequencing of information, and approach. The approach used by the researcher reflects his or her underlying interpretive scheme. Interpretive schemes are often presented as a "story" in which main themes and subtexts unfold as the story is told. Consider the following examples:

In her ethnography of children diagnosed with leukemia, Bluebond-Langner[6] presented her analysis of the children's experiences in the form of a play with acts and scenes. The characters in the play represented a composite of the children, families, and medical personnel she had interviewed and observed. In this way, Bluebond-Langner was able to creatively and immediately immerse the reader into the worlds of dying children, their parents, and medical staff. Her approach showed the sequence of events experienced by children as they moved through stages of diagnosis, remission, relapse, and finally death, highlighting the interactions between children and parents, physicians, and nursing staff. The style of reporting reflected the way in which the children presented themselves to the investigator.

In contrast, in a study of 26 African American women with breast disease, Mathews et al.[7] began their report with an excerpt from an interview with one of their informants. The authors provided a brief overview of the theoretical foundation for understanding narratives and the relationship between personal accounts and cultural systems. The rest of the report was structured more traditionally and included "Background for the Study," "Profile of the Patient Population and Description of Methodology," "Results of the Narrative Analysis," and "Conclusions."

Another important aspect of reporting in naturalistic inquiry is the inclusion of a section that describes the researcher's personal biases and feelings in conducting the study. Bluebond-Langner,[6] for example, included an appendix entitled, "Doing the Fieldwork: a Personal Account." Other researchers discuss their personal perspective on conducting the study as part of the introduction to their report.

Although the report in naturalistic inquiry may be structured in many different ways, it contains some of the same basic elements used in report writing for experimental-type research. Using the language of naturalistic research, Box 22-2 provides the basic sections for writing a report. Reporting in naturalistic research may not follow the sections in the sequence as shown, but each report usually contains these basic elements.

The introduction in naturalistic design contains the purpose for conducting the research. An investigator may include personal purposes, as well as a purpose related to the development and advancement of professional knowledge.

The query, epistemological foundation, and theoretical framework may appear separately or combined in one section of the report. As described in previous

---

BOX 22-2
BASIC SECTIONS OF A NATURALISTIC INQUIRY REPORT

1. Introduction
2. Query
3. Epistemological foundation
4. Theoretical framework(s)
5. Research process
6. Information
7. Analysis
8. Meaning and implications

chapters, these thinking and action processes are integrated throughout the conduct of naturalistic research and therefore can be presented as such. However, consistent with the principle of clarity in presentation, investigators need to select a format that is clear and easily understood by the target audience and consistent with the purpose of the study and report.

By now you may have noticed that we have not listed literature review as part of the reporting process. Consistent with the naturalistic research tradition, literature may be presented as a conceptual foundation for the query or as evidence that supports the data or main interpretations presented by the investigator. In most reports the literature is used to ground the research in a body of knowledge, to support the main findings, or to examine competing interpretations of the findings.

Reporting naturalistic research departs from experimental-type reporting in the presentation of the research process and information. Naturalistic investigators rely heavily on the narrative to report their data.[8] Quotations from informants may be woven throughout the narrative text. Visual and numerical display of information, such as taxonomic charts and content analyses, are also used in naturalistic reporting, depending on the query, epistemological foundation, purpose, and intended audience. Let us now consider how the reports from different naturalistic designs may be structured.

Ethnography

Although there are divergent approaches to ethnography, the primary function of this approach is to identify patterns and characterize a cultural group. Therefore the report tells a story about the underlying values, roles, beliefs, and normative practices of the culture. It is not unusual for ethnographers to begin with "method"; that is, the investigator frequently begins by reporting how he or she gained access to the cultural setting. The report may be developed chronologically, and literature, other sources of information, and conclusions are interspersed throughout and summarized in the end. Liebow[9] exemplifies this structure in *Tally's Corner*.

In *Living and Dying at Murray Manor,* Gubrium's approach is another example of how interpretation is integrated throughout, as reflected in the way he describes what it is like to live in a nursing home.[10] Each chapter builds on the previous one but focuses on a different aspect of life in the nursing facility (e.g., "The Setting," "Top Staff and Its World"). The entire book represents his findings. He introduces formal literature through the use of footnotes, which are designed either to support his points or to lead the reader to other literature for more discussion of a particular concept that is introduced.

A written report in ethnography is usually lengthy because of the expansiveness of the domain and nature of narrative data.

Phenomenology

Because the focus in phenomenological research is on the unique experience of one or more persons, the report is often written in the form of a story. If specific points about the lived experience of the informants are made, they are fully supported with information from the informants themselves, frequently in the form of direct quotes from the field notes. Because the length of phenomenological studies varies extensively, they may appear as full-length journal articles, books, or other literary styles between these formats. The reports highlight life experience and its interpretation by those who experience it, and they minimize interpretations imposed by the investigator.

The nature and purpose of phenomenological designs differ from those of ethnography, as does the reporting format. In both cases, form follows function. In ethnography the function of the investigator is to make sense of what he or she has observed, whereas in a phenomenological study the investigator reports how others make sense of their experience. These differences are clearly reflected in the written report.

In summary, naturalistic researchers use a variety of reporting action processes to share their findings. Although there is a heavy reliance on narrative data, the naturalistic investigator has the option of using numerical and visual representations, as well as other media. All reports contain the basic sections (see Box 22-2), but the order and emphasis differ among naturalistic designs and the preferences and personal styles of the investigator.[8,11,12]

WRITING AN INTEGRATED REPORT

Because integrated reports have made a relatively recent appearance in the research world, there are no guidelines for language and format.[13] In addition, the nature and structure of the report depend on the level of integration, types of designs used, purpose of the work, and audience who will receive the report. We can, however, offer two principles that may help your writing action process. First, you should include the components of a complete research report (see Boxes 22-1 and 22-2). Regardless of its length, organization, or complexity, your report should contain a statement of purpose, review of the literature, methodology section, presentation of findings, and conclusions. Second, because integrated design is not as well established as designs that are distinctly experimental type or naturalistic, it is often useful to include an evaluation of the methodology in the report and the justification for the use of each design, as well as the way in which each complements the other.

ACCESSIBILITY

In addition to guidelines for writing, there is another important reporting principle. Communicating knowledge brings with it an important obligation, that of providing knowledge in accessible formats for all groups who may benefit. *Accessible* is a term that describes the usability of a product or service. In the case of communicating research, the "product" is the research report.

In the past several years, two approaches to expanding information access have emerged: accommodative and universal. Accommodative strategies refer to those that adapt and customize information to meet condition or group-specific needs.[14] Universal approaches (often called "universal design" or "universal access") are distinct from group-specific approaches in that they provide information in forms that all people, to the extent possible and regardless of group-specific diversity characteristics, can access without the need for adaptation.[15] Vanderheiden (in Preiser and Ostrow) suggests that because of the huge range of human diversity, universal design is a "process" rather than a tangible outcome:

Universal design is more a function of keeping all of the people and all of the situations in mind and trying to create a product that is as flexible as is commercially practical.[16]

To the extent possible and purposive, we believe that it is incumbent on researchers to plan communication so that it can be accessed by all who can benefit. Universal approaches to communication of information provide the framework for this goal (see later discussion on dissemination).

LINGUISTIC SENSITIVITY

The third principle we discuss in reporting research concerns how language is used in a particular context, or linguistic sensitivity. By *linguistic sensitivity* we mean having knowledge about the target audience and the meaning of language to that group. Our point can be best illustrated by two recent incidents that occurred to colleagues.

> In a recent trip to Egypt to study and teach, our colleague was surprised to find that despite the arrangements to teach in English, few people, including her intended students, spoke English with sufficient fluency to be able to benefit from her lectures. She called the sponsor, who was an Egyptian woman who spoke fluent English, to discuss how to address the language barrier. She began the conversation with the statement, "No one speaks English here," to which she received an immediate reply, "What do you expect? You are in Egypt teaching Egyptians." Although her immediate reaction was anger at the flip comment, on further reflection she realized that her statement had been misunderstood and her words placed in a context different from the one she intended.
>
> Another colleague made this observation at a conference on employment law and disability for attorneys and researchers. He noticed that in the research presentations, the attorneys looked rather bored, and that in the law presentations, the researchers expressed skepticism about claims made by the attorneys, claims that were supported only by individual and anecdotal stories about clients.

In both situations, much can be learned about communication and the meaning of words, or language. The Egyptian experience illustrates that people who speak the same language do not necessarily speak the same "meaning." The conference incident demonstrates that credibility varies between and within groups. That is to say, the language of evidence that is convincing to one group or individual may not be believable or even interesting to another. Keep these stories in mind as you plan and implement the action strategies of sharing knowledge.

As suggested throughout this book, there are multiple research languages and structures. Likewise, there are multiple ways in which you may choose to present and structure the reporting and disseminating of your research. The reporting language and structure you use must be congruent with the epistemological framework of your study; it must fit the purpose for dissemination and the target audience. In all types of communication, keep in mind the important points made earlier about diversity in meaning, differing perceptions of the criterion for credibility, and universal access. Also, remember that research reporting and disseminating are analogous to telling a story. As Richardson states:

> Whenever we write science, we are telling some kind of story, or some part of a larger narrative. Some of our stories are more complex, more densely described, and offer greater opportunities as emancipatory documents; others are more abstract, more distanced from lived experience, and reinscribe existent hegemonies.[8]

DISSEMINATION

Many ways are available to you for disseminating your research. Let us examine three popular modes of disseminating.

Sharing Written Reports

Sharing a written report is one of the most common ways of disseminating research findings. As discussed, written reports may reflect different formats, depending on the purpose of the report and the audience. Journal articles may be the most popular outlet for disseminating a written report, but many other valuable formats are available. These include research briefs in periodicals and newsletters, summary articles in professional newsletters, local newspapers, and university newsletters, as well as reports to fund-

ing agencies, master's and doctoral theses, chapters in edited books, and full-length books. Once you have written a report, the next action process is publication.

Publishing Your Work

The process of publishing your work is exciting but sometimes frustrating if you are new to the process. The first step in considering publication is to ensure that your work is high quality and meets the rigorous standards for research discussed in previous chapters. However, writing a sound report does not ensure publication. If you are attempting to publish your first piece of written work, we suggest that you consult with someone who is knowledgeable about the process.

It is critical to select a medium that is compatible with the design, purpose, focus, and level of development of your work. Each publication has a set of guidelines and requirements for authors that are usually available in one or more of the yearly issues of the publication. Scholarly and professional journals usually publish instructions for authors at least twice a year. These guidelines include a list of the required format for writing, typing and notation style, and submission processes. For refereed journals, once you submit your work, it is sent out to several (usually three) reviewers for comment and evaluation. This process takes between 3 and 6 months. Do not be surprised if your work is rejected. Most journals have many more submissions than they can publish, and rejection does not mean your work is poor. It is not unusual for journal editors to suggest alternative journals that may accept your work. If your written report is accepted, frequently it will be accompanied with requested revisions from the reviewers or the editor. After revisions, the work is placed in an issue, and galley proofs are sent to you for your review. These galleys are typeset models of your work. Be vigilant in reviewing them to ensure that no mistakes have occurred in the typesetting process.

Celebrate your work as you read it in publication. You have met the research criterion of "usefulness"!

Sharing Your Research Through Other Methods

Written dissemination is not the only method for sharing your work. There are many other outlets, including presentations at professional and scholarly conferences, oral presentations in other forums, continuing and in-service education, collaborative work with colleagues, and presentations on the World Wide Web. Sharing your work not only is useful to others, but also helps you receive constructive criticism that will advance your own thinking and conceptual development.

SUMMARY

Disseminating your research is a major and essential part of the research process. Sharing your work provides knowledge to others to inform practice, tests existing knowledge and theory, develops new knowledge and theory, and ultimately promotes the collective advancement of knowledge in health and human services.

EXERCISES

1. Find a research article reported in a professional research journal. Also, identify a research report published in a practice-oriented newsletter for a professional association. Compare the style of writing and the basic elements of the research process in light of the intended audiences.

2. Identify a published research study using an experimental-type design and a study using a naturalistic design. Compare the style of writing, the basic elements of the report, and particularly the presentation of data.

REFERENCES

1. Gitlin LN, Lyons KJ: *Successful grant writing: strategies for health and human service professionals,* ed 2, New York, 2004, Springer.
2. Babbie E: *The basic of social research,* ed 3, Belmont, Calif, 2005, Wadsworth.
3. Grinnell RM: *Social work research and evaluation,* ed 6, Itasca, Ill, 2000, Peacock.
4. Ary H, Jacobs LC, Razavieh A: *Introduction to research in education,* Belmont, Calif, 2002, Wadsworth.
5. Moher D, Schulz KF, Altman DG: The CONSORT statement: revised recommendations for improving the quality of reports of parallel-groups of randomized trials, *Lancet* 357:1911-1914, 2001.
6. Bluebond-Langner M: *The private worlds of dying children,* Princeton, NJ, 1978, Princeton University Press.
7. Mathews HF, Lannin DR, Mitchell JP: Coming to terms with advanced breast cancer: black women's narratives from eastern North Carolina, *Soc Sci Med* 38(6):789-800, 1994.
8. Richardson L: *Writing strategies: reaching diverse audiences,* Newbury Park, Calif, 1990, Sage.
9. Liebow E: *Tally's corner,* Boston, 1967, Little, Brown.
10. Gubrium JF: *Living and dying at Murray Manor,* New York, 1975, St Martin's Press.
11. Emerson RM, Fretz RI, Shaw LL: *Writing ethnographic fieldnotes,* Chicago, 1995, University of Chicago Press.
12. Wolcott HF: *Writing up qualitative research,* Newbury Park, Calif, 1990, Sage.
13. Tashakkori A, Teddue C: *Handbook of mixed methods in social sciences,* Thousand Oaks, Calif, 2002, Sage.
14. DePoy E, Gilson SF: *Evaluation practice,* Belmont, Calif, 2003, Brooks-Cole.
15. Center for Universal Design, North Carolina State, http://www.design.ncsu.edu/cud/univ_design/ud.htm, accessed 1997.
16. Vanderheiden G: Fundamentals and priorities for design information and telecommunication technologies. In Preiser W, Ostrow E: *Universal design handbook,* New York, 2001, McGraw Hill.

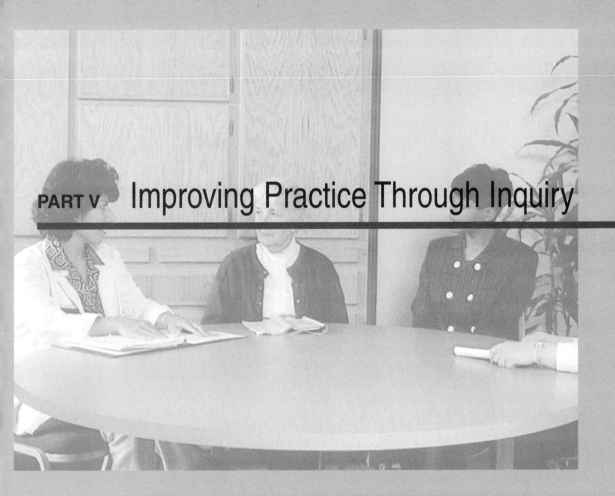

PART V Improving Practice Through Inquiry

We have finally arrived at the part of the book that answers the question, "So now that I am familiar with the thinking and action processes of both research traditions and their integration, how do I use this learning to improve my own practice and contribute to practice knowledge?" We now depart from the conceptual framework that we have used throughout the book to locate experimental-type, naturalistic, and mixed methods of research in the larger context of practice examination, efficacy, and our own practice experience. In Part V we examine specific professional applications of what you have studied throughout the text.

Because case study has been used as a method to evaluate the process and outcome of professional health and human service intervention, we include it here to illustrate an important way to apply inquiry to individuals and groups as single units of focus.

As you enter Part V, congratulate yourself on your learning, and see now what research can be all about in your health and human service practice.

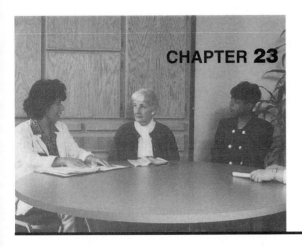

CHAPTER 23 Case Study Designs

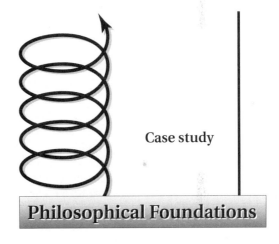

Case study

Philosophical Foundations

extensively on case study and whose perspective is consistent with ours.

WHAT IS A CASE STUDY?

Let us begin to understand case methodology by examining the definition advanced by Yin,[2] who defines *case study* in two technical parts:

Part One: "An empirical inquiry that…investigates a contemporary phenomenon within its real life context; especially when the boundaries between phenomenon and context are not clearly evident."

Part Two: "Copes with the technically distinctive situation in which there will be many more variables of interest than data points, and as one

In the past, case study designs have been viewed as inferior to group or nomothetic designs (discussed in Chapter 8). However, the value and flexibility of case study designs are increasingly asserted by researchers and practitioners. Case study designs represent a methodology that can be quite complex.[1] In this chapter we examine case study methodology and suggest guidelines for its use. We draw much of our discussion from the work of Yin, who has written result, relies on multiple sources of evidence, with data needing to converge in a triangulating fashion, and as another result, benefits from the prior development of theoretical propositions to guide data collection and analysis."[2]

It is usually assumed that case study is a design in which a single subject is investigated. However, you might have noticed that this element of case study designs does not even appear in Yin's definition. The view that all case studies are investigations that focus on a single person is misleading. Rather, case study designs may involve multiple persons or units. The key element of case study design as illuminated by Yin is that it is an approach that is used to investigate a "single phenomenon" in context. A single phenomenon may be a single subject, a single part, or many subparts. For example, an investigator may be interested in a single family as the "case." Because a family is composed of more than one individual, case study design may involve more than one person, where all the individuals make up one unit of analysis, the family.

Yin's definition does not limit case study to a particular research tradition or design strategy; that is, a case study approach does not exclusively belong to experimental-type or naturalistic research. Rather, the approach is flexible; it can be conducted in either research tradition, or it can integrate both traditions. The purpose of a case study can be to describe phenomena, examine relationships, or make predictions.

Furthermore, a critical element of case study research is its reliance on multiple methods of data collection to capture the complexity of a case. *Triangulation* (more recently referred to as crystallization;[3] see Chapters 17 and 20), or collecting information using different strategies to examine a phenomenon, is a basic strategy in case study designs.[2] In keeping with the flexibility of case study research, one can gather information using experimental-type or naturalistic techniques or their combination. Box 23-1 summarizes the four basic characteristics of case study.

STRUCTURE OF CASE STUDIES

There are many variations of case study designs that are labeled as single-subject, single-system, or "N of 1" single-case experimental trial (N refers to the size

---

BOX 23-1
CHARACTERISTICS OF CASE STUDY DESIGNS

■ Flexibility
■ Used by either experimental-type or naturalistic tradition
■ Multiple purposes
■ Multiple data collection methods

---

of the sample). A case study approach is useful in the following circumstances: (1) when it is not possible or desirable to randomize, (2) when it is not possible or desirable to study a particular population as a group with similar characteristics, (3) when it is desirable to determine intervention outcomes or change in a behavior over time as a consequence of one or multiple interventions, or (4) when it is desirable to obtain pilot information in a cost-efficient way. Moreover, case study is an excellent theory-generating tool, since the findings of a single case can be theoretically explained and then tested through other types of design strategies.

To understand the different approaches to case study designs, we use Yin's description of its structural components. Yin[2] classifies case studies into four categories created through combining two dimensions: the structure of the unit of analysis (holistic or embedded) and the number of cases (single or multiple) (Figure 23-1). Let us examine each dimension now in more detail.

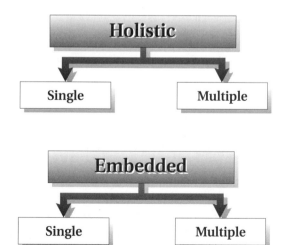

Figure 23-1 Four types of case study design.

Structural Dimension

Two elements make up the structural dimension, holistic and embedded. Holistic case studies are those in which the unit of analysis is viewed as one global phenomenon. For example, if we were to select family function as our object of study, a holistic case study approach would treat the family as a single unit. In contrast, the embedded study would treat the family as multiple subparts or as subparts placed within larger contexts. Consider the following example:

> You are interested in studying family violence. The investigator who believes that family violence is a cultural phenomenon may select a holistic single-case study design to analyze the response of the total family to cultural sanctions for violence. The family would therefore be observed and tested as a whole. In the embedded approach, individual members of the family are observed and tested as subparts of the single-family case study. This type of case study would be the design of choice for the investigator who is attempting to determine the dynamics among individual family members that may potentially provoke family violence.

When considering holistic versus embedded designs, the investigator must examine the nature of the phenomenon that is of interest as the basis for deciding how to proceed. Does the unit of analysis have natural parts that will reveal relevant information? If "yes," then an embedded approach would be used. Does the "whole" provide the most informative approach? If "yes," then a holistic approach is used.

Number of Cases

Now that you understand a holistic versus embedded approach, let us consider the differences between single-case and multiple-case designs. In a *single-case design,* only one study of a single unit of analysis is conducted. In a *multiple-case design,* more than one study of single units of analysis is conducted. It logically follows, therefore, that the holistic single-case study is conducted only once on one case. The holistic multiple-case study examines several global units of analysis more than once. Likewise, an embedded single-case study focuses on multiple

parts of a single case using only one case. On the other hand, an embedded multiple-case study examines more than one case in which each case contains many subparts.

The decision to conduct a single-case or multiple-case study depends on several considerations. First, the aim of the research must fit the structure that is selected. Multiple-case studies enable the investigator to examine the same phenomenon across several different cases. It is somewhat analogous to the concept of "replication" in group (or nomothetic) designs. Thus, if an investigator wants to repeat a study to strengthen theory or test the findings of a single case on other cases, a multiple-case study approach is preferred. However, if the purpose of the research is to generate theory, explicate an atypical phenomenon, or describe the progress of an individual over time, a single-case study approach is warranted.

> You are a hospice social worker who is working in the homes of clients with acquired immunodeficiency syndrome (AIDS). In your client group, you find one individual who seems unusual in her ability to cope with terminal illness. To understand this individual better and to discover the factors that contribute to coping strategies, you conduct a single-case study. This "deviant" case study approach can illuminate distinctions in coping strategies. However, if you are interested in characterizing the experience of persons with AIDS in their communities, it may be more appropriate to select a multiple-case study design.

The reason an investigator would select a multiple-case study design instead of a more traditional group design lies in the definition of case study designs. Case study, whether single or multiple, is ideal for describing persons in depth and over time in their contemporary context without sacrificing or reducing the complexity of human experience.

DESIGN SEQUENCE

Assume you plan to conduct a case study and have decided on its basic structure and size; that is, you have determined whether you will use a holistic or embedded, single-case or multiple-case approach. Deciding on basic structure and size is one of the first thinking processes involved in implementing a case study design. The second thinking process involves determining the sequence of the design.

Many types of case study design sequences can be used, depending on the purpose of the study. Each design sequence has specific strengths and weaknesses. Some design sequences are more consonant with the naturalistic research tradition, in which the sequence is flexible and may change in the process of collecting and analyzing information. Alternatively, the design sequence may be linear and fixed, similar to experimental-type designs.

Experimental-Type Approach

Let us examine some of the more frequently used case study designs that follow an experimental-type structure. There are many different strategies in this genre of single-subject research. Each strategy is based on the premise that the individual serves as his or her own control. Bloom et al.[4] refer to the elements in single-subject design as "phases." They note that phases consist of distinct parts of intervention research, beginning with the baseline phase, in which no intervention occurs, proceeding to the intervention phase, and then ending with the follow-up phase. Many variations of these phases, including multiple intervention and follow-up phases, can be found in the case study research literature.

AB Design

Single-subject case study designs that follow experimental-type traditions have their own notation system similar to experimental-type design. However, different symbols are used. Rather than denoting the phases with X and $O,$ case study uses A and $B;$ A depicts the observation, and B indicates the intervention or independent variable. The most basic design is called the "AB design," where A represents the baseline phase and B represents the intervention phase. Although this type of design cannot predict, it can explain what happens during an intervention.

During the baseline period (A), repeated measures are obtained on specified variables. The investigator should obtain as many measurements as possible, typically from six to nine observation points, to establish a stable baseline. However, the number of measurements may vary depending on whether the

observed behavior is stable. If, for example, observed scores are highly variable, many repeated measures may be necessary to detect a baseline pattern of behavior. It is important to establish a baseline pattern before introducing the intervention phase.

After a baseline pattern has been established, the intervention is introduced, followed by repeated measurement. The A phase represents the measures that form the control measures. The B phase represents the measures that are obtained after intervention. The B phase measures are compared with those of the A phase. It is recommended that a similar number of observations be obtained in both the A phase and the B phase to examine the stability of change over time.

Let us now look at how investigators organize their data for analysis in AB designs. After conducting the AB assessments, the investigator plots each score and performs a visual analysis to detect a change in the pattern of scoring between the A and B phases. Typically, a *celeration line* is drawn through the baseline data to facilitate visual inspection of observed scores. This line represents the "best fit" of the baseline data points. The same line is then drawn along the data points in phase B to determine whether there is a difference in the direction and placement of scores (Figure 23-2).

Variations. There are many variations on the AB design, such as the ABA and $ABAB$ designs. In the "ABA design" a baseline period (A) is followed by an intervention period (B), which is then followed by the withdrawal of the intervention (A). In the "$ABAB$ design" the previous sequence is followed, and then the intervention is reapplied.

Many more options can be introduced into designs that use phases A and B. For example, there may be multiple B phases in which each B phase may involve different therapeutic strategies. The structure of the ABA design is stronger than a simple AB sequence when there are questions regarding the extent to which change is produced as an outcome of an intervention.

Time Series Design

The *time series design*, another type of single-subject design, is used to follow one subject over time (see Chapter 9). Consider the following example:

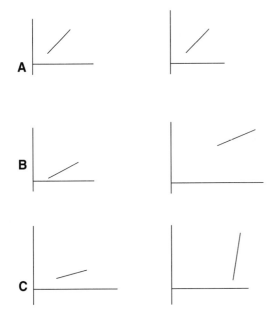

Figure 23-2   Celeration lines. **A,** No change: pattern returns to baseline and assumes the same trajectory. **B,** No change: pattern of change assumes the same trajectory. **C,** Change: pattern changes between first set of measurements and second set of measurements; trajectory is visibly different.

You want to determine if an innovative intervention with a chronically depressed population decreases levels of depression. Because you are unable to test a group of subjects, you select a single-subject design. For the first three sessions, you administer a depression inventory. You then conduct the intervention and follow up with three administrations of the same instrument. If, based on visual inspection, you observe a difference between the observed scores immediately preceding and immediately after the intervention, you can surmise that a change occurred and that this change may be a consequence of the intervention. With this type of design, you cannot claim that the intervention is the cause of the improvement. However, you have demonstrated that a change occurred. You have credible evidence to support the need for further investigation to determine the effectiveness of the intervention.

Data Collection and Analysis

Now that we have discussed the basics of structure, size, and sequence, let us further explore the nature of data collection in single-case designs. As suggested by Yin,[2] even when your study is consistent with the experimental-type tradition, multiple data collection strategies strengthen the credibility of findings in case study research. Ideally, the use of several measures at both baseline and follow-up phases should be used.

You are interested in ascertaining the extent to which a group approach improved the socialization skills of nursing home residents. You select an embedded single-case study. The unit of analysis is the group in whom the subparts are the participants. To test socialization before the initiation of the group, you establish a counting system to measure the amount or extent to which interaction occurs among the participants of the group. You complete this measure on six occasions to obtain a baseline. Additionally, you administer a self-report of socialization to ascertain the extent to which your observations and the perceptions of the subjects are similar. You continue data collection using the two strategies throughout the intervention and after its termination. Your results therefore provide two measures of socialization to inform you about the change in the frequency of socialization.

Data analysis of experimental-type case study designs is controversial. Although many consider it inappropriate to use statistical techniques to analyze single-subject data, other researchers disagree. Those who suggest that group analyses are not appropriate call our attention to sampling logic. For most statistical analyses, an underlying assumption is that a sample is selected to represent a population and that every effort is made to minimize bias that can be introduced through inadequate sampling. Because group sampling logic (discussed in Chapters 12 and 19) does not guide the selection of a case, statisticians suggest that the use of group analysis techniques is contraindicated. On the other end of the spectrum, investigators may subject multiple-case studies to group analyses. These investigators argue that group analysis of multiple cases is analogous to meta-analysis, where investigators aggregate the findings of replicated studies and conduct secondary analysis of the data, even though the studies are not originally planned as part of the larger investigation.

Our position is that each of these perspectives is neither right nor wrong. The choice to use group analytical techniques for case study designs needs to be explicated, and a clear rationale for doing so should lie in the purpose and nature of the research question and the investigator's view of knowledge. We suggest, however, that analytical strategies such as descriptive statistics, visual presentation of changes in quantitative measures, and inductive analyses of narrative information are the most useful analytical tools in case study designs. We urge investigators to consider these techniques before others in which the fit between design and analytical strategy may be tenuous.

A major concern in case study research is "generalizability." There is a limitation to the external validity of a case study. However, its limited external validity is in part overcome by the ability to generalize findings to theory through replication, or the repetition of systematic single-subject studies, and the evaluation of each of these efforts as a whole.

Naturalistic Approach

Now let us look at case studies that are consistent with the naturalistic tradition. This approach to case study would be used when you are seeking (1) to generate theory in the absence of research literature, (2) to develop alternative theory, (3) to identify and develop lexical and operational definitions of important constructs for further measurement, or (4) to examine the complexity of your case in its natural context. As you would expect, these studies are flexible in structure, size, and sequence. It is possible to move between holistic and embedded designs or from single to multiple cases, depending on the emergence of insights as the study proceeds. What characterizes naturalistic case study and distinguishes it from other naturalistic designs is its logic structure, that is, the identification of a "case" as the phenomenon of interest. Let us return to our example of socialization in a nursing home facility to illustrate.

Suppose you not only wanted to know the frequency of socialization that your intervention produced, but were interested in the nature of the socialization as well. In a naturalistic case study, you might observe participants at various times throughout the day, recording field notes to examine the interactions. Proceeding inductively in your analysis, you would search for patterns and meanings.

Mixed-Method Approach

Consistent with Yin,[2] we suggest that mixing experimental-type and naturalistic traditions in a single study is the best approach to designing and conducting case study research. The use of multiple measures of socialization combined with the findings from your field notes will tell you much more than either strategy could yield if used alone.

SUMMARY

Case study represents an approach to systematic inquiry that can incorporate experimental-type, naturalistic, or mixed-method thinking and action processes. The case study approach is particularly helpful when little is known about a phenomenon and when aggregating or grouping responses across subjects does not allow sufficient insight into the phenomenon of interest. A variety of design structures and sequences are available to the researcher. Also, multiple data collection methods can be used and are desirable across the range of case study approaches.

The ability to use different design structures, methodologies, and data collection approaches makes the case study a flexible research option. A case study approach is useful under a variety of circumstances, especially to explicate in-depth understandings of a phenomenon, to examine change over time in one or more individuals, or to develop and examine a theoretical construct.

EXERCISES

1. Find a research study that uses a case study approach. Identify its underlying structure using Yin's classification scheme. Redesign the study using a different structural approach. Compare and contrast the strengths and weaknesses of each structure.

2. Choose a setting in which a direct health or human service might be delivered to a client. The setting can be an outpatient department, a senior center, a community organization, or another context. Design a case study that examines the delivery of a service in that setting.

REFERENCES

1. Stake RE: *The art of case study research,* Thousand Oaks, Calif, 1995, Sage.
2. Yin RK: *Case study research: design and methods,* ed 3, Newbury Park, Calif, 2002, Sage.
3. Denzin NK, Lincoln YS: *Handbook of qualitative research,* ed 2, Thousand Oaks, Calif, 2000, Sage.
4. Bloom M, Fisher J, Orme J: *Evaluating practice: guidelines for the accountable professional,* ed 4, Englewood, Calif, 2002, Prentice Hall.

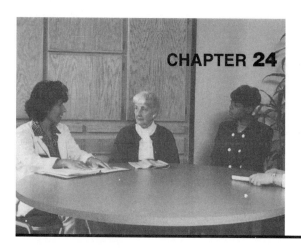

CHAPTER 24

Practice Efficacy

KEY TERMS

Blinding
Clinical trial
Double-blind trial
Evaluation practice
Evidence-based practice
Phase I clinical trial
Phase II clinical trial
Phase III clinical trial
Randomized controlled trial
Reflexive intervention
Single-blind trial
Translational phase
Treatment fidelity

CHAPTER OUTLINE

You now have some level of comfort with the thinking and action processes involved in the experimental-type and naturalistic research traditions. These processes serve as your working tools to apply to a health or human service practice arena. In this chapter we turn to the action of "application," or applying research principles to the practice arena, and discuss three approaches that attempt to bridge the research-practice gap: evidence-based practice, clinical trial methodology, and evaluation practice.

EVIDENCE-BASED PRACTICE

If you are a practicing health or human service professional, you most likely have heard of *evidence-based practice*. Most professional organizations highly espouse this practice as a critical way of basing treatment and clinical practices in research evidence. If you are not involved in a practice arena, you may be asking, "What's all the fuss about?" After all, you probably assume that all health and human service practices are based in or derived from evidence or knowledge that has been systematically obtained, rather than from hearsay, trial and error, or casual decision making. However, this has not exactly been the case. At issue are the definition of evidence and what constitutes "adequate evidence" for informing practice decisions.

Evidence-based practice is not a research method or design. Rather, it is a model of professional practice that draws heavily on research and uses particular methodologies to draw conclusions from research literature. Major aspects of evidence-based practice include how to organize a clinical setting to engage in this form of practice, how to teach this approach, and the barriers to its implementation. However, our focus here is how evidence is defined in this approach and how evidence-based practice uses research principles to draw evidentiary-based conclusions to inform practice. We begin our discussion with a brief history, then define and provide critical comments on this contemporary practice approach.

Definitions and Models

Since early in the twentieth century, policy makers, scholars, and practitioners have been debating the nature and role of research in professional practice.[1] Numerous terms have been used in these discussions to describe professional activity that in some way uses or generates knowledge based on the principles of scientific inquiry. In part the disagreements about what constitutes science (and by extension, scientific inquiry) and how or even if science should form the foundation of professional practice have contributed to the conflict about scientifically driven practice.[2] Remember that we define science as follows:

1. It is theory based or theory generating.
2. It is developed according to the rigor criteria of systematic use of inductive, abductive, and deductive logic structures in all phases of thinking and action processes.
3. It involves detailing the explicit evidence and reasoning on which knowledge claims are based.

Keep these definitional elements in mind as you learn more about evidence-based practice, since they form both its strengths and its limitations. Many different terms are used to discuss models of scientific inquiry in professional practice. In general, all models posit the value of scientifically derived knowledge to support professional decision making and to examine the extent to which desired outcomes have been achieved.

Public health and education were the first professional fields to emphasize the importance of systematic evaluation for practice accountability.[3,4] In the early 1950s, proliferation of federally supported programs resulted in the expansion of evaluation

into a field unto its own, with its focus on fiscal accountability.[5] Concurrently, debates emerged between those who espoused "empiricism" and those who opposed it in a "value-based" practice context.[6] As evaluation was espoused by health and human service fields, debate increased about whether to conduct empirical inquiry to support practice. Discussion shifted away from polar arguments to a more expansive and complex analysis of the nature of evidence, when evidence is appropriate, and methods to generate it.[7]

The following definitions of evidence-based practice are from medicine,[8,9] nursing,[10] and occupational therapy[11]:

> The conscientious, explicit and judicious use of current best evidence in making decisions about the care of individual patients. The practice of evidence based medicine means integrating individual clinical expertise with the best available external clinical evidence from systematic research.[8]
>
> The conscientious and judicious use of current best evidence from clinical care research in the management of individual patients.[9]
>
> [The] process by which nurses make clinical decisions using the best available research evidence, their clinical expertise and patient preferences, in the context of available resources.[10]
>
> [A]n ethical, conscientious, discriminative process of applying the best research-based evidence to decisions regarding client care.[11]

As you can see, each definition emphasizes the use of research evidence in the context of clinical expertise, although they all differ slightly. According to Mullen,[12] two primary models are reflected in these definitions. In one model, intervention is selected from an array of efficacious, empirically supported practices. In the second model, practitioner and client consider best evidence to make decisions together.

Existing models of evidence-based practice are based on a particular understanding of evidence as ranging along a continuum from anecdotal experience of providers and consumers, organizational guidelines, consensus groups, single-study review, and then to highly structured systematic review of the literature (meta-analysis). Most important, the traditional approach is grounded in the assumption of a "hierarchy of evidence" in which judgment about the value of knowledge is based on the methods of inquiry. The *randomized controlled trial* (RCT) is considered the highest level of evidence to support intervention efficacy, and other forms of knowledge are typically devalued. Thus the true-experimental design to support claims about the efficacy of interventions remains as the methodological pinnacle of desirability, whereas other design approaches (e.g., quasi-experimental, naturalistic inquiry) tend to receive less acclaim, or they are not systematically considered in the evaluation of evidence.[8]

In general, all evidence-based practice models can be defined by their use of "best evidence" to guide practice decisions, thereby creating standard, valid interventions to the extent possible for specific conditions, diagnoses, and problem areas that are well researched.

Approaches to Identifying Evidence

As stated earlier, evidence-based practice is not a methodology, but it does utilize methodologies for systematically reviewing evidence and linking the evidence to actual practice decisions. There are four methodological steps in applying evidence to clinical practice in this framework: reviewing the literature, rating the evidence, developing clinical guidelines, and applying or translating guidelines to a clinical case.

The key research action process in this form of practice is systematically reviewing published scientific literature, including clinical practice guidelines, meta-analysis (both qualitative and experimental type), and web-based searches for relevant research-generated information. That is, key to the success of basing a clinical decision on the evidence is how investigators review the literature (see Chapter 5), including how they bound the topic or query through the selection of key terms and how they tailor the search. As in a search for any research inquiry, it is critical to know the limitations of the databases that are searched and how the bounding rules constructed will shape the evidence obtained. Given the complexity and time-consuming nature of conducting a comprehensive and adequate literature review, new search engines have been created, such as PubMed, which gives free access to MEDLINE databases (www.ncbi.nlm.nih.gov/PubMed), or SumSearch (http://sumsearch.uthscsa.edu),

which searches databases that contain sources for evidence-based guidelines.

Once relevant research articles have been identified and retrieved, the next methodological step is applying a systematic rating to each type of research study and form of evidence retrieved (Box 24-1). Then, based on the ratings that are derived, a series of clinical guidelines can be articulated (Box 24-2). The final step involves translating the evidence and guidelines to a particular clinical group or case. In this step the researcher must ask numerous critical questions (Box 24-3). It is particularly important to determine whether differences exist between study populations and the particular clinical population

---

BOX 24-1
EXAMPLES OF RATING SYSTEMS IN EVIDENCE-BASED PRACTICE

"ABCD" SYSTEM

A = Evidence from well-defined meta-analysis.

B = Evidence from well-designed controlled trials (randomized and nonrandomized) with results that consistently support a specific action.

C = Evidence from observational studies (correlational, descriptive) or controlled trials with inconsistent results.

D = Evidence from expert opinion or multiple case reports.

"1-2-3" SYSTEM

1 = Generally consistent findings in a majority of studies.

2 = Based on either a single acceptable study or a weak or inconsistent finding in multiple acceptable studies.

3 = Limited scientific evidence that does not meet all criteria of acceptable studies.

"I-II-III-IV" SYSTEM

I = Evidence from at least one properly randomized controlled trial.

II-A = Evidence from well-designed controlled trials without randomization.

II-B = Evidence from well-designed cohort or case-control analytical studies.

III = Evidence obtained from comparisons between times or places with or without the intervention.

IV = Opinions of respected authorities based on clinical experience, descriptive studies, or reports of expert committees.

BOX 24-2

SAMPLE OF CLINICAL GUIDELINES BASED ON RATING THE EVIDENCE

■ Best to individualize music selection in accordance with patient preferences (evidence grade = B).
■ Best to intervene 30 minutes before a person's peak level of agitation (evidence grade = B).
■ Music intervention session should last about 30 minutes (evidence grade = B).
■ Use of headphones may be confusing (evidence grade = D).

Modified from National Guideline Clearinghouse (www.guideline.gov), 2002.

BOX 24-3

APPLYING EVIDENCE TO PRACTICE

■ What were the results?
■ How large are treatment effects
■ Are results valid?
■ Will results help me in caring for my cases/clients/community?
■ Can results be applied?
■ Were all outcomes of clinical significance considered?
■ Are treatment benefits worth the potential harms and costs?
■ Are there specific characteristics of the group/persons with whom I am working that differ from the study populations so as to affect treatment outcome?

---

or case and whether these may diminish the treatment response or change the risk/benefit ratio. This translational step draws on clinical knowledge and judgment.

Limitations of Evidence-Based Practice

From our discussion thus far and what you have learned in this book, what do you see as some of the important limitations of an evidence-based practice approach?

First, as an empirically based approach borrowed principally from medicine, its application to health and social service practices can be problematic for several reasons. Health and human service professionals engage in practice to address a wide range of human problems for which knowledge through systematic inquiry is necessary. However, the knowledge required to understand human problems is not necessarily amenable to RCTs. Also, other forms of knowledge may be of equal importance in understanding, for example, dynamic processes between therapist and client and how best to involve a clinical population in a disease prevention activity. Health and human service practice extends far beyond the focus on medical intervention or single treatments and the "magic bullet" medicine approach amenable to randomized design strategies.

A second significant limitation of this model of practice is that it is based on the assumption that the RCT is the only valid design to generate knowledge that is useful in clinical practice. Only one type of research (the RCT and empirical evidence) is upheld as valuable in evidence-based practice and thus is viewed as the cornerstone of practice.[13,14] This approach diminishes other forms of knowledge, such as that derived from the naturalistic tradition or other experimental-type design strategies that can contribute different types of knowledge.

A related point is that evidence-based practice involves the application of nomothetically derived knowledge to idiographic concerns.[5,15] In this case the issue for the evidence-based practitioner becomes how best to translate group data to the individual case. Given the growing emphasis on diversity and multicultural competence, knowledge of central tendencies (nomothetically generated research) does not necessarily capture a full range of diverse and unique experiences and needs and may not be appropriate to inform individual circumstance. The assertion that "design rigor and structure determine knowledge quality" is a myth that limits the critical assessment of knowledge for use in professional practice.

The nature of evidence continues as an important area of debate. Because practice theories in so many health and human service professions[16-18] stress use of self and the relationship between client and practitioner, students and practitioners often identify the incompatibility of logical, systematic thinking with the relational foundations of practice. Recent acceptance of faith and spirituality in professional theory and practice are even more incongruent with positivist approaches to understanding human experience and human need as currently used in evidence-based practice.[19] Thus, although we believe that different forms of evidence are credible for different professional and other stakeholder interest groups,[5] evidence-based practice approaches discount this view and are often antithetical to the professional commitment to respect for diversity as it applies to acceptable evidence for practice process and outcome.

We see major limitations of current models of evidence-based practice for supporting professional practice, but we do not want to "throw out the baby with the bathwater." As we have throughout this book, we encourage you to be critical thinkers and fully evaluate for which clinical challenges this approach is important and whether and how evidence-based practice may be useful in your daily practice.

CLINICAL TRIAL METHODOLOGY

As discussed in Chapter 9, most quantitative investigators and scientific journals consider the true-experimental design, also referred to as the *clinical trial* (or RCT), as the design of choice to answer specific questions related to the efficacy of behavioral or biomedical interventions, including drugs, treatments, service programs, and devices. Also, as just discussed, the RCT is upheld as the most important design structure from which evidence can be deduced. Thus, we now focus on the application of the true-experimental design to clinical practice.

Although seemingly straightforward, the traditional two-group randomized controlled design is actually rather complex, and many action processes have been developed to structure this study design and ensure rigor. Because of its importance in health and human service research and its prominence in scientific journals, let us examine some key critical issues in implementing a clinical trial in an applied setting, such as the clinic, community center, or home. Because it is not possible to cover every aspect of the RCT in this text, we highlight here the key language that sets clear rules and expectations for the adequacy of the RCT design and research procedures.

Phases of Clinical Trials

Clinical trials are designed to address three different levels of development for interventions. A *Phase I*

clinical trial is the first type of randomized design that is usually conducted. The purpose of the Phase I study is to test a new behavioral or biomedical intervention not previously evaluated in a small group of people (20 to 80) to determine its acceptability, feasibility of implementation, and safety (e.g., side effects, safe dosage range for drugs). The next step, a *Phase II clinical trial,* is conducted to study the efficacy of an intervention in a larger group of people (several hundred) to determine efficacy and further evaluate safety. The final step, a *Phase III clinical trial,* may have a threefold purpose: (1) evaluate effectiveness further in a much larger group of persons (several hundred to thousands), (2) compare the intervention to other standard or experimental interventions to determine its added value or significance, and (3) evaluate how the intervention can be implemented safely in a larger community.

Each clinical trial phase may use randomization procedures and strict adherence to various protocols, but their goals differ. For Phase I the goal is "proof of concept," for Phase II it is "efficacy," and for Phase III it is "effectiveness and safety" related to real-world implementation. These phases tend to fit best with classic pharmacological drug trial research, for which many of the procedures discussed in relation to clinical trial methodology have been developed. Nevertheless, these terms continue to be applied to behavioral and other clinical-type interventions and are noted here because they are used frequently by the experimentalist.

An additional phase is specific to behavioral interventions that are most relevant to health and human service and involves the "translation" of a proven or evidence-based intervention into a service or clinical setting. Most intervention protocols that are tested using clinical trial methodology require additional modification or translation to fit into and be effective in an applied setting or with a different target population than those involved in the initial testing. The *translational phase* may or may not involve a randomized two-group design, but it does require an evaluative approach to determine the acceptability and benefit. In this translational phase, it is important to ensure that the core components of a proven intervention remain intact. However, small changes that may have a large impact in the new setting or with a different target population may be necessary to ensure cultural appropriateness and acceptability.

For example, suppose you want to implement a proven group-exercise conditioning program. However, the population you want to target does not typically engage in formal exercise programs. Thus, you may need to modify specific aspects of the program to enhance its acceptability and preserve its effectiveness. A small change that would not affect the fidelity of the tested program might involve naming and framing the program differently or offering a wider range of exercise options. However, changing the frequency of the exercise regimen or offering it as a private versus group activity would alter the integrity of the intervention and possibly its effectiveness. Let us examine how you might enact each phase of your clinical trial.

You have an idea for a new therapeutic regimen to enhance community reintegration for persons with traumatic head injury. You first conduct a Phase I study with a small group of patients, about 30 people, who fit highly specified inclusion and exclusion criteria. In this first phase your goal is to evaluate whether your intervention approach is acceptable to patients, the extent to which participants comply with the innovative regimen, and the initial impact on treatment outcome (magnitude of change). Your main outcome is "life satisfaction," as measured by self-report, and the "ability to live alone safely," as measured by professional observation of daily self-care. You decide to use a two-group design and randomize 15 persons to receive the intervention program and 15 persons to a "usual care" control group. The control group receives a traditional rehabilitation program or usual care, and those in the intervention receive your treatment program.

Assume this first phase is successful. You have evidence of treatment effect; 10 of the 15 persons randomized to treatment are able to perform self-care independently and safely, compared with 5 of 15 persons in the control group. Also, persons who received the treatment seemed to enjoy the therapeutic regimen and attended all skill classes and one-on-one sessions such that compliance was close to 95%. Based on this evidence, you design a Phase II trial involving many more persons, perhaps over 150, recruited from two rehabilitation facilities. In Phase II, you seek to achieve statistically significant treatment effects and continue to monitor acceptability and participation, as well as safety (e.g., unsafe

incidents from attending classes, living alone). Again, you find that your results from this phase are very promising, with small to medium treatment effects, high compliance, and no adverse or unsafe events related to treatment.

Your next step is to develop a Phase III study, which might involve participation by numerous rehabilitation centers across the country and an attempt to implement the intervention in multiple sites. With the success of the intervention at each stage, there is great interest in using your intervention in rehabilitation.

However, another translational step is necessary to integrate your treatment in the current structure of rehabilitation. The intervention, as tested, is too labor intensive, and third-party intermediaries may not reimburse every component. Thus you develop a translational phase in which you modify aspects of the intervention while preserving its essential elements, to integrate it successfully into clinical practice and obtain reimbursement for at least some of its therapeutic components.

Blinding (Masking)

Another key language structure of clinical trials is blinding or masking techniques. Remember that the procedures put into place in RCTs are designed to reduce bias. This is important for the RCT structure because its main intent is to determine the impact or effect of a specific treatment regimen or intervention on a set of outcomes. Thus, critical to this design is the minimization of any competing reasons (e.g., Type I and II errors) that could explain a particular outcome.

Potential sources of bias are the tester, investigator, or interventionist.

You are an interviewer in a large study that is testing the efficacy of social support groups for persons undergoing cancer treatments. You are responsible for conducting both the pretest and the posttest interviews to evaluate whether group support impacts a person's well-being. However, you are aware of a person's assignment to intervention or control as you interview. You may be favorably predisposed to observing positive changes in the intervention group. Or, because of your enthusiasm and investment in the intervention, you may inadvertently set a tone or ask questions that introduce a source of bias.

Thus, to minimize partiality or the possibility of introducing any form of bias, most clinical trials implement some type of *blinding* procedures. One simple approach to blinding, or masking, is to minimize who among the research team in contact with study participants is informed of group assignment. It is usually possible to mask interviewers to group assignments.

Blinding works best in medical trials. A *single-blind trial* means that the persons enrolled in the study do not know what group or treatment they have been assigned to, but the investigative team does know. In a *double-blind trial,* neither study participants nor investigators (nor anyone else on the research team) are aware of group assignments. As you can see, this level of blinding is difficult to achieve in behavioral-oriented treatments that are being evaluated in an RCT.

Randomization Scheme

The language of randomization is also essential to the clinical trial design structure. The way in which study participants are randomized to the experimental and control group conditions can take different forms and is scrutinized by institutional review boards, data and safety monitoring boards, and scientific journals (see Chapter 12).

There are many different ways to randomize to ensure that subjects are assigned to experimental and control groups by chance. In complex designs or large clinical trials, a statistician is usually responsible for establishing a randomization scheme. Once a randomization format has been developed, assignments are typed up on single sheets of paper, and each is sealed in opaque double envelopes so that the investigators or research team members cannot see the paper until it is opened and cannot influence the group assignment.

A related consideration is whether simple randomization alone is sufficient to ensure comparability between the experimental and control groups.

Suppose you are testing a mental health intervention involving counseling and activity engagement for persons with functional limitations. The dependent or outcome variable is a measure of depressive symptoms. You know that gender is highly related to depressive symptoms, with women reporting higher scores than men. Given the strong association between gender and your treatment outcome, you might want to consider a method of randomization to ensure that an equal number of men and women will be assigned to both the experimental and the control condition.

One approach would be to "stratify" randomization by gender (male, female) to ensure that the two groups will be balanced with respect to this factor. This involves setting up a separate or independent randomization scheme for both males and females. Within each stratum (male and female), randomization would occur by the method of "random permuted blocks" to control for possible changes over time in the subject mix. A blocking number is usually developed by a statistician and is not disclosed to the investigators or members of the project team. The statistician generates randomization lists for each of the two strata and then prepares two sets of randomization envelopes (double-enveloped), one set for males and the other for females. Each subject is randomized by opening the next envelope with the appropriate stratum.

Treatment Fidelity

Clinical trial methodology involves the systematic evaluation of an intervention. A critical aspect of such trials is the assurance that the intervention is delivered to study participants assigned to the experimental group as it is intended and as specified by a written protocol. Attention to the integrity of implementing the intervention is referred to as *treatment fidelity.*[20,21] Actions that an investigator can take to enhance treatment fidelity include (1) creating a detailed manual of the intervention so that it can be delivered consistently, is reproducible, and is independent of interventionist style; (2) providing careful training in the intervention; (3) providing constant oversight of its delivery through direct observation of treatment sessions or review of audio or video recordings of its delivery; and (4) tracking adherence and reasons for nonparticipation.

One way of understanding treatment fidelity is by a model used in psychotherapeutic intervention studies.[20,21] This model posits three components (domains) of treatment fidelity that need to be

TABLE 24-1		
Three Domains of Treatment Fidelity		
Domain	Enhancement Strategy	Monitoring and Data Collection Strategy
Delivery	Systematic training of interventionists Manual of procedures	Frequency of contact and intensity

Receipt	Use of different implementation strategies
	    (e.g., video, hands-on instruction, role playing)
		Participant's acknowledgment of participation and receipt
		    of intervention materials
		Evidence of receipt (e.g., knowledge test, improved
		    understanding)

Enactment	Identification of how and when to implement strategies Recording forms	Evidence of integration, use of knowledge, skills or intervention strategies Participant's feedback as to use Enhanced proximal outcomes

enhanced and monitored: delivery, receipt, and enactment (Table 24-1). Basically, for an intervention to be effective, it must be delivered consistently, it must be received and be acceptable to participants, and finally, intervention strategies must be enacted or used. Although the definition of each component is still evolving, this model provides a helpful tool for thinking about the procedures that need to be considered and put into place to ensure the integrity of an intervention.

EVALUATION PRACTICE

New models to bridge the research-practice gap are emerging that apply systematic strategies to evaluating practice and integrating research into practice. One approach, the RE-AIM model (see www.RE-AIM.org), facilitates the systematic translation of proven behavioral and health promotion interventions into practice settings.[22,23]

Another new model, "evaluation practice," infuses everyday practice with an evaluative and systematic knowledge-generating framework. In their model of *evaluation practice,* DePoy and Gilson[5] define "evaluation" as the conduct of three major thinking and action processes: problem and need clarification, reflexive intervention, and outcome assessment. All rely on the systematic thinking and action processes presented throughout this book. These processes are now being applied to the context of practice.

Problem and Need Clarification

Because of the complexity of defining and understanding health and social problems, methods to address and alleviate them are often unclear. As we frequently see in professional practice, why a particular approach to intervention is needed and to what problem it responds are often omitted from the thinking and action processes of many health and human service efforts. Without a clear understanding of what problem is being addressed, and without evidence supporting the method needed to address it, we cannot demonstrate the value of our practices.

Clarification of the problem is critical to any professional effort because how a problem is conceptualized, who owns it, who is affected by it, and what needs to be done about it are all questions based in political-purposive and ideological arenas. Thus the problem forms the basis from which all subsequent systematic evaluative activity takes place, and it provides the ultimate foundation for the implementation and continuation of interventions. In all arenas of practice, a clear and well-supported understanding of "problem" and "need" is essential. Without problem and need clarification, interest groups may define problems differently and thus expect different outcomes from the same intervention.

In the model of evaluation practice, a clear understanding of need must be based on credible evidence. Although we may make claims on what type of intervention is needed to resolve problems, accountability in making informed professional decisions depends on the presence and organization of empirical evidence of need. Setting goals and objectives for intervention derives directly from need.

Reflexive Intervention

As discussed in previous chapters, reflexivity is an important construct, defined as self-examination for the purpose of ascertaining how the researcher's perspective influences the interpretation of data. In the model of evaluation practice, the term is expanded to denote the set of thinking and action processes that we believe should take place throughout interventions. The term *reflexive intervention* reminds us that the intervention action processes, resources, and influences are essential parts of evaluation practice and are thus subject to the same systematic scrutiny as needs assessment. Thus the objective of reflexive thinking processes in evaluation practice is not limited to an individual; rather, it is applied to the sum total of the intervention and scope of influences on the process and outcome of intervention.

Reflexive intervention involves three important foci: monitoring process, resource analysis, and consideration of indirect influences on the intervention.

Monitoring (Process Assessment)

Monitoring, or process assessment, is the element of evaluation that examines if and how the intervention is proceeding. Monitoring is an essential evaluation practice action in which the actual implementation of an intervention is systematically studied and characterized. Monitoring processes not only examine the scope of the intervention, but also scrutinize the intervention processes to determine who they affect, assess the degree to which goals and process objectives are efficaciously reflected in the intervention, and provide feedback for revision based on empirical evidence. The primary purpose of monitoring is to ascertain if an intervention was delivered as planned

> To systematically monitor funding, transportation, and elder involvement in activity, you set up a tracking system. You can determine what was done, who participated, and the frequency of participation. Without this information, you would not know what was done and could not attribute any chances in outcome to your program.

so that attribution of outcome can be positioned properly (similar to the concept of treatment fidelity in clinical trials).

Resource Analysis

Similar to monitoring, resource analysis occurs throughout the intervention and requires reflection. When we think of resource analysis, cost in dollars for services rendered is the resource most often examined. In evaluation practice, however, resource analysis includes the full host of human and nonhuman resources used to conduct an intervention and related to its need and outcome.

Consideration of Influences on the Intervention

Part of the process of reflexive intervention must be a consideration of factors external to the intervention that affect both process and outcome. Without widening the scope of examination, it is difficult to determine why change is occurring (or why it is not occurring) in the desired direction. What if you neglected to look at community influences and a local church had implemented a community program for elders serving your same population? You can see how this unplanned influence might change your expectations and attribution of outcomes.

Outcome Assessment

Outcome assessment is the action process of evaluation practice that is most familiar. It answers the question, "To what extent did the desired outcomes occur?" Outcome assessment also examines the parts of an intervention and the intervention context that relate to outcome, as well as differential outcomes resulting from other influences (e.g., intervention processes, target populations, complexity of outcome expectations). Although its aim seems obvious—to judge the value of an intervention in its achievement of goals and objectives—outcome assessment serves many other important purposes. Outcome assessment provides empirical information on which to make programmatic, policy, and resource decisions that influence and shape social and human services at multiple levels.[24]

Evaluation practice provides a systematic framework by which to develop a knowledge base of professional practice. Documenting your systematic thinking and action processes throughout every practice sequence provides credible evidence from which to support practice claims and improve practice. Thus, evaluation practice provides a systematic and "doable" link between practice and research.

SUMMARY

The current model of interjecting evidence into practice is the evidence-based model generated primarily from medicine. This has led to difficulties in application, primarily because of its underlying assumptions of a hierarchy of knowledge, dismissal of all forms of research-generated knowledge except that derived from true-experimental designs, and attempt to enforce nomethetically generated knowledge on ideographic contexts. The randomized clinical trial is the design of choice when evaluating an innovative treatment approach or a new device, technology, or service program. The language structure of a clinical trial is important to know given its primacy in evidence-based practice and scientific journals. Nevertheless, evidence-based models and randomized trials cannot address every important aspect of health and human service questions and queries. The new model of evaluation practice illustrates the application of the thinking and action processes learned throughout this book to the practice arena.

EXERCISES

1. Find an evidence-based literature review on a topic of interest to you and examine its use in informing your practice. Would you seek additional information to make sound practice decisions? Why or why not? What information might you acquire beyond the research evidence presented in the literature review?
2. Identify a practice issue or problem and develop a randomized control trial. Then develop an evaluation practice design that includes all elements of this new model.

REFERENCES

1. Sonnert G: *Ivory bridges: connecting science and society,* Cambridge, Mass, 2002, MIT Press.
2. Gieryn TF: *Cultural boundaries of science: credibility on the line,* Chicago, 1999, Chicago University Press.
3. Brownson RC et al: *Evidence-based public health,* Oxford, 2003, Oxford University Press.
4. Thyer B: *The handbook of social work research methods,* Thousand Oaks, Calif, 2001, Sage.
5. DePoy E, Gilson SF: *Evaluation practice,* Belmont, Calif, 2003, Brooks-Cole.
6. Gordon WE: Toward a social work frame of reference, *J Soc Work Educ* 1:19-26, 1965.
7. Grinell R: *Social work research and evaluation: quantitative and qualitative approaches,* Itasca, Ill, 2000, Peacock.
8. Sackett DL et al: *Evidence-based medicine: how to practice and teach EBM,* ed 2, New York, 2000, Churchill Livingstone.
9. Guyatt GH, Sackett DL, Cook DJ: Users' guides to the medical literature, II: How to use an article about therapy or prevention, A. Are the results of the study valid?, Evidence-Based Medicine Working Group. *JAMA* 270:2598-2601, 1993.
10. DiCenso A, Cullum N, Ciliska D: Implementing evidence-based nursing: some misconceptions, *Evidence-Based Nursing,* 1:38-40, 1998.
11. Lloyd-Smith W: Evidence-based practice and occupational therapy, *BJOT* 60: 474-478, 1997.
12. Mullen E: *Evidence-based knowledge: designs for enhancing practitioner use of research findings (a bottom up approach).* Presented at 4th International Conference on Evaluation for Practice, University of Tampere, Tampere, Finland, 2002.
13. Guyatt GH, Sackett DL, Cook DJ: Users' guides to the medical literature, II. How to use an article about therapy or prevention. B. What were the results and will they help me in caring for my patients? Evidence-Based Medicine Working Group. *JAMA* 271:59-63, 1993.
14. Gibbs L, Gambrill E: *Critical thinking for social workers: exercises for the helping professions,* Thousand Oaks, Calif, 1999, Pine Forge.
15. Rosen A: *Evidence-based social work practice: challenges and promises.* Presented at Society for Social Work and Research, San Diego, 2002.
16. Kirst-Ashman KK, Hull GH: *Understanding generalist practice,* ed 2, Chicago, 1999, Nelson Hall.
17. Toseland RW, Rivas RF: *An introduction to group work practice,* ed 4, Boston, 2002, Allyn & Bacon.
18. Woods ME, Hollis F: *Casework: a psychosocial therapy,* Columbus, 1999, McGraw-Hill.
19. Ellor J, Netting FE, Thibault JM: *Religious and spiritual aspects of human service practice (social problems and social issues),* Columbia, 1999, University of South Carolina Press.
20. Lichstein KL, Riedel BW, Grieve R: Fair tests of clinical trials: a treatment implementation model, *Adv Behav Res Ther* 16:1-29, 1994.
21. Burgio L et al: Judging outcomes in psychosocial interventions for dementia caregivers: the problem of treatment implementation, *Gerontologist* 41:481-489, 2001.
22. Glasgow, RE, et al: The future of health behavior change research: What is needed to improve translation of research into health promotion? *Ann Behav Med* 27:3-12, 2004.
23. Dzewaltowski, DA et al: Behavior change research in community settings: How generalizable are the results? *Health Promo Int,* 19(2) 235-245, 2004.
24. Unrau VA: Using client exit interviews to illuminate outcomes in program logic models: a case example, *Evaluation and Program Planning* 24:353-361, 2001.

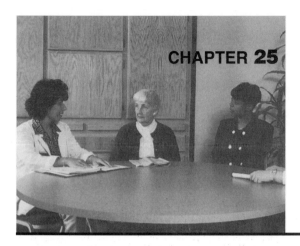

CHAPTER 25

Stories from the Field

Here we are at the end of our book but certainly not, we hope, at the end of your involvement in research. The beauty of research is that you learn from doing, and it is a never-ending process. At each step of the process, new, more refined, and complex queries and questions will emerge and whet your appetite.

We have introduced you to what some may believe are "heavy" philosophical thoughts, technical language, and logical ways of thinking and acting. These are your tools to creatively explore the challenges you identify in your practice, daily life, or professional experience and in your reading of the literature. As you apply these thinking and action tools to health and human service–related issues,

you will discover both the artistry and the science involved in research and its application to your professional practice.

Research, like any other human activity, has its low and high points, its tedium and thrill, its frustrations and challenges, its drastic mistakes, and its clever applications of research principles. Research is foremost a thinking process. If you think about what you are doing and reflect on what you have done, you can learn from mistakes, and you can keep refining your skill as an investigator.

We would like to share with you some of our own stories from the research field to highlight the twists and turns of research and how human this activity really is.

Just Beginning

It was an urban anthropology class, and we were split into groups to conduct urban ethnographies on health practices by different ethnic groups in the city. The big assignment? The Chinese community. The research group? A hippie-type woman, a rock musician, and a topless go-go dancer who dressed the part day and night. The threesome entered the Chinese community, a relatively self-contained 5- by 10-block area of the inner city. As you can imagine, we were quite a sight. How would we ever be able to "enter" the world of this community and engage in passive observation and active participation in community activities? We started out by walking around and scoping out the area. We made observations of the physical environment and spent some great times eating lunch and dinner in various restaurants.

We became Chinese restaurant experts for friends and family, but we had no breakthrough. No Chinese family agreed to meet with us or to be interviewed. Young people were curious and asked lots of questions about us, but their parents remained removed, detached, and unavailable. We caused quite a stir in the community. We split up a couple of times to see if one of us could gain access, but we had no luck.

Then one day we happened to pass a small building with an announcement for a Chinese Political Youth Club. The sign was posted in Chinese and English (a sign of a new acculturated generation?), and we walked directly to the address of the club. We were welcomed and engaged in long discussions of the political climate in the university and the dilemmas confronting the community. Bingo! This was a beginning. Although our access to the community remained through the ears, eyes, and thoughts of this radical subgroup, we were able to delineate health practices and health issues as perceived by this group. This was a lesson in nonreactive research, gaining access, and the impact of key informants on the type of information and understandings that are obtained.

"I'll Do It for You, Sweetie"

It was my first important research position. I was working with a gerontological research institute and learning the ropes of how to coordinate a large, federally funded research grant. I was responsible for putting together a rather lengthy face-to-face interview that included questions generated by me and the research team, as well as an arsenal of standardized instruments used in gerontology. Finally, we were ready for pretesting. We pretested the battery with five older adults, who immediately became bored and uninterested and found the interview questions tedious and irrelevant. "I'll do it for you, sweetie," became the constant song. I was devastated but assured by my mentors that this is a common response and that the interview schedule was indeed comprehensive and asked what was intended. This was my first big disillusionment with standardized questionnaires.

In Search of Significance!

Five years of intensive interviewing, data entry, data cleaning, and sophisticated statistical analyses, but where is the significance? Accepting no significance when you want to find statistically significant differences between an experimental and a control group can be difficult. Nonsignificance can be as an important finding as obtaining significant differences, but it can also present a challenge to get the findings published.

Is Health Care Effective?

In our research class, students are required to develop a research question or query and a proposal that describes how they intend to answer the problem. Our most frustrating but popular "research question" is the one posed by many beginning students in research, "Is nursing effective?" or "Is occupational therapy effective?"

Is this a researchable question? Can you explain what is wrong with the way this question is posed?

Elevator Insight

The values of occupational therapy students in a particular program were studied by administering a values test to incoming students, first-year students, and second-year students. It was hypothesized that a change in values would occur, which would indicate that students had acquired the professional values that were intricate components of the curriculum.

After the test was administered, some of the students were talking about it on the elevator without realizing that the investigator was present. The students discussed the content of the questions; they were comparing responses and hoped that they had answered them correctly! The investigator realized at that incredible, serendipitous moment that the students had answered the questions as they thought they should. They thought it was a test with only one set of correct answers. Their responses did not reflect how they actually felt or believed but what was socially and professionally desirable.

A "Good" Research Subject

We established what we believed were clear, objective criteria by which to identify eligible subjects from a pool of older adults who were in rehabilitation for a stroke, a lower limb amputation, or an ortho-pedic deficit. The purpose of the study was to identify the initial perceptions and attitudes of older patients toward the assistive devices they received in the hos-pital and whether these issued devices were used at home after hospitalization.

As the recruitment process began, periodic meet-ings were held with therapists who were responsible for identifying potential study subjects. At one of these initial meetings, we asked how recruitment was pro-ceeding and if everyone understood the study criteria. Therapists relayed that all was going well, and that they were very pleased they had been able to identify the first few subjects who would "do very well" in this study. The therapists were asked what they meant by "doing well." We learned that therapists had referred patients to the study who they believed greatly valued their assistive devices and would use them at home. Therapists were systematically referring only the "good" patients and were ignoring the potential study eligibility of those patients whom they did not like or whom they suspected would be noncompliant to device use.

This represented a fatal flaw in the recruitment process that would have contaminated the entire data collection effort and study results. We immediately changed the recruitment process and examined the hospital census records to determine who may have been available for study participation but systemati-cally excluded by the therapists at this initial study phase.

A "Bad" Research Subject

In a study of family caregiving, an eligible subject enrolled in the study and was randomly assigned to receive an experimental intervention. The experimen-tal intervention involved in-home occupational ther-apy visits designed to help the caregiver modify the home environment to support caregiving efforts. This particular subject had very unusual religious beliefs and social practices that upset the member of the research team providing the experimental interven-tion. Initially, the interventionist was unable to handle these value differences and suggested to the investiga-tors that the subject was inappropriate for the study and should be considered ineligible. In actuality, there were no objective criteria for excluding this caregiver

from the study. The caregiver fit all eligibility criteria. Additionally, the individual had agreed to participate in the study and had signed an informed consent form.

It is for this very reason that criteria for subject selection are developed. Furthermore, oversight of their implementation and protection of the protocol must be maintained by the investigator. Subjective reasons for excluding individuals from study partic-ipation are a serious source of bias. In this case the investigators worked with the interventionist to alle-viate her anxiety and to proceed with the implemen-tation of the intervention according to protocol.

Native American?

Because we were interested in the ethnic background of our sample of elder women, we added an item on our survey seeking that information. We were sur-prised when we found that 98% of the respondents had checked "Native American." Living in Maine, and knowing that almost all persons in our sample were Caucasian, we were perplexed. So we asked our respondents why they checked Native American. One woman replied, "Well, what else would I check? I was born here, lived here all my life, and expect that I will die in America."

The Pearson, or the Moral of the Coding, Story

A student was almost finished with her dissertation when the crisis occurred. She had measured two con-structs: years that faculty members were teaching and their attitudes toward their jobs. She coded years in actual numbers of years teaching from 0 and then ascending. She coded attitudes, measured with interval level data from 1 to 5, with *1* denoting most positive and *5* denoting least positive. When she conducted her analysis, she calculated a Pearson *r* value of −.7 and interpreted it as a strong association between years teaching and positive attitudes. She finished her conclusion section based on this finding. Because the Pearson value was negative, however, the student's faculty advisor told her that she would have to rewrite the findings section. So she missed her desired graduation date. But who was correct? The student was correct. What are the morals of the story?

Code clearly. If you choose to code as this student did, be clear in your discussion of findings. And if you are a faculty advisor, read carefully, and think!

If You Can't Deliver, Don't Ask

We were embarking on a needs assessment study in which we convened a series of focus groups composed of individuals who were receiving long-term care services. We wanted to know what could be improved in the service system. When we arrived, all the focus group members were present. One by one, each spoke and clearly told us that if we could not deliver what they requested, we should not take their time by conducting another group interview.

Don't Ask if You're Not Prepared to Answer

In a randomized controlled trial to evaluate an intervention to support family caregivers, we were concerned that families assigned to the "no treatment" control group would lose interest in the study and decide to withdraw. We thus decided to conduct monthly telephone check-in calls to control group caregivers to maintain their interest in the study and enhance retention. The problem, however, was what to say to this group of highly stressed and emotionally vulnerable population. We learned quickly that a simple statement (e.g., "Hello, Mrs. Smith; how are you today?") elicited clinically revealing statements about the person's psychological and physical health. Some caregivers began to cry, expressed feeling extremely depressed and not knowing who to turn to, and revealed serious health complaints and incidents of physical abuse. We were ethically bound to respond appropriately, and this quick check-in telephone call to maintain study contact turned into a meaningful clinical intervention.

No Detail Too Small

To set up a randomization scheme based on stratification by gender, a blocking scheme was developed for both men and women and provided to a research assistant to create envelopes with appropriate group assignment sheets (experimental or control). As study participants were enrolled, we noticed that the first 10 women to enter the study were assigned to control and all four men were assigned to intervention. With the blocked randomization scheme we were using, this was not possible, so an investigation was done.

It was discovered that the research assistant had placed only control sheets in the envelopes for women and only intervention sheets in the envelopes for men. This required official notification of the institutional review board and the data and safety monitoring board, as well as a plan of action to determine how best to preserve the original randomization scheme and manage the errors to date. The lesson learned? Even the smallest details, such as reading a person's handwriting and stuffing envelopes, can have profound methodological implications for a study.

Wow, You Got It!

Your heart starts to beat, you feel a rush; it all clicks, falls into place; you uncovered a pattern, a finding, something really striking, and it is significant. The data are right before your eyes. The result has the potential of having an impact on how professionals practice, on how clients feel, and on their health and well-being! Wow, you got it! You feel great.

This is so important—you have to do it again.

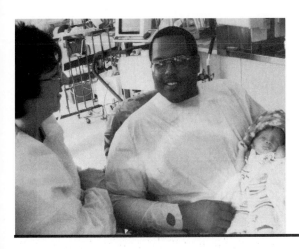

Appendix

- Sample Informed Consent Document for Human Subjects Research
- Informed Consent
- Informed Consent Checklist
- Sample Informed Consent Form
- Sample Relative Permission Form
- Patient/Participant Release Form: Audiotape, Photographs, Videotape, or Film

Thomas Jefferson University
Informed Consent Document for Human Subjects Research

CAREGIVER PERMISSION

Department:_____Community and Homecare Research Division_____

Principal Investigator:_____Laura N. Gitlin, Ph.D._____**Telephone**:_____

Co-Investigator(s):_____Laraine Winter, Ph.D._____**Telephone**:_____

Medical Title:_____Tailored Activity to Improve Affect in Dementia_____

Lay Title: _____Simplifying Meaningful Activities for Persons with Memory Loss_____

What Is an Informed Consent?

You are being asked to take part in a clinical research study. Before you can make an informed decision whether to participate, you should understand the possible risks and benefits associated with this study. This process is known as *informed consent* and means that you will:

- Receive detailed information about this research study.
- Be asked to read, sign, and date this informed consent, once you understand the study and wish to participate. If you don't understand something about the study or if you have questions, please be sure to ask for an explanation before you sign this form.
- Be given a copy of this signed and dated form to keep for your own records.

You should understand that your relationship with the study occupational therapy interventionist is different than your relationship with other health professionals. The study interventionist treats all study participants according to a research plan to obtain information about the program being studied and with the understanding that you may or may not benefit from your participation in the study.

Introduction and Study Purpose

You have been asked to participate in a research study, "Tailored Activity to Improve Affect in Dementia," that is being conducted by the Community and Homecare Research Division, Jefferson College of Health Professions, Thomas Jefferson University. The purpose of this study is to evaluate the benefits of introducing meaningful activities to your family member with memory loss. A total of 60 family caregivers will be enrolled in this study.

Procedures/Treatment

If you agree to participate in this study, the following procedures will be performed over an 8-month period:

(1) First, a personal interview lasting up to 2 hours will occur in your home at a time that is convenient for you. You will be asked questions about your health, how you are feeling, and some of the difficulties you may be having taking care of your family member with memory loss. You will also be asked questions about your family member's health and everyday behaviors. You do not have to answer questions that you object to.

(2) The interviewer will also administer to the family member you are caring for a brief 15-minute questionnaire (the Mini-Mental Status Exam to assess cognitive status and the Cornell Index to assess affect).

(3) On a randomized (like flipping a coin) basis you will be assigned to one of two groups.

(4) If assigned to Group A, within the next 4 months, you will receive up to 6 in-home visits of $1^{1}/_{2}$-hour duration each and 2 follow-up telephone contacts of up to 20 minutes each by an occupational therapist interventionist (a total of up to 9 hours and 40 minutes). The interventionist will provide educational materials about dementia and the importance of taking care of oneself as a caregiver. The interventionist will ask you questions about the previous roles, habits, interests and past and current daily routines of your family member. Also, the interventionist will briefly meet with your family member in your presence and introduce a simple activity to evaluate your family member's motor abilities, comprehension, and memory. Based on this simple assessment, the interventionist will work with you to identify and introduce activities that may be meaningful to your family member and in which he/she may be able to participate in. This may also involve helping you to simplify your home, communicate effectively, or simplify everyday tasks that your family member is involved in.

At the end of the 4-month period, you will be interviewed again in your home by a member of the research team. This follow-up interview will take approximately 2 hours and will be similar to the first interview. If assigned to Group A, the duration of the study will be 4 months.

(5) If assigned to Group B, at the end of 4 months from your initial interview, you will be interviewed again in your home by a member of the research team. This follow-up interview will take approximately 2 hours and will be similar to the first interview.

After this second interview you will then receive the same intervention as Group A that is described above (6 home visits and 2 telephone contacts for up to 9 hours and 20 minutes of contact with an interventionist). At the end of the intervention or 4 months later (8 months from your initial interview), you will be interviewed again in your home by a member of the research team. This follow-up interview will take approximately 2 hours and will be similar to the first interview. If assigned to Group B, the duration of the study will be 8 months.

Risks/Discomforts

There are minimal risks associated with participation in this study. One risk is that you or your family member may experience fatigue in having project staff call or visit your home. Also, some questions may be upsetting to you. However, these risks are minimal and a trained interviewer and interventionist will be able to help you should you feel this way. Also, you can stop at any point if you feel too tired to continue with the interviews or home visits. There is also the minimal risk of the inadvertent release of personal information. However, all information collected as part of this study is stored in locked filing cabinets in the Community and Homecare Research Division, Thomas Jefferson University.

Subject Intitials:_____
(Date)_____

Do Not Write Below This Line

For IRB Stamping

Alternative Treatments

Your alternative is not to participate in this study. Education materials and support on the topic of caregiving for persons with progressive memory loss are available from community organizations. We know of no other treatment or service similar to this research project.

Confidentiality

You have rights regarding the privacy of your health information collected prior to and in the course of this research. This health information, called "protected health information" (PHI), includes demographic information (your name, address) and your self-rated health. You have the right to limit the use and sharing of your PHI, and you have the right to see your research study records and know who else is seeing them.

While the research is in progress, you will not be allowed to see your health information that is created or collected during the course of the research. After the research is finished, however, you may see this information.

By signing this consent form, you are allowing the research team to have access to your PHI. The research team includes the investigators listed on this consent form and other personnel involved in this specific study. Your PHI will also be shared, as necessary, with the University's Division of Human Subjects Protections, the Institutional Review Board (a University committee that reviews, approves, and monitors research involving human subjects), and with any person or agency required by law. All of the above entities are obligated to protect your PHI.

Your PHI may also be shared with the National Institutes of Mental Health which sponsors this research and is providing funds to Thomas Jefferson University to conduct this research. This organization does not have the same obligation to protect your PHI. However, any information provided will only have an identification code and will not contain your name.

The PHI that may be used or disclosed and the purposes for those uses or disclosures are as follows:

- Demographic and self-rated health data for statistical analyses purposes only.
- Social Security number which will be submitted to Thomas Jefferson University Sponsored Programs for you to receive payment for study participation. You may choose not to provide your social security number for this purpose. However, you will not be able to receive payment for study participation.

All the above information is being collected to test the benefits of in-home programs designed to help family members caring for individuals with memory problems. If you do not sign this consent form, you will be ineligible to participate in the research study for which this consent is being requested.

You may revoke this authorization to use and share your PHI (demographic and self-reported health data) at any time by contacting the principal investigator, in writing. If you revoke this authorization, you will no longer be able to participate in this research study and the use or sharing of future PHI will be stopped. However, the PHI that has already been collected may still be used.

Subject Intitials:_____
(Date)_____
_____ Do Not Write Below This Line
For IRB Stamping

The results of the interviewers and intervention assessments performed as part of this research may be published in scientific journals or presented at scientific meetings, but you will not be personally identified in these publications and presentations.

The information collected in each interview will contain only an identification code and will be kept in a locked file drawer in the Community and Homecare Research Division located at 130 S. 9th Street, Philadelphia, PA. Interview information will be stored separately from any documentation containing names or other identifying information.

Parts of the home interview and/or sessions with a health professional may be audio-taped strictly for research purposes. These tapes will also be kept confidential, with identification codes only and locked in file cabinets at Thomas Jefferson University.

Compensation in the Case of Injury

In the event that you experience a research-related injury, comprehensive medical and/or surgical care (including hospitalization) to the extent needed and available will be provided. However, Thomas Jefferson University cannot assure that this comprehensive medical and/or surgical care will be provided without charge, and the costs incurred for this care may ultimately be your responsibility. A research-related injury is a physical injury or illness resulting to you as a direct result of the experiments, treatment(s) and/or procedure(s) used in this study that you would not have incurred if you had not participated in this study. No other financial compensation is available.

Benefits to Subject

You may not benefit directly from your participation in this study. However, there may be a benefit to society, in general, from the knowledge gained in connection with your participation in this study. Possible benefits from your participation in this study may include an understanding of ways to handle difficult caregiving problems, an understanding of memory loss and needs of caregivers, the capabilities of your family member, and activities that you can introduce for your family member. Any information obtained in this study, and which may be important to your or your relative's health or disease progression, will be shared with you.

Payment

You will receive $20 for completion of each home interview.

Contact Information

If you have any questions or concerns about this research, or if you experience a research-related injury, call the Principal Investigator, Dr. Laura Gitlin at (XXX) XXX-XXXX or the Project Director, Nancy Chernett, at (XXX) XXX-XXXX. Should you have any questions regarding your rights as a research participant,

Subject Intitials:_____
(Date)_____

_____ Do Not Write Below This Line _____
For IRB Stamping

you may contact Thomas Jefferson University's Institutional Review Board, which is concerned with the protection of participants in research studies, at telephone: (XXX) XXX-XXXX.

Significant New Findings

As the research progresses, any significant new finding(s), beneficial or otherwise, will be told to you and explained as they relate to the course of your participation.

Voluntary Consent and Subject Withdrawal

You voluntarily consent to participate in this research investigation. You have been told what your participation will involve, including the possible risks and benefits. Your participation in this research project may be terminated if the study procedures are determined to be inappropriate for you. You may also be terminated from participation at any time, at the study principal investigator's discretion, for any reason(s) she deems appropriate.

You may refuse to participate in this investigation or withdraw your consent and discontinue participation in this study without penalty and without affecting your future care or your ability to receive medical treatment at Thomas Jefferson University.

Non-Waiver of Legal Rights Statement

By your agreement to participate in this study, and by signing this consent form, you are not waiving any of your legal rights.

You affirm that you have read this consent form. You have been told that you will receive a copy.

Subject Intitials:_____
(Date)_____

_____ Do Not Write Below This Line _____
For IRB Stamping

Signatures:

_____(Date)
Your Name *(please print or type)*

_____(Date)   _____(Date)
Your Signature   Witness Signature
                                                         (Only required if subject understands and speaks
                                                         English, but cannot read English—delete if
                                                         inapplicable)

_____(Date)
Name of Person Conducting Consent Interview

_____(Date)
Signature of Person Conducting Consent Interview

_____(Date)
Signature of Principal Investigator, Dr. Gitlin, or
Co-Investigator, Dr. Winter, or Project Director,
Ms. Nancy Chernett

Subject Intitials:_____
(Date)_____
_____ Do Not Write Below This Line _____
For IRB Stamping

INFORMED CONSENT

Except where specifically waived or altered by the IRB under Section III.D.3-4 of the University of Maine's *Policies and Procedures for the Protection of Human Subjects of Research,* all human subjects research will require written informed consent. For projects exempt from further review, documentation (signature) of informed consent is not required, but the same basic elements of an informed consent should be applied. The following two paragraphs were taken from the Office for Human Research Protections (NIH) website on the protection of human subjects of research (http://ohrp.osophs.dhhs.gov/humansubjects/guidance/ictips.htm).

"Informed consent is a process, not just a form. Information must be presented to enable persons to voluntarily decide whether or not to participate as a research subject. It is a fundamental mechanism to ensure respect for persons through provision of thoughtful consent for a voluntary act. The procedures used in obtaining informed consent should be designed to educate the subject population in terms that they can understand. Therefore, informed consent language and its documentation (especially explanation of the study's purpose, duration, experimental procedures, alternatives, risks, and benefits) must be written in 'lay language', (i.e., understandable to the people being asked to participate). The written presentation of information is used to document the basis for consent and for the subjects' future reference. The consent document should be revised when deficiencies are noted or when additional information will improve the consent process."

"Use of the first person (e.g., 'I understand that …') can be interpreted as suggestive, may be relied upon as a substitute for sufficient factual information, and can constitute coercive influence over a subject. Use of scientific jargon and legalese is not appropriate. **Think of the document primarily as a teaching tool not as a legal instrument**."

NOTE: For non-exempt studies, approval and expiration dates will be affixed to the approved informed consent document. Copies of the dated documents must be used in obtaining consent. This procedure helps ensure that only the current, IRB-approved informed consent documents are presented to subjects and serves as a reminder to the investigators of the need for continuing review.

INFORMED CONSENT CHECKLIST

Include these items in the form: (NOTE: The form should be written at no higher than an eighth grade reading level.)

☐ 1) A statement that the potential subject is being asked to participate in a research project. Include the name of the person who is conducting the research and his/her title/department.

☐ 2) An explanation of the purpose of the research.

☐ 3) A description of the procedures to be followed. Include sample questions from any instruments that may be used (not required for mail surveys where the questionnaire is enclosed).

☐ 4) An estimate of the amount of time it may take to participate.

☐ 5) A risk statement (reasonably foreseeable risks or discomforts). Examples: in some studies, answering questions may cause people to become uncomfortable; for studies involving standard blood draws, the possibility of bruising exists. For studies that have no foreseeable risks, examples include, "There is no more risk to you in participating than in everyday living," or "Except for your time and inconvenience, there are no foreseeable risks to you in participating in this study."

☐ 6) A description of any potential benefits to the subject or to others that may reasonably be expected from the research. List course credit as a benefit. It is possible that a study will have no direct benefit to the participant (e.g., "While this study will have no direct benefit to you, this research will help us learn more about …").

☐ 7) For treatment studies only, include a description of appropriate alternative procedures or courses of treatment that might be advantageous to the subjects.

☐ 8) A description of confidentiality. Will names be associated with the data? Will the data be coded and linked to a master list of names? Who will have access to the data? Where will the data be stored (e.g., locked office)? Explain the retention of the data: a) If coded, when will the key be destroyed? and b) How long will the data be kept (e.g., destroyed at the end of the study, after x years, etc.)? Is the study anonymous? Don't confuse anonymity and confidentiality. If you have collected names (even if you have coded the data), you can't tell participants that their identity will remain anonymous. You can only guarantee anonymity if you have not collected names or any other identifying information.

☐ 9) A statement that participation is voluntary. If subjects choose to participate, they may stop at any time or skip any questions they do not wish to answer. If the study involves benefits such as payment or course credit, make sure it is clear what happens to the benefit if they drop out (e.g., do they have to complete the entire study to receive the benefit, is there partial benefit for completing part of the study, or do they receive the benefit regardless of the length of participation ("you may stop at any time without loss of benefit"). For an anonymous mail survey, include the statement, "return of the questionnaire implies consent to participate."

☐ 10) An explanation of who to contact for answers to questions about the research (include name, address, phone, e-mail). If a student is the principal investigator, also include the same information for the faculty advisor. Also include a statement directing people to Gayle Anderson, Office of Research and Sponsored Programs, XXX-XXXX, if they have questions about their rights as a research participant.

☐ 11) A statement that their signature (if not exempt) indicates they have read and understand the information. Indicate that they will receive a copy of the form.

Other suggestions:

- Use familiar words (e.g., "cholesterol" instead of "blood lipids").
- Avoid using scientific, medical, or legal terms; if you must use them, define them.
- Avoid abbreviations or acronyms.

SAMPLE INFORMED CONSENT FORM

You are invited to participate in a research project being conducted by (name), a (faculty member, graduate student, etc.) in the Department of (name) at the University of Maine. The purpose of the research is _____.

What Will You Be Asked to Do?

If you decide to participate, you will be asked to (describe procedures, give examples of sample questions if applicable). It may take approximately (amount of time) to participate.

Risks

- There is the possibility that you may become uncomfortable answering the questions.
- Except for your time and inconvenience, there are no foreseeable risks to you in participating in this study.

Benefits

- You will receive $X for participating in this study.
- You will receive $X for completing the first part of this study and $X for the remaining part.
- You will receive 1 hour of research credit for participating in this study.

Confidentiality

Your name will not be on any of the documents. A code number will be used to protect your identity. Data will be kept in the investigator's locked office. (List others who may have access to data, such as faculty advisor and/or others working on the project.) The key linking your name to the data will be destroyed after data analysis is complete, and all data will be destroyed after X years (or the investigator will keep the data indefinitely).

(OR)

This study is anonymous. Please do not write your name on the questionnaire. There will be no records linking you to the data.

Voluntary

Participation is voluntary. If you choose to take part in this study, you may stop at any time during the study (without loss of benefits if applicable). You may skip any questions you do not wish to answer.

(For a mail survey: Return of the survey implies consent to participate.)

Contact Information

If you have any questions about this study, please contact me at (phone, address, email). You may also reach the faculty advisor on this study at (phone, address, e-mail). If you have any questions about your rights as a research participant, please contact Gayle Anderson, Assistant to the University of Maine's Protection of Human Subjects Review Board, at XXX-XXX (or e-mail _____).

(If applicable)

Your signature below indicates that you have read and understand the above information. You will receive a copy of this form.

_____   _____

Signature   Date

THOMAS JEFFERSON UNIVERSITY
RELATIVE PERMISSION

Department:_____ Community and Homecare Research Division _____

Principal Investigator:_____ Laura N. Gitlin, Ph.D. _____ **Telephone**: _____

Co-Investigator: _____ Laraine Winter, Ph.D. _____ **Telephone**: _____

Project Director: _____ Nancy Chernett _____ **Telephone**: _____

Medical Title: Tailored Activity to Improve Affect in Dementia _____

Lay Title: Simplifying Meaningful Activities for Persons with Memory Loss _____

What Is an Informed Consent?

Your relative, _____, is being asked to take part in a research study. Before you can make an informed decision about whether you would like your relative to participate, you should understand the possible risks and benefits associated with this study. This process is known as *informed consent* and means that you will:

- Receive detailed information about this research study.
- Be asked to read, sign, and date this proxy informed consent form on behalf of your relative, once you understand the study and choose that your relative can participate. If you don't understand something about the study or if you have questions, please be sure to ask for an explanation before you sign this form.
- Be given a copy of this signed and dated form to keep for your own records.

Introduction and Study Purpose

You have been asked your permission for your family member to participate in a research study entitled "Tailored Activity to Improve Affect in Dementia," which is being conducted by the Community and Homecare Research Division, Thomas Jefferson University. The purpose of this study is to evaluate the benefits of introducing meaningful activities.

Procedures/Treatment

If you give consent for your family member to participate in this study, you as the caregiver will be asked to provide information about your family member who is experiencing memory problems. There will also be a direct assessment of your family member. He/she will be asked to take a brief test. The test is called the Mini-Mental Status Exam (MMSE). Also, he/she will be asked a few questions about how he or she is feeling. Both assessments will only take a total of about 15 minutes.

Subject Intitials:_____
(Date)_____

During one of your in-home visits with the occupational therapist interventionist, a brief (10-minute) activity (leather lacing) will be introduced to your family member to assess his/her approach to learning a new task. The results of all of these tests will provide an assessment of your relative's overall capabilities.

Your relative will be given the MMSE and activity assessment once. Your relative will be asked how he or she is feeling at each follow-up interview.

Risks/Discomforts

You have been told that there are minimal risks associated with participation in this study. One risk is that your relative may experience fatigue in taking the test or participating in the brief activity. Also, some questions may be upsetting. However, these risks are very minimal, and a trained interviewer and interventionist will be able to help your relative should this occur. Your relative can stop at any point if he/she feels too tired to continue with either the interview or the activity.

Alternative Treatments

Your alternative is to not have you or your relative participate in this study.

Confidentiality

You have rights regarding the privacy of the health information you provide regarding your family member that is collected in the course of this research. This health information, called "protected health information" (PHI), includes demographic information (your family member's name), and your rating of their health and cognitive status. You have the right to limit the use and sharing of your family member's PHI, and you have the right to see his/her research study records and know who else is seeing them.

While the research is in progress, you will not be allowed to see your family member's health information that is created or collected during the course of the research. After the research is finished, however, you may see this information.

By signing this consent form, you are allowing the research team to have access to this PHI. The research team includes the investigators listed on this consent form and other personnel involved in this specific study. Your family member's PHI will also be shared, as necessary, with the University's Division of Human Subjects Protections, the Institutional Review Board (a University committee that reviews, approves and monitors research involving human subjects) and with any person or agency required by law. All of the above entities are obligated to protect your PHI.

Your family member's PHI may also be shared with the National Institutes of Mental Health, which sponsors this research and is providing funds to Thomas Jefferson University to conduct this research. This organization does not have the same obligation to protect your family member's PHI. However, any information provided will only have an identification code and will not contain your name.

Subject Intitials:_____
(Date)_____

The PHI that may be used or disclosed and the purposes for those uses or disclosures are as follows:

Demographic data for statistical analysis purposes only.

Cognitive and affective status to help identify meaningful activities for statistical analysis purposes only.

All the above information is being collected to test the benefits of in-home programs designed to help family members caring for individuals with memory problems. If you do not sign this consent form, you will be ineligible to participate in the research study for which this consent is being requested.

You may revoke this authorization to use and share your family member's PHI (demographic and self-reported health data) at any time by contacting the principal investigator, in writing. If you revoke this authorization, you will no longer be able to participate in this research study, and the use or sharing of future PHI will be stopped. However, the PHI that has already been collected may still be used.

The results of the interviewers and intervention assessments performed as part of this research may be published in scientific journals or presented at scientific meetings, but you will not be personally identified in these publications and presentations.

The information collected in each interview will contain only an identification code and will be kept in a locked file drawer in the Community and Homecare Research Division located at 130 S. 9th Street, Philadelphia, PA. Interview information will be stored separately from any documentation containing names or other identifying information.

Parts of the home interview and/or sessions with a health professional may be audio-taped strictly for research purposes. These tapes will also be kept confidential, with identification codes only and locked in file cabinets at Thomas Jefferson University.

Compensation in the Case of Injury

There is no risk of physical injury or illness as a result of your relative's participating in this study. However, in the event of physical injury or illness resulting to your relative as a direct result of the procedure(s) used in this investigation, comprehensive medical and/or surgical care (including hospitalization) to the extent needed and available will be provided. However, Thomas Jefferson University cannot assure that this comprehensive medical and/or surgical care will be provided without charge, and the costs incurred for this care may ultimately be your relative's responsibility.

Benefits to Subject

Your relative may not benefit directly from his/her participation in this study. However, there may be a benefit to society, in general, from the knowledge gained in connection with his/her participation in this study. A possible benefit from your family member's participation is being able to engage in meaningful activities. Any information obtained from this research study, and which may be important to your relative's health, will be shared with you.

Subject Intitials:_____

(Date)_____

New Findings

Significant new findings developed during the course of the research that may relate to your willingness for your relative to continue participation will be provided to you by a member of the research team.

Payment

Your relative will not receive payment for participating in this study.

Additional Information

If you or your relative have any questions or concerns about this research, either of you are free to ask questions about these procedures and to ask for additional information from the person identified on this consent form as the Principal Investigator, Dr. Laura N. Gitlin, at (XXX) XXX-XXXX, or the Project Director, Ms. Nancy Chernett, at (XXX) XXX-XXXX. Should you have any questions regarding your rights as a research participant, you may contact Thomas Jefferson University's Institutional Review Board, which is concerned with the protection of participants in research studies, at (XXX) XXX-XXXX.

Disclosure of Financial Interest

The sponsor of this research study, the National Institute of Mental Health, is paying Thomas Jefferson University to conduct this study.

Voluntary Consent and Subject Withdrawal

You voluntarily consent for your relative to participate in this research investigation. You have been told what your relative's participation will involve, including the possible risks and benefits. Your relative's participation in this research project may be terminated if the procedure is determined to be inappropriate for him/her. You and your relative may refuse to participate in this investigation or withdraw your consent and discontinue participation in this study at any time without penalty and without affecting you or your relative's future care or ability to receive medical treatment at Thomas Jefferson University.

Subject Intitials:_____
(Date)_____

Non-Waiver of Legal Rights Statement

By your agreement for your relative to participate in this study, and by signing this consent form, you are not waiving any of your relative's legal rights.

You affirm that you have read the preceding or it has been read to you and discussed with you. A copy of this consent form will be given to you. Your signature below means that you have freely agreed for your relative to participate in this project.

<u>***Signatures:***</u>

_____(Date)
Your Name *(please print or type)*

_____(Date)
Signature of Next of Kin/Patient's Surrogate

_____(Date)
Your Signature

_____(Date)
Witness Signature
(Only required if subject understands and speaks English, but cannot read English—delete if inapplicable)

_____(Date)
Name of Person Conducting Consent Interview

_____(Date)
Signature of Person Conducting Consent Interview

_____(Date)
Signature of Principal Investigator (Laura N. Gitlin, Ph.D.),
Co-Investigator (Laraine Winter, Ph.D.), or Project Director (Nancy Chernett, MPH)

Subject Intitials:_____
(Date)_____

Thomas Jefferson University
Patient/Participant Release Form:
Audiotape, Photographs, Videotape, or Film

TITLE OF STUDY   <u>Simplifying Meaningful Activities for Persons with Memory Loss</u>

PRINCIPAL
INVESTIGATOR   Laura N. Gitlin, Ph.D.

TELEPHONE #   _____

DESCRIPTION OF AUDIOTAPE, PHOTOGRAPHY, VIDEOTAPE OR FILM

<u>Select interview and intervention sessions may be audiotaped to help monitor the study and assure quality. Photographs may be taken for instructional purposes and research presentations.</u>

You hereby agree and consent to be audiotaped, photographed, videotaped or filmed on the premises of Thomas Jefferson University as a part of this study. You have been told that these recorded materials will be used only for research, educational or regulatory purposes. You waive all claims for any compensation for your agreement herein and hold Thomas Jefferson University and the sponsor (if applicable, state name) harmless from any claim, demands or damages related to such filming, taping or photographing.

If you later decide to withdraw your consent, the recorded materials will be kept for regulatory pupuses only, as required by law.

You give permission for your name to be used in association with these recorded materials:
☐ Yes ☐ No

You have been told that you will receive a copy of this release form.

_____
Printed Name of Patient/Participant

_____   _____
Signature of Patient/Participant   Date

_____   _____
Signature of Next of Kin/Patient's Surrogate   Date
(if appropriate)

_____   _____
Signature of Investigator   Date

Glossary

Abductive reasoning Patterns and concepts that emerge from an examination of information or data, which in some cases may relate to available theories and in other cases may not.

Abstract Research report that appears before the full report and briefly summarizes or highlights the major points made in each subsequent section.

Abstraction Symbolic representation of an observable or experienced referent.

Accessible Comprehensible to the user.

Accidental sampling See *Convenience sampling.*

Action processes Set of actions that researchers follow to implement a design; include setting boundaries of the study, collecting and analyzing information, and reporting and disseminating study findings.

Action research Inquiry undertaken to generate knowledge to inform action.

Adequacy Satisfactory according to rigor criteria.

Analysis of covariance Statistical technique that removes the effect of the influence of another variable on the dependent or outcome variable.

Analysis of variance Parametric statistic used to ascertain the extent to which significant group differences can be inferred to the population.

Artifact review Data collection technique in which the meaning of objects in their natural context is examined.

Assent Agreement to participate in a study of subject who cannot legally consent.

Associational statistics Set of procedures designed to identify relationships between multiple variables; determines whether knowledge of one set of data allows inference or prediction of the characteristics of another set of data.

Attention factor Phenomenon in which research subjects may experience change simply from the act of participating in a research project; also known as *Hawthorne effect* or *halo effect.*

Audit trail Path of a person's thinking and action processes that enables others to follow the logic and manner in which knowledge was developed.

Axial coding Set of procedures whereby data are put back together in new ways after open coding by making connections between categories (see Chapter 18).

Bias Potential unintended or unavoidable effect on study outcomes.

Bimodal distribution Distribution in which two values occur with the same frequency.

Boundary setting One of the first action processes of research in which the investigator establishes the conceptual limits of the study, as well as the types of information and study participants that will be included.

Breakdowns Points in data collection in naturalistic inquiry in which the expectation of the researcher does not match the observation or information gathered.

Call for proposals Announcements and requests from federal foundations and other sources for investigators to submit research plans for potential funding.

Case study Detailed, in-depth description of a single unit, subject, or event.

Categories Basic analytical step used in naturalistic inquiry in which the investigator groups phenomena according to similarities and labels the groups.

Celeration line Approach to the visual analysis of data points obtained in single-subject designs; drawn across pretest and posttest data points, reflects the central tendency of the data.

Chi-square Nonparametric statistic used with nominal data to test group differences.

Cleaning data Action process whereby the investigator checks the inputted data set to ensure all data have been accurately represented.

Clinical trial Research designed to investigate treatment efficacy.

Closed-ended question Data-gathering strategy in which a question is formed and the study participant is asked to choose a response among prescribed sets of answers.

Cluster sampling Random sampling technique whereby the investigator begins with large units, or clusters, in which smaller sampling units are contained, then randomly selects elements from these clusters.

Codebook Record of variable names for each variable in experimental-type research; record of categories, codes, and line placement in naturalistic inquiry.

Coding of categories Repeated review and examination of the narrative in naturalistic data analysis.

Cohort study   Research that examines specific subpopulations as they change over time.

Concept   Symbolic representations of an observable or experienced referent.

Concept matrix   Two-dimensional organizational system that presents all information that the investigator reviews and evaluates.

Conceptual definition   Stipulates the meaning of concepts or constructs with other concepts or constructs; also known as *lexical definition*.

Concurrent validity   Extent to which an instrument can discriminate the absence or presence of a known standard.

Confidence interval   Estimated range of values in which an unknown population parameter is likely to exist.

Confidence level   The probability value associated with a confidence interval; usually represented as percentage.

Confidentiality   Assurance, on the part of the investigator, that no one other than the research team can have access to a respondent's information unless those who see the data are identified to the person before participation; the information cannot be linked to a person's identity.

Confirmable   One of the four basic characteristics of research (see Chapter 1); the researcher must clearly and logically identify the strategies used in a study, enabling others to follow the sequence of thoughts and actions and to derive similar outcomes and conclusions.

Confirming cases   Naturalistic boundary-setting strategy in which the investigator purposely selects participants to support an emerging interpretation or theory.

Confounding variables   See *Intervening variables.*

Constant comparison   Naturalistic data analysis technique in which each datum is compared and contrasted with previous information to fit all the pieces together inductively into a bigger puzzle.

Construct   Symbolic representation of shared experience that does not have an observable or directly experienced referent.

Construct validity   Fit between the constructs that are the focus of the study and the way in which these constructs are operationalized.

Content validity   Degree to which an indicator seems to agree with a validated instrument measuring the same construct.

Context specific   One of the central features of naturalistic inquiry; refers to the specific environment or field in which the study is conducted and information is derived.

Contextualization   Placement of data into a larger perspective (see Chapter 18).

Contingency table   Two-dimensional frequency distribution primarily used with categorical data.

Continuous variables   Variables that take on an infinite number of values.

Control   Set of action processes that directs or manipulates factors to minimize extraneous variance in order to achieve an outcome.

Control group   Group in experimental-type design in which the independent variable is withheld; thus the control group represents the characteristics of the experimental group before being changed by participation in the experimental condition.

Convenience sampling   Boundary-setting action process that involves the enrollment of available subjects as they enter the study until the desired sample size is reached; also known as *accidental sampling, opportunistic sampling,* or *volunteer sampling.*

Correlational analysis   Method of determining relationships among variables.

Counterbalance design   Variation on experimental design in which more than one intervention is tested and in which the order of participation in each intervention is manipulated.

Credibility   Truthfulness and accuracy of findings in naturalistic inquiry; also referred to as *truth value.*

Criterion validity   Correlation or relationship between a measurement of interest and another instrument or standard that has been shown to be accurate.

Critical theory   Worldview that suggests both an epistemology and a social change purpose for conducting research; complex set of strategies united by commonality of sociopolitical purpose designed to know about social justice and human experience as a means to promote social change.

Critical value   Numerical value that indicates how high the sample statistic must be at a given level of significance to reject the null hypothesis.

Cronbach's alpha   Statistical procedure used to examine the extent to which all items in the instrument measure the same construct.

Crossover design   Variation on true-experimental design in which one group is assigned to the experimental group first and to the control condition later, and then the order for the other group is reversed.

Cross-sectional studies   Studies that examine a phenomenon at one point in time.

Crystallization   See *Triangulation.*

Culture   Explicit and tacit rules, symbols, and rituals that guide patterns of human behavior within a group.

Data   Set of information obtained through systematic investigation; data can refer to information that is numerical or narrative; singular, *datum.*

Data reduction Procedures used to summarize raw data into more compact and interpretable forms.

Data set Set of raw numbers generated by experimental-type data collection.

Database management Set of actions necessary to develop and maintain the raw data and statistical control files that are developed in experimental-type studies.

Deductive reasoning Moving from a general principle to understanding a specific case.

Degrees of freedom Values that are free to vary in a statistical test.

Dependent variable Presumed effect of an independent variable.

Descriptive questions See *Level 1 questions and query.*

Descriptive research Research that yields descriptive knowledge of population parameters and relationships among those parameters.

Descriptive statistics Procedures used to reduce large sets of observations into more compact and interpretable forms.

Design Plan, or blueprint, that specifies and structures the action processes of collecting, analyzing, and reporting data to answer a research question or query.

Deviant case Naturalistic boundary-setting strategy in which the investigator selects participants who have experiences that deviate or are vastly different from the mainstream.

Directional hypothesis Type of hypothesis in which the direction of the effect of the independent variable on the dependent variable is clearly articulated.

Disconfirming cases Naturalistic boundary-setting strategy in which the investigator selects participants who challenge an emerging interpretation or theory.

Discrete variables Variables with a finite number of distinct values.

Dispersion Summary measure, such as range or standard deviation, that describes the distribution of observed values; also referred to as *variability.*

Effect size Strength of differences in the sample values that the investigator expects to find.

Embedded case study Design in which the cases are conglomerates of multiple subparts, or are subparts themselves, placed within larger contexts.

Emic perspective "Insider's" or informant's way of understanding and interpreting experience.

Endogenous research Inquiry that is conceptualized, designed, and conducted by researchers who are "insiders" of the culture, using their own epistemology and structure of relevance.

Epistemology Branch of philosophy that addresses the nature of knowledge and how one comes to know.

Ethics Integrity of the scientific process, with specific concerns for the behavioral conduct of the investigator throughout the research process and for the ethical involvement of human subjects in research.

Ethnography Primary research approach in anthropology concerned with description and interpretation of cultural patterns of groups, as well as the understanding of the cultural meanings people use to organize and interpret their experiences.

Etic perspective Systematic understanding of phenomena developed by those who are external to a group.

Evidence-based practice A model of practice in which decisions are supported by research.

Exempt status Institutional review status in which a study protocol is exempt from formal review from either the full board or its subcommittee.

Ex post facto design One type of nonexperimental, passive observation design in which the phenomena of interest have already occurred and cannot be manipulated in any way.

Experimental group Group in experimental design that receives the experimental condition.

Experimental-type research Designs that are based in a positivist philosophical foundation and that yield numerical data for analysis.

Explanatory research Research designed to predict outcomes.

Exploratory research Studies conducted in natural settings with the explicit purpose of discovering phenomena, variables, theory, or combinations thereof.

External validity Capacity to generalize findings and develop inferences from the sample to the study population.

Extraneous variables See *Intervening variables.*

Extreme or deviant case Naturalistic boundary-setting technique in which the investigator selects a case that represents an extreme example of the phenomenon of interest.

Factorial design Variation on true-experimental design in which the investigator evaluates the effects of two or more independent variables (X_1 and X_2) or the effects of an intervention on different factors or levels of a sample or study variables.

Field notes Naturalistic recordings written by the investigator that are composed of two basic components: (1) recordings of events, observations, and occurrences and (2) recordings of the investigator's own impressions of events, personal feelings, hunches, and expectations.

Field study Research conducted in natural settings.

Flexible design One of the central characteristics of designs in naturalistic inquiry; refers to the unfolding nature of designs in which data collection decisions are based on an interactive process of simultaneously collecting and analyzing information.

Focus group design Naturalistic design that uses a small group process to facilitate data collection and analysis.

Frequency distribution Distribution of values for a given variable and the number of times each value occurs.

Full disclosure Adequacy of information provided to research participants; necessary for them to make informed decisions about the degree of their participation in a study.

Full integration Method that integrates multiple purposes and thus combines design strategies from different paradigms, enabling each to contribute knowledge to the study of a single problem to derive a more complete understanding of the phenomenon under study.

Funder Agency or organization providing financial support for research.

Gaining access Naturalistic action process of entering the context of a field study.

Grounded theory Method in naturalistic research used to generate theory, primarily employing the inductive process of constant comparison.

Guttman scale Unidimensional or cumulative scale in which the researcher develops a small number of items (four to seven) that relate to one concept and then arranges them so that endorsement of one item means an endorsement of items below it.

Halo effect See *Attention factor.*

Hawthorne effect See *Attention factor.*

Health Insurance Portability and Accountability Act (HIPAA) Legislation protecting the privacy of individuals' health information.

Heuristic design Research approach that encourages investigator to discover and methods that enable further investigation; design strategy that involves complete immersion of the investigator into the phenomenon of interest and self-reflection of the investigator's personal experiences.

History Effect of external events on study outcomes.

Holistic Philosophical approaches that view individuals as creating their own subjective realities that cannot be understood by "atomizing," or separating, experience into discrete parts.

Holistic case study Design in which the unit of analysis is seen as only one global phenomenon.

Homogeneous selection Naturalistic action process of boundary setting in which the investigator attempts to reduce variation in study participants, thereby simplifying the number of experiences, characteristics, and conceptual domains that are represented among study participants.

Human subject protection Legislated methods to reduce harm and preserve privacy of human research participants.

Hypothesis Testable statements that indicate what the researcher expects to find, based on theory and level of knowledge in the literature.

Idiographic Pertaining to uniqueness of individuals.

Inclusion and exclusion criteria Sets of criteria that determine who can and cannot participate in a study.

Independent variable Presumed cause of the dependent variable, sometimes referred to as the "predictor variable."

Inductive reasoning Human reasoning that involves a process in which general rules evolve or develop from individual cases or from observation of a phenomenon.

Inference Extent to which the samples reflect the population at both pretest and posttest times.

Inferential statistics Type of statistics used to draw conclusions about population parameters, based on findings from a sample.

Informants Participants in a research study who play an active role of informing the investigator as to the context and its cultural rules.

Informed consent Official statement developed by the researcher that informs study participants of the purpose and scope of the study.

Institutional review board (IRB) Board of experts that must be established at each institution involved in a research process to oversee the ethical conduct of research.

Integrated design Structure used to strengthen a study by selecting and combining designs and methods from both paradigms so that one complements the other to benefit the whole or contribute to an understanding of the whole.

Interactive effect Changes that occur in the dependent variable as a consequence of the combined influence or interaction of taking the pretest and participating in the experimental condition.

Interactionist Specific philosophical approach in naturalistic inquiry; assumes that human meaning evolves from the context of social interaction; human phenomena are therefore understood through interpreting the meanings in social discourse and exchange.

Internal validity Ability of the research design to answer accurately the research question.

Interpretation Analytical step in naturalistic inquiry in which the investigator examines the derived categories and themes and develops a conceptual understanding of the phenomenon.

Interquartile range Measure of variability in experimental-type research that refers to the range of scores that compose the middle 50% of subjects, or the majority responses.

Interrater reliability Test involving the comparison of two observers measuring the same event.

Interrupted time series design Quasi-experimental design involving repeated measurement of the dependent variable, both before and after the introduction of the independent variable, and no control or comparison group.

Interval numbers Numbers that share the characteristics of ordinal and nominal measures but also have the characteristic of equal spacing between categories.

Intervening variables Phenomena that have an effect on the study variables but are not necessarily the object of the study; also known as *confounding variables* or *extraneous variables.*

Interview Information-gathering action process conducted through verbal communication and occurring face-to-face or by telephone; process may be structured or unstructured and usually is conducted with one individual.

Investigator involvement One of the principal characteristics of most forms of naturalistic inquiry in which the investigator becomes fully immersed in the data collection and analytical process.

Judgmental sampling See *Purposive sampling.*

Kuder–Richardson formula (K–R 20) Statistical procedure used to examine the extent to which all the items in the instrument measure the same construct.

Laboratory study Research implemented in controlled environments.

"Learning the ropes" Ongoing naturalistic action process that involves negotiation and renegotiation with members of a field site or with the individual or groups of individuals who are the focus of the study.

Level 1 questions Experimental-type research questions that aim to describe phenomena; also known as *descriptive questions.*

Level 2 questions Experimental-type research questions that explore relationships among phenomena that have already been studied at the descriptive level; also known as *relational questions.*

Level 3 questions Experimental-type research questions that test concepts by manipulating one to affect the other; also known as *predictive questions.*

Levels of abstraction Four levels that guide theory development and testing: concept, construct, relationships, and propositions or principles.

Levels of significance Probability that defines how rare or unlikely the sample data must be before the researcher can reject the null hypothesis.

Lexical definition See *Conceptual definition.*

Life history Type of naturalistic inquiry concerned with eliciting life experiences and with how individuals interpret and attribute meanings to these experiences; a research approach designed to reveal the nature of the "life process traversed over time."

Likert scale Type of scale most frequently scored on a 5- to 7-point range, indicating the subject's level of positive or negative response to an item.

Linguistic sensitivity Having knowledge about the target audience and the meaning of language to that group.

Literature review chart Approach to organizing a literature review in which research studies are summarized in a table format along key categories, such as type of design, measures, and outcomes.

Logical deduction Human process of reasoning that begins with an abstraction and then focuses on discrete parts of phenomena or observations.

Logical positivism Philosophical school of thought characterized by a belief in a singular, knowable reality that exists separate from individual ideas and reductionism.

Logical process One of the four criteria of research (see Chapter 1); suggests that research must be clear and conform to accepted norms of deductive, inductive, or abductive reasoning and proceed systematically and logically through the thinking and action processes.

Longitudinal study Research design in which data collection occurs at discrete points over long periods of time.

Main effects Direct effects of one variable on another.

Manipulation Action process of maneuvering the independent variable so that the effect of its presence, absence, or degree on the dependent variable can be observed.

Maximum variation Boundary-setting strategy that involves seeking individuals for study participation who are extremely different along dimensions that are the focus of the study.

Mean Average score calculated by adding the objects or items and then dividing the sum by the number of objects or items.

Measure of variability Degree of dispersion among scores.

Measurement Translation of observations into numbers.

Measures of central tendency Numerical information regarding the most typical or representative scores in a group.

Median Point in a distribution at which 50% of the cases fall above and 50% below.

Member checking Technique whereby the investigator "checks out" his or her assumptions with informants.

Memoing Particular approach to coding segments of narrative that is used in naturalistic forms of analysis; investigator indicates personal notations as to emerging hypotheses and subsequent directions for analysis.

Meta-analysis Analysis technique of data and/or information aggregated from more than one source.

Mixed-method design Combination of multiple strategies or designs that answers a series of research questions.

Mode Value that occurs most frequently in a data set.

Mortality Subject attrition, or dropping out of a study before its completion.

Multiple comparisons Statistical tests used to determine which group is greater than the others.

Multiple regression Equation based on correlational statistics in which each predictor variable is entered into the equation to determine how strongly it relates to the outcome variable and how much variation in the outcome variable can be predicted by each independent variable.

Multiple-case study Design in which more than one study on single units of analysis are conducted.

Narrative Set of words, derived from stories, interviews, written journals, and other written documents, which forms the data set in naturalistic inquiry.

Naturalistic inquiry Set of research approaches that are based in holistic-type philosophical frameworks and that use inductive and abductive forms of reasoning to derive qualitative information.

Networking See *Snowball sampling.*

Nominal numbers Numbers used to name attributes of a variable.

Nomothetic Referring to group characteristics.

Nondirectional hypothesis Type of hypothesis in which the research indicates an expected effect but not the direction of that effect.

Nonequivalent control group designs Quasi-experimental designs in which there are at least two comparison groups, but subjects are not randomly assigned to these groups.

Nonexperimental designs Experimental-type designs in which the three criteria for true experimentation do not exist.

Nonparametric statistics Formulas used to test hypotheses when (1) normality of variance in the population is not assumed, (2) homogeneity of variance is not assumed, (3) data generated from measures are ordinal or nominal, and (4) sample sizes may be small.

Nonprobability sampling Sampling in which nonrandom methods are used to obtain a sample.

Nonrandom error See *Systematic error.*

Nonreactive methodology See *Unobtrusive methodology.*

Null hypothesis Hypothesis of no difference.

One-shot case study Pre-experimental design in which the independent variable is introduced and in which the dependent variable is then measured in only one group.

Ontology Term of philosophy that refers to a person's view or definition of reality.

Open-ended questions Form of asking questions in which the response is open and in which participants are free to formulate specific verbal responses, rather than choose among fixed response options.

Operational definition Definition that reduces the abstraction of a concept to a concrete observable form by specifying the exact procedures for measuring or observing the phenomenon.

Opportunistic sampling See *Convenience sampling.*

Ordinal numbers Numerical values that assign an order to a set of observations.

Panel study Similar to cohort design, except that the same set of people is studied over time.

Parametric statistics Mathematical formulas that test hypotheses based on three assumptions: (1) samples come from populations that are normally distributed, (2) there is homogeneity of variance, and (3) data generated from the measures are interval level.

Participant observation Naturalistic data collection strategy in which the researcher takes part in the context under scrutiny.

Participants Individuals who provide information in naturalistic studies.

Participatory action research Approach that directly involves study participants in each of the 10 research essentials; that is, it involves study participants that contribute to formulating the research question or query, study design, and approach to analysis.

Passive observation designs Nonexperimental designs used to investigate phenomena as they naturally occur and to ascertain the relationship between two or more variables.

Pearson product-moment correlation Statistic of association using interval level data and yielding a score between −1 and +1.

Peer debriefing Use of more than one investigator as a participant in the analytical process, followed by reflection on other possible competing interpretations of the data.

Phase I clinical trial Study of a small sample to test a new behavioral or biomedical intervention not previously evaluated.

Phase II clinical trial Study of the efficacy and safety of an intervention in a larger group of people.

Phase III clinical trial Study to evaluate comparative effectiveness and safety of an intervention in a large group of persons (several hundred to thousands).

Phenomenology Form of naturalistic inquiry used to uncover the meaning of how humans experience phenomena through the description of those experiences as they are lived by individuals.

Philosophical foundation   Formal belief system guiding the research approach.

Pluralism   Central characteristic of naturalistic inquiry that suggests there are multiple realities that can be identified and understood only within the natural context in which human experience and behavior occur.

Population   Group of persons, elements, or both with common characteristics that are defined by the investigator.

Post hoc comparisons   Statistical tests used to determine which group is greater than the others.

Posttest   Observation or measurement subsequent to the completion of the experimental condition.

Practice evaluation   Application of research methods to examining practice process and outcome.

Practice research   Investigation of human experience in the context of health care and human service institutions, agencies, or settings.

Predictive questions   See *Level 3 questions.*

Predictive validity   Extent to which an instrument can predict or estimate the occurrence of a behavior or event.

Pre-experimental designs (experimental-type designs)   Designs in which two of the three criteria necessary for true experimentation are absent.

Pretest   Observation or measurement before introduction of the experimental condition.

Principles   See *Propositions.*

Probability sampling   Sampling plans that are based on probability theory.

Probe   Statement that is neutral, designed to encourage the study participant to provide additional information or elaboration.

Problem statement   Statement that identifies the phenomenon to be explored and the reason(s) it needs to be examined or why it is a problem or issue.

Proposal   Formal description of an intended research project.

Propositions   Statements that govern a set of relationships and give them a structure; also called *principles.*

Prospective studies   Studies that describe phenomena, search for cause-and-effect relationships, or examine change in the present or as the event unfolds over time.

Purpose statement   Statement that articulates the specific purpose of or reason for conducting the research study; identifies the particular goals of the study.

Purpose statement   Articulation of the reasons for conducting and using research.

Purposive sampling   Deliberate selection of individuals by the researcher based on certain predefined criteria; also known as *judgmental sampling.*

Quasi-experimental design   Experiments that have treatments, outcome measures, and experimental units but do not use random assignment to create comparison from which treatment-caused change is inferred; instead, the comparisons depend on nonequivalent groups who differ from each other in many ways other than the presence of the treatment being tested (see Chapter 8).

Query   Broad statement that identifies the phenomenon or natural field of interest in naturalistic forms of inquiry.

Question   Interrogative statement that a study is designed to answer. See *research question.*

Questionnaires   Written instruments that may be administered either face-to-face, by proxy, or through the mail; may vary as to the structure of questions (closed or open) that are included.

Quota sampling   Nonrandom technique in which the investigator purposively obtains a sample by selecting sample elements in the same proportion that they are represented in the population.

Random error   Error that occurs by chance.

Randomization   Selection or assignment of subjects based on chance.

Range   Difference between the highest and lowest observed value in a collection of data.

Ratio numbers   Numbers that have all the characteristics of interval numbers but also have an absolute 0 point.

Raw data file   Set of numbers in a computer file that is entered from a questionnaire or other data collection instrument used in experimental-type research; its creation is the first action step in the process of preparing data for statistical analysis.

Reflexivity   Process of self-examination.

Regression   Statistical phenomenon in which extreme scores tend to regress or cluster around the mean (average) on repeated testing occasion.

Relational questions   See *Level 2 questions.*

Reliability   Stability of a research design.

Research   Multiple, systematic strategies to generate knowledge about human behavior, human experience, and human environments in which the thought and action processes of the researcher are clearly specified so that they are (1) logical, (2) understandable, (3) confirmable, and (4) useful.

Research design   Plan that specifies and structures the action processes of collecting, analyzing, and reporting data to answer a research question.

Research question   Statement that guides an experimental-type investigation; must be concise and framed in such a way that systematic inquiry can be carried out; establishes the boundaries or limits as to what concepts, individuals, or phenomena will be examined.

Research topic   Broad area of inquiry from which the investigator develops a more specific question or query.

Retrospective studies   Describe and examine phenomena after the fact or after the phenomena have occurred.

Reviewers (review committee)   Individuals who read and consider the efficacy and worth of a proposed study.

Sample   Subset of the population participating or included in the study.

Sampling error   Difference between the values obtained from the sample and those that actually exist in the population.

Sampling frame   Listing of every element in the target population.

Saturation   Point at which an investigator has obtained sufficient information from which to obtain an understanding of the phenomena.

Scales   Tools for the quantitative measurement of the degree to which individuals possess a specific attribute or trait.

Secondary data analysis   Analysis of a data set that has been developed in a previous study or by another investigator; usually conducted to explore specific research questions that were secondary to the primary study purpose.

Semantic differential   Scaling technique in which the researcher develops a series of opposites or mutually exclusive constructs that ask the respondent to give a judgment about something along an ordered dimension, usually of 7 points.

Significance level   Extent to which group differences are a function of chance.

Simple random sampling (SRS)   Probability sampling technique in which a sample is randomly selected from a population.

Single-case study   Design in which only one study on a single unit of analysis is conducted.

Snowball sampling   Obtaining a sample through asking subjects to provide the names of others who may meet study criteria; also known as *networking*.

Solomon four-group design   True-experimental design that combines true experimentation and posttest-only designs into one design structure.

Spearman rho   Statistic of association using ordinal level data and yielding a score between −1 and +1.

Split-half technique   Reliability technique in which instrument items are split in half and a correlational procedure is performed between the two halves.

Standard deviation   Indicator of the average deviation of scores around the mean.

Static group comparison   Pre-experimental design in which a comparison group is added to the one-shot case study design.

Statistic   Number derived from a mathematical procedure as part of the analytical process in experimental-type research.

Statistical conclusion validity   Power of an investigator's study to draw statistical conclusions.

Statistical power   Probability of identifying a relationship that exists, or the probability of rejecting the null hypothesis when it is false or should be rejected.

Stratified random sampling   Technique in which the population is divided into smaller subgroups, or strata, from which sample elements are then chosen.

Subjects   Participants in experimental-type studies.

Sum of squares   Descriptive statistic for interpreting variability; derived by squaring the difference between each score from the mean, which are then summed.

Survey designs   Nonexperimental designs used to measure primarily characteristics of a population, typically conducted with large samples through mail questionnaires, telephone, or face-to-face interview.

Systematic error   Systematic bias or an error that occurs consistently with an instrument; impacts the extent to which an instrument is valid or represents the underlying construct or concept; also known as *nonrandom error*.

Systematic random sampling   Technique in which a sampling interval width *(K)* is determined based on the needed sample size, and then every Kth element is selected from a sampling frame.

Target population   Group of individuals or elements from which the investigator is able to select a sample.

Taxonomic analysis   Naturalistic data analysis technique in which the researcher organizes similar or related categories into larger categories and identifies differences between sets of subcategories and larger or overarching categories.

Ten essentials   Ten thinking and action processes that compose any type of research that is experimental type, naturalistic, or integrated (see Chapter 2).

Test-retest reliability   Reliability test in which the same test is given twice to the same subject under the same circumstances.

Theme   Analytical process used in naturalistic inquiry in which the investigator identifies patterns and topics from which a theme is derived.

Theoretical sensitivity   Researcher's ability to detect and give meaning to data.

Theory   Set of interrelated constructs, definitions, and propositions that presents a systematic view of phenomena by specifying relations among variables, with the purpose of explaining or predicting phenomena (see Chapter 1).

Theory-based selection Approach in naturalistic inquiry wherein key informants or study participants are selected, based on their ability to illuminate the particular theoretical construct that is being explored.

Theory generating One of the primary purposes of many forms of naturalistic inquiry; use of naturalistic approaches to link each piece of datum from which concepts, constructs, relationships, and propositions are generated or derived.

Theory testing One of the primary purposes of many forms of experimental-type research; use of experimental methodologies to test formally a set of propositions of a theory.

Thinking processes Logical thought processes of research that involve deductive, inductive, or abductive thinking; include identifying a philosophical foundation and theoretical framework, framing a question or query, substantiating the research approach, and developing a design structure.

Time series design Quasi-experimental design that involves repeated data collection over time for a single group.

Transcription Typed narrative derived from an audiotape or a video image of an interview with an individual or group; represents an action process primarily used in naturalistic inquiry as the first step in the analysis and interpretation of narrative.

Treatment fidelity Attention to the integrity of implementing an intervention.

Trend study Research examining a general population over time to see changes or trends that emerge as a consequence of time.

Triangulation Use of multiple strategies or methods as a means to strengthen the credibility of an investigator's findings related to the phenomenon under study; also known as *crystallization*.

True-experimental design Classic two-group design in which subjects are randomly selected and randomly assigned *(R)* to either an experimental or a control group condition; before the experimental condition, all subjects are pretested or observed on a dependent measure *(O)*; in the experimental group, the independent variable or experimental condition is imposed *(X)*, and it is withheld in the control group; subjects are then posttested or observed on the dependent variable *(O)* after the experimental condition.

Truth value Term used in naturalistic inquiry to refer to the accuracy of interpretation or how closely the analytical scheme reflects the natural context or focus of the investigation; also referred to as *credibility*.

t-Test Parametric test to ascertain the extent to which any significant differences between the means of two sample groups can be inferred from the sample to the population.

Type I error Rejecting the null hypothesis when it is true.

Type II error Failing to reject the null hypothesis when it is false.

Typical case Naturalistic boundary-setting strategy in which the investigator selects participants who are typical or representative of the particular event or experience that is the focus of the inquiry.

Understandable criteria One of the four criteria of research (see Chapter 1); refers to the requirement that a study makes sense and that all study procedures are precisely articulated.

Univariate statistics Descriptive data reduction approaches for one variable.

Unobtrusive methodology Observation and examination of documents and objects that bear on the phenomenon of interest; also known as *nonreactive methodology*.

Useful criteria One of the four criteria of research (see Chapter 1); refers to the requirement that a research study contributes to knowledge building.

Validity Extent to which an investigator's findings are accurate or reflect the underlying purpose of the study.

Variability See *Dispersion*.

Variable Concept or construct to which a numerical value is assigned; by definition, it must have more than one value, even if the investigator is interested in only one condition.

Variable label Applied to each variable in a computer file; follows certain conventions that are based on the particular statistical software used by the investigator.

Variance Descriptive statistic that reflects a measure of variability; reflects the mean or average of the sum of squares; the larger the variance, the larger the spread of scores.

Voluntary participation Informed decision to be a subject or study participant.

Volunteer sampling See *Convenience sampling*.

Vulnerable populations Participants in studies considered to be vulnerable or at risk; require special set of ethical procedures to ensure their protection; examples include pregnant women, fetuses, children, individuals with cognitive impairments or mental illness, and prisoners.

Index